Current
Dermatologic
Diagnosis & Treatment

Current Dermatologic
Diagnosis & Treatment

Edited by

Irwin M. Freedberg, MD

Chairman
Ronald O. Perelman Department of Dermatology
New York University School of Medicine
New York, New York

Miguel R. Sanchez, MD

Associate Clinical Professor
Ronald O. Perelman Department of Dermatology
New York University School of Medicine
New York, New York

Current Medicine, Inc., Philadelphia

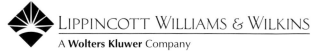

A **Wolters Kluwer** Company

Philadelphia • Baltimore • New York • London
Buenos Aires • Hong Kong • Sydney • Tokyo

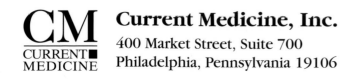

Current Medicine, Inc.
400 Market Street, Suite 700
Philadelphia, Pennsylvania 19106

Developmental Editor: Bill Edelman
Editorial Assistant: Nicole Garron
Cover Design, Design and Layout: John McCullough and Jennifer Knight
Assistant Production Manager: Simon Dickey

ISBN 0-7817-3531-9

Although every effort has been made to ensure that the drug doses and other information are presented accurately in this publication, the ultimate responsibility rests with the prescribing physician. Neither the publishers nor the authors can be held responsible for errors or for any consequences arising from the use of the information contained herein. Products mentioned in this publication should be used in accordance with the manufacturer's prescribing information. No claims or endorsements are made for any drug or compound at present under clinical investigation.

Distributed worldwide by Lippincott Williams & Wilkins

Manufactured in Hong Kong
Printed by Paramount
5 4 3 2 1

Macrene Alexiades-Armenakas, MD, PhD
Teaching Assistant
Ronald O. Perelman Department of Dermatology
New York University School of Medicine
New York, New York

Robin Ashinoff, MD
Clinical Assistant Professor
Ronald O. Perelman Department of Dermatology
New York University School of Medicine
New York, New York

Robert Auerbach, MD
Clinical Professor
Ronald O. Perelman Department of Dermatology
New York University School of Medicine
New York, New York

Marisa Baldassano, MD
Assistant Professor
Ronald O. Perelman Department of Dermatology
New York University School of Medicine
New York, New York

Rebecca Baxt, MD, MBA
Clinical Instructor
Ronald O. Perelman Department of Dermatology
New York University School of Medicine
New York, New York

Samuel Beck, MD
Fellow
Ronald O. Perelman Department of Dermatology
New York University School of Medicine
New York, New York

Dina Began, MD
Assistant Professor
Ronald O. Perelman Department of Dermatology
New York University School of Medicine
New York, New York

Arthur P. Bertolino, MD
Clinical Associate Professor
Ronald O. Perelman Department of Dermatology
New York University School of Medicine
New York, New York

Mary Ellen Brademas, MD
Clinical Assistant Professor
Ronald O. Perelman Department of Dermatology
New York University School of Medicine
New York, New York

Ronald R. Brancaccio, MD
Clinical Professor
Ronald O. Perelman Department of Dermatology
New York University School of Medicine
New York, New York

Rena Brand, MD
Clinical Assistant Professor
Ronald O. Perelman Department of Dermatology
New York University School of Medicine
New York, New York

Lance H. Brown, MD
Clinical Instructor
Ronald O. Perelman Department of Dermatology
New York University School of Medicine
New York, New York

Bruce Burgreen, MD
Clinical Assistant Professor
Ronald O. Perelman Department of Dermatology
New York University School of Medicine
New York, New York

Jean-Claude Bystryn, MD
Professor
Ronald O. Perelman Department of Dermatology
New York University School of Medicine
New York, New York

Mary W. Chang, MD
Assistant Professor
Dermatology and Pediatrics
Ronald O. Perelman Department of Dermatology
New York University School of Medicine
New York, New York

Jeanie Chung-Leddon, MD, PhD
Teaching Assistant
Ronald O. Perelman Department of Dermatology
New York University School of Medicine
New York, New York

Lesley Clark-Loeser, MD
Fellow
Ronald O. Perelman Department of Dermatology
New York University School of Medicine
New York, New York

David E. Cohen, MD, MPH
Assistant Professor
Ronald O. Perelman Department of Dermatology
New York University School of Medicine
New York, New York

Michael Cohen, MD
Clinical Instructor
Ronald O. Perelman Department of Dermatology
New York University School of Medicine
New York, New York

Doris J. Day, MD
Instructor
Ronald O. Perelman Department of Dermatology
New York University School of Medicine
New York, New York

Bruce Deitchman, MD
Clinical Assistant Professor
Ronald O. Perelman Department of Dermatology
New York University School of Medicine
New York, New York

Jonathan Dosik, MD
Clinical Instructor
Ronald O. Perelman Department of Dermatology
New York University School of Medicine
New York, New York

Rhett Drugge, MD
Clinical Instructor
Ronald O. Perelman Department of Dermatology
New York University School of Medicine
New York, New York

Wendy Epstein, MD
Clinical Assistant Professor
Ronald O. Perelman Department of Dermatology
New York University School of Medicine
New York, New York

Joshua P. Fogelman, MD
Teaching Assistant
Ronald O. Perelman Department of Dermatology
New York University School of Medicine
New York, New York

Paul Frank, MD
Teaching Assistant
Ronald O. Perelman Department of Dermatology
New York University School of Medicine
New York, New York

Andrew Franks, Jr., MD
Clinical Associate Professor
Ronald O. Perelman Department of Dermatology
New York University School of Medicine
New York, New York

Linda K. Franks, MD
Clinical Assistant Professor
Ronald O. Perelman Department of Dermatology
New York University School of Medicine
New York, New York

Paul Friedman, MD
Teaching Assistant
Ronald O. Perelman Department of Dermatology
New York University School of Medicine
New York, New York

Alvin Friedman-Kien, MD
Professor
Dermatology and Microbiology
Ronald O. Perelman Department of Dermatology
New York University School of Medicine
New York, New York

Casey Gallagher, MD
Teaching Assistant
Ronald O. Perelman Department of Dermatology
New York University School of Medicine
New York, New York

Contributors

Sharon Galvin, MD
Clinical Assistant Professor
Ronald O. Perelman Department of
Dermatology
New York University School of Medicine
New York, New York

Ellen Gendler, MD
Clinical Associate Professor
Ronald O. Perelman Department of
Dermatology
New York University School of Medicine
New York, New York

Roy Geronemus, MD
Clinical Professor
Ronald O. Perelman Department of
Dermatology
New York University School of Medicine
New York, New York

Barry Goldman, MD
Clinical Instructor
Ronald O. Perelman Department of
Dermatology
New York University School of Medicine
New York, New York

Elizabeth K. Hale, MD
Teaching Assistant
Ronald O. Perelman Department of
Dermatology
New York University School of Medicine
New York, New York

Patrick Hennessey, MD
Clinical Associate Professor
Ronald O. Perelman Department of
Dermatology
New York University School of Medicine
New York, New York

Sumayah Jamal, MD, PhD
Instructor
Ronald O. Perelman Department of
Dermatology
New York University School of Medicine
New York, New York

J.E. Jelinek, MD
Clinical Professor
Ronald O. Perelman Department of
Dermatology
New York University School of Medicine
New York, New York

Brian Jiang, MD
Clinical Instructor
Ronald O. Perelman Department of
Dermatology
New York University School of Medicine
New York, New York

Edwin Joe, MD
Teaching Assistant
Ronald O. Perelman Department of
Dermatology
New York University School of Medicine
New York, New York

Hideko Kamino, MD
Associate Professor
Clinical Dermatology
Ronald O. Perelman Department of
Dermatology
New York University School of Medicine
New York, New York

Arielle Kauvar, MD
Clinical Associate Professor
Ronald O. Perelman Department of
Dermatology
New York University School of Medicine
New York, New York

Paul Kechijian, MD
Clinical Associate Professor
Ronald O. Perelman Department of
Dermatology
New York University School of Medicine
New York, New York

Leonard Kim, MD
Teaching Assistant
Ronald O. Perelman Department of
Dermatology
New York University School of Medicine
New York, New York

Alfred W. Kopf, MD
Clinical Professor
Ronald O. Perelman Department of
Dermatology
New York University School of Medicine
New York, New York

Marina Kuperman Beade, MD
Fellow
Ronald O. Perelman Department of
Dermatology
New York University School of Medicine
New York, New York

Sheri Lagin, MD
Clinical Assistant Professor
Ronald O. Perelman Department of
Dermatology
New York University School of Medicine
New York, New York

Jo-Ann Latkowski, MD
Instructor
Ronald O. Perelman Department of
Dermatology
New York University School of Medicine
New York, New York

Jacob Lau, MD
Student
Ronald O. Perelman Department of
Dermatology
New York University School of Medicine
New York, New York

Vicki J. Levine, MD
Assistant Professor
Ronald O. Perelman Department of
Dermatology
New York University School of Medicine
New York, New York

George Lipkin, MD
Professor
Ronald O. Perelman Department of
Dermatology
New York University School of Medicine
New York, New York

Cynthia Loomis, MD, PhD
Assistant Professor
Dermatology and Cell Biology
Ronald O. Perelman Department of
Dermatology
New York University School of Medicine
New York, New York

Erick Mafong, MD
Teaching Assistant
Ronald O. Perelman Department of
Dermatology
New York University School of Medicine
New York, New York

Kenneth A. Mark, MD
Teaching Assistant
Ronald O. Perelman Department of
Dermatology
New York University School of Medicine
New York, New York

Jeffrey Marx, MD
Clinical Associate Professor
Ronald O. Perelman Department of
Dermatology
New York University School of Medicine
New York, New York

Thomas Meola, MD
Clinical Assistant Professor
Ronald O. Perelman Department of
Dermatology
New York University School of Medicine
New York, New York

Janet Moy, MD
Clinical Assistant Professor
Ronald O. Perelman Department of
Dermatology
New York University School of Medicine
New York, New York

Narayan S. Naik, MD
Teaching Assistant
Ronald O. Perelman Department of
Dermatology
New York University School of Medicine
New York, New York

Christopher Nanni, MD
Clinical Instructor
Ronald O. Perelman Department of
Dermatology
New York University School of Medicine
New York, New York

Rhoda Narins, MD
Clinical Professor
Ronald O. Perelman Department of
Dermatology
New York University School of Medicine
New York, New York

Allen Natow, MD
Clinical Assistant Professor
Ronald O. Perelman Department of
Dermatology
New York University School of Medicine
New York, New York

Steven Natow, MD, MBA
Clinical Instructor
Ronald O. Perelman Department of
Dermatology
New York University School of Medicine
New York, New York

Philip Orbuch, MD
Clinical Associate Professor
Ronald O. Perelman Department of
Dermatology
New York University School of Medicine
New York, New York

Seth J. Orlow, MD, PhD
Associate Professor
Dermatology and Cell Biology
Ronald O. Perelman Department of
Dermatology
New York University School of Medicine
New York, New York

Ira A. Pion, MD
Clinical Assistant Professor
Ronald O. Perelman Department of
Dermatology
New York University School of Medicine
New York, New York

David Polsky, MD, PhD
Assistant Professor
Ronald O. Perelman Department of
Dermatology
New York University School of Medicine
New York, New York

Miriam Pomeranz, MD
Assistant Professor
Ronald O. Perelman Department of
Dermatology
New York University School of Medicine
New York, New York

Rhonda J. Pomerantz, MD
Clinical Assistant Professor
Ronald O. Perelman Department of
Dermatology
New York University School of Medicine
New York, New York

Paul Possick, MD
Clinical Associate Professor
Ronald O. Perelman Department of
Dermatology
New York University School of Medicine
New York, New York

David Ramsay, MD, MEd
Clinical Professor
Ronald O. Perelman Department of
Dermatology
New York University School of Medicine
New York, New York

Michael Reed, MD
Clinical Assistant Professor
Ronald O. Perelman Department of
Dermatology
New York University School of Medicine
New York, New York

Peter Reisfeld, MD
Clinical Assistant Professor
Ronald O. Perelman Department of
Dermatology
New York University School of Medicine
New York, New York

M. Joyce Rico, MD
Adjunct Associate Professor
Ronald O. Perelman Department of
Dermatology
New York University School of Medicine
New York, New York

Perry Robins, MD
Clinical Professor
Ronald O. Perelman Department of
Dermatology
New York University School of Medicine
New York, New York

Stanley Rosenthal, PhD
Clinical Associate Professor
Ronald O. Perelman Department of
Dermatology
New York University School of Medicine
New York, New York

Jeremy Rothfleisch, MD
Teaching Assistant
Ronald O. Perelman Department of
Dermatology
New York University School of Medicine
New York, New York

Deborah S. Sarnoff, MD
Clinical Assistant Professor
Ronald O. Perelman Department of
Dermatology
New York University School of Medicine
New York, New York

Chrysalyne Delling Schmults, MD
Teaching Assistant
Ronald O. Perelman Department of
Dermatology
New York University School of Medicine
New York, New York

Judith Shapiro, MD
Clinical Assistant Professor
Ronald O. Perelman Department of
Dermatology
New York University School of Medicine
New York, New York

Jerome Shupack, MD
Clinical Professor
Ronald O. Perelman Department of
Dermatology
New York University School of Medicine
New York, New York

Roy L. Stern, MD
Clinical Instructor
Ronald O. Perelman Department of
Dermatology
New York University School of Medicine
New York, New York

Nicholas A. Soter, MD
Professor
Ronald O. Perelman Department of
Dermatology
New York University School of Medicine
New York, New York

Bruce E. Strober, MD, PhD
Teaching Assistant
Ronald O. Perelman Department of
Dermatology
New York University School of Medicine
New York, New York

Diane Tanenbaum, MD
Clinical Associate Professor
Ronald O. Perelman Department of
Dermatology
New York University School of Medicine
New York, New York

Sara L. Tarsis, MD, PhD
Clinical Instructor
Ronald O. Perelman Department of
Dermatology
New York University School of Medicine
New York, New York

Cheryl Thellman, MD
Clinical Instructor
Ronald O. Perelman Department of
Dermatology
New York University School of Medicine
New York, New York

Louis Vogel, MD
Clinical Assistant Professor
Ronald O. Perelman Department of
Dermatology
New York University School of Medicine
New York, New York

Ken Washenik, MD, PhD
Assistant Professor
Ronald O. Perelman Department of
Dermatology
New York University School of Medicine
New York, New York

Samuel Weinberg, MD
Clinical Professor
Ronald O. Perelman Department of
Dermatology
New York University School of Medicine
New York, New York

Katherine L. White, MD
Teaching Assistant
Ronald O. Perelman Department of
Dermatology
New York University School of Medicine
New York, New York

Michael Whitlow, MD, PhD
Clinical Associate Professor
Ronald O. Perelman Department of
Dermatology
New York University School of Medicine
New York, New York

Dimitris Zouzias, MD
Clinical Assistant Professor
Ronald O. Perelman Department of
Dermatology
New York University School of Medicine
New York, New York

The Ronald O. Perelman Department of Dermatology of New York University School of Medicine has a long, illustrious history in the field of dermatologic education and patient care. In *Current Dermatologic Diagnosis & Treatment*, the active members of the Department present their approach to dermatologic disease and its care at the beginning of the 21st Century. The authors appreciate that there are many sources of dermatologic knowledge, in print, recorded, and digital forms. Their goal was to prepare a volume that the busy clinician can use, efficiently and effectively, when faced with a patient who has a dermatologic problem.

We have presented each chapter in a uniform way, throughout the volume, so that the care provider can rapidly assess the signs, symptoms, appropriate investigations, and complications on the first page of each two-page chapter, with treatment options, both pharmacological and nonpharmacological, on the second page. Differential diagnosis, etiology, epidemiology, treatment aims, prognosis, and references are discussed, wherever appropriate, in the sidebars that frame the primary presentations. Illustrations from the extensive photographic collection of the Department are included throughout the text. Special sections review our approaches to dermatologic compounding, topical and systemic therapy, and unique dermatologic modalities, such as cryotherapy and phototherapy.

It is only you, the readers of *Current Dermatologic Diagnosis & Treatment*, who can tell us whether we have met our goals well and offer us suggestions for improvement in future editions. We look forward to hearing from you.

Irwin M. Freedberg, MD
Miguel Sanchez, MD
New York, New York

Dedication

To all those who have gone before us at the Skin and Cancer Unit of the Department of Dermatology of NYU, epitomized by their past leaders, George Miller MacKee (1927–1949), Marion B. Sulzberger (1949–1961) and Rudolf L. Baer (1961–1981).

Contents

Contents

Contents by specialty

Contents by specialty

This book provides current expert recommendations on the diagnosis and treatment of all major disorders throughout medicine in the form of tabular summaries. Essential guidelines on each of the topics have been condensed into two pages of vital information, summarizing the main procedures in diagnosis and management of each disorder to provide a quick and easy reference.

Each disorder is presented as a "spread" of two facing pages: the main procedures in diagnosis on the left and treatment options on the right.

Listed in the main column of the **Diagnosis** page are the common symptoms, signs, and complications of the disorder, with brief notes explaining their significance and probability of occurrence, together with details of investigations that can be used to aid diagnosis.

The left shaded side column contains information to help the reader evaluate the probability that an individual patient has the disorder. It may also include other information that could be useful in making a diagnosis (*e.g.*, classification or grading systems, comparison of different diagnostic methods).

Disorder

Diagnosis

Signs

- xxxxxxxxxxxxxxxxxxxxxxxxxxxxxxxxxxxxxxxxxxxx
xxxxxxxxxxxxxxxxxxxxx
xxxxxxxxxxxxxxxxxxxxxx
xxxxxxxxxxxxxxxx
xxxxxxxxxxxxxxxxxx
xxxxxxxxxxxxxxxxxxxx
xxxxxxxxxxxxxxxxxxxxx

Symptoms

- xxxxxxxxxxxxxxxxxxxxxxxx
xxxxxxxxxxxxxxxxxxxxxxx
xxxxxxxxxxxxxxxxxx
xxxxxxxxxxxxxxx
xxxxxxxxxxxxxxxxxx
xxxxxxxxxxxxxxx
xxxxxxxxxxxxxxx
xxxxxxxxxxxxxx xxxxxxxxxxxxx

Investigations

- xxxxxxxxxxxxxxxxxxxxxxxxxxxxxxxxxxxxxxxx
xxxxxxxxxxxxxxxxxxxxxxxxxxxxx
xxxxxxxxxxxxxxxxxxxxxxxxxxxxxxxxxx

Complications xxxxxxxxxxxxxxxxxxxxxxxxxx
xxxxxxxxxxxxxxxxxxxxxxxx
xxxxxxxxxxxxxxxxxxxxx
xxxxxxxxxxxxxxxxxxxxxx

XXXXXXXXXX
xxxxxxxxxxxxxxxxxxxx
xxxxxxxxxxxxxxxxxxx
xxxxxxxxxxxxxxxxxx
xxxxxxxxxxxxxx
xxxxxxxxxxxxxx
xxxxxxxxxxxxxxxx
xxxxxxxxxxxxxxxx
xxxxxxxxxxxxxxxxxx
xxxxxxxxxxxxxxxxxx

XXXXXXXXXX
- xxxxxxxxx
xxxxxxxxxxxxxxxx
xxxxxxxxx
xxxxxxxxxxxxxxxx
xxxxxxxxxxxxxxxx
xxxxxxxxxxxxxx

XXXXXXXXXX
- xxxxxxxxxxxxxxxx
xxxxxxxxxxxxxxxx
xxxxxxxxxxxxxxxx
- xxxxxxxxxxxxxxxx
xxxxxxxxxxxxxxxx
xxxxxxxxxxxxxxxx
xxxxxxxxxxxxxxxx

xxx

Disorder

Treatment

Diet and Lifestyle

- xxxxxxxxxxxxxxxxxxxxxxxxxxxxxxxxxxxxxxxx
- xxxxxxxxxxxxxxxxxxxxxxxxxxxxxxxxxxxxxxx
- xxxxxxxxxxxxxxxxxxxxxxxxxxxxxxx

Pharmacological treatment
-
xxxxxxxxxxxxxxxxxxxxxxxxxxxxxxxxxxxxxx
x
xxxxxxxxxxxxxxxxxxxxxxxxxxxxxxxxxxxxxx
xxx •
x
xxxxxxxxxxxxxxxxxxxxxxxxxxxxxxxxxxxxxx
xxxxxxxxxxxxxxxxxxxxxxxxxxxxxxxxxxxx
xxxxxx

xxxxxxx xxxxxxxxxxx
xxxxxxx xxxxxxxxxxxxxxxxxx
xxxxxxx xxxxxxxxxxxxxx
xxxxxxx xxxxxxxxxxxxxxxx
xxxxxxxxxx xxxxxxxxxxx
-
xxxxxxxxxxxxxxxxxxxxxxxxxxxxxxxxxxxxxx
xxxxxxxxxxxxxxxxxxxxxxxxxxxx

XXXXXXXXXX
xxxxxxxxxxxxxxxx
xxxxxxxxxxxxxxxxxxxxxxx
xxxxxxxxxxxxxxxxxxxxxxxxx
xxxxxxxxxxxxxx
xxxxxxxxxxxxxxx
xxxxxxxxxxxxxxxxxxxxxxxxx

XXXXXXXXXX
- xxxxxxxxxxxxxxxxx
- xxxxxxxxxxxxxx

XXXXXXXXXX
xxxxxxxxxxxxxxxx
xxxxxxxxxxxxxxxxxxxxxxx
- xxxxxxxxxxxxxxxx
xxxxxxxxxxxxxxxxxxxxxxx

XXXXXXXXXX
xxxxxxxxxxxxxxxx
xxxxxxxxxxxxxxxxxxxxxxx
xxxxxxxxxxxxxxxx
xxxxxxxxxxxxxxxxxxxxxxx

XXXXXXXXXX
xxxxxxxxxxxxxxxxxxxxxx
xxxxxxxxxxxxxxxx
xxxxxxxxxxxxxxxx
xxxxxxxxxxxxxxxx

xxx

On the **Treatment** page, the main column contains information on lifestyle management and nonspecialist medical therapy of the disorder, with general information on specialist management when this is the main treatment.

Whenever possible under "Pharmacological treatment," guidelines are given on the standard dosage for commonly used drugs, with details of contraindications and precautions, main drug interactions, and main side effects. In each case, however, the manufacturer's drug data sheet should be consulted before any regimen is prescribed.

The main goals of treatment (*e.g.*, to cure, to palliate, to prevent), prognosis after treatment, precautions that the physician should take during and after treatment, and any other information that could help the clinician to make treatment decisions (*e.g.*, other nonpharmacological treatment options, special situations or groups of patients) are given in the right shaded side column. The key and general references at the end of this column provide the reader with further practical information.

Diagnosis

Signs

Acanthosis nigricans (AN): Dry and rough, gray-brown or black pigmentation and palpable thickening of the skin with small papillomatous elevations, giving a velvety texture. Commonly seen on the axillae, back and sides of neck, anogenital region, and groin and less often on other flexures, the inframammary region, and umbilicus. In the malignant form, almost the entire body can be involved. As the lesions progress, the skin becomes more thickened, the skin lines are further accentuated, the surface becomes mamillated, and verrucous excrescences develop.

Variants: acral acanthotic anomaly develops in the dorsa of the palms and soles of dark-skinned persons. Unilateral (nevoid) AN develops unilaterally and may enlarge before stabilizing.

Confluent reticulated papillomatosis (CRP): Confluent, verrucous, dry planar papules, up to 5 mm in diameter. Lesions first appear between the breasts and in the midline of the back and gradually extend over the breasts, sometimes reaching the shoulders and the sides of the neck.

Symptoms

• Both **AN** and **CRP** are usually asymptomatic, but may be pruritic.

Investigations

AN: Diagnosis is clinical. Biopsy shows papillomatosis and hyperkeratosis, but only slight, irregular acanthosis, and usually no hyperpigmentation. Evaluation in obese patients and adolescents with limited involvement is unnecessary in the absence of systemic symptoms (other than screening for diabetes with measurement of glycosylated hemoglobin level or glucose tolerance test). If rapid progression occurs and malignancy is suspected, imaging studies and endoscopy are indicated (for adenocarcinoma of gastrointestinal or genitourinary tract).

CRP: Biopsy shows mild hyperkeratosis and papillomatosis. Focal acanthosis is limited to the valleys between elongated papillae.

Complications

AN: Types 1 through 4 are benign. Type 5 may precede other symptoms of malignancy, by 5 years.

CRP: None

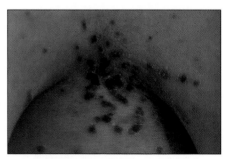

Lesions of confluent reticulated papillomatosis in netlike pattern on inframammary area.

Differential diagnosis

AN: CRP, pityriasis versicolor, X-linked ichthyosis, retention hyperkeratosis, linear epidermal nevus, reticulate pigmented anomaly of the flexures (Dowling-Degos disease), pellagra, hemochromatosis, or Addison's disease.

CRP: AN, tinea versicolor, Darier's disease, hereditary reticulate dyschromatosis.

Etiology

AN: There are five types of AN.

Type 1: Hereditary benign; onset during childhood or puberty.

Type 2: Benign; various endocrine disorders associated with insulin resistance: type 1 diabetes, hyperandrogenetic states, Cushing's disease, Addison's disease, hypothyroidism.

Type 3: Pseudo; complication of obesity, which produces insulin resistance; more common in patients with darker pigmentation.

Type 4: Drug-induced; nicotinic acid in high doses, stilbestrol, oral contraceptives, methyltestosterone, fusidic acid, triazinate, and insulin.

Type 5: Malignant (paraneoplastic); 91% are abdominal, and 69% of these are stomach and less commonly genitourinary cancers and lymphomas.

CRP: Genetic defect of keratinization or abnormal response to colonization by *Pityrosporum orbiculare* or follicular bacteria has been proposed.

Epidemiology

AN: Overall incidence is 7.1% in children. Overall, 13% in blacks, 5.5% in Hispanics, and <1% in whites, usually in obese, hirsute, and hyperandrogenic adults. Malignant AN is exceptionally rare.

CRP: Most cases are sporadic, some are familial. Median age at onset is 21 years. Female:male ratio is 2.5:1. Black:white ratio is 2:1.

Treatment

Diet and lifestyle

AN: Weight loss can resolve type 3 AN and has a beneficial effect on the other types.

• Controlled low-fat or low-carbohydrate diet may help control associated insulin resistance.

• Reportedly successful but suspect supplements include dietary fish oils, thyroid-stimulating hormone, thyroglobulin, and methyl thiouracil.

Pharmacological treatment

• In AN, combinations of topical agents—such as keratolytics, tretinoin, and corticosteroids—are typically used, as are applications of podophyllin resin.

Topical, for AN or CRP

• Salicylic acid 5% to 10% in hydrophilic petrolatum.

• Urea 10% to 40% cream or lotion.

• Hydroquinone 2% to 8% cream.

• Imidazole antifungal creams.

• Tretinoin 0.1% cream (often effective in CRP).

• Fluorouracil 5% cream.

• High-potency corticosteroids.

• Podophyllin resin 25%, applied every 2–4 weeks.

• Selenium sulfide 2.5%.

Systemic

CRP: Minocycline, 100–200 mg/d for 1–3 months.

AN or CRP: Isotretinoin, 2 mg/kg/day, and acitretin, 25–50 mg/day, 1–3 months, have been reported to be effective, anecdotally.

AN type 5: Cyproheptadine may inhibit release of tumor factors.

Nonpharmacological treatment

Supportive methods

• Oral antihistamines and topical antipruritic agents for pruritus.

• Lipid-controlling (statins) and diabetic controlling (*eg*, sulfonylureas, insulin) medications have been reported to clear AN.

Physical modalities (for AN and CRP).

• Trichloroacetic acid peels, 25%–90%.

• Dermabrasion.

• Cryosurgery with 10–30-second thaw time.

• Erbium:YAG or CO_2 laser resurfacing.

Surgery

AN: Indicated if there is an underlying malignancy.

Treatment aims

To improve appearance of skin and, for AN, to determine cause.

Prognosis

AN: Type 1: Accentuated at puberty and, at times, regresses when older.

Type 2: Stable.

Type 3: May regress after significant weight loss.

Type 4: Resolves when therapy with causative drug is discontinued.

Type 5: Regression follows removal of malignancy, but prognosis is poor.

CRP: Often responds to treatment but can recur.

General references

Schwartz RA: Acanthosis nigricans. *J Am Acad Dermatol* 1994, **31**:1–19.

Lee MP, *et al.*: Confluent and reticulated papillomatosis: response to high-dose oral isotretinoin therapy and reassessment of epidemiologic data. *J Am Acad Dermatol* 1994, **31**:327–331.

Montemarano AD, *et al.*: Confluent and reticulated papillomatosis: response to minocycline. *J Am Acad Dermatol* 1996, **34**:253–256.

Steven Natow and Allen Natow

3

Acne vulgaris and hidradenitis suppurativa

Diagnosis

Signs

Acne vulgaris (AV): Characteristic lesion: open or closed comedone; other: inflammatory papule, papulopustule, pustule, cyst, scar. Usually on face; back, upper chest, scalp. Adults: Facial periphery, chin often involved. **Acne conglobata**: Chronic, highly inflammatory; widespread polyporous comedones, pustules, large tender nodules, abscesses, draining sinus tracts, hypertrophic scars; back, buttocks, chest, less often on abdomen, shoulders, neck, face, upper arms, thighs. Most common in young men. Musculoskeletal symptoms include sacroiliitis. **Acne fulminans**: Nodulocystic lesions become necrotic, ulcerate. Fever, malaise, myalgias, arthritis, weight loss, anemia, leukocytosis, elevated erythrocyte sedimentation rate. Typically white male adolescents. Follicular occlusion triad syndrome: acne conglobata, hidradenitis suppurativa, dissecting folliculitis of scalp. **Hidradenitis suppurativa (HS)**: Chronic, recurrent erythematous, subcutaneous nodules, abcesses; usually rupture, drain purulent malodorous discharge; often hypertrophic scarring. Fistulas, sinus tracts in subcutaneous honeycomb pattern. In women, more common on axilla, then inguinal region, breasts. In men, perianal, anogenital areas more common than axillae. Either gender: buttocks, periumbilical skin, scalp, popliteal fossa, zygomatic, malar areas of face.

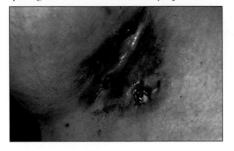

Inflamed, erythematous axillary skin with nodules, elliptical abscesses, sinuses draining seropurulent fluid, and fibrotic bands in a patient with hidradenitis suppurativa.

Symptoms

Acne (A): Skin often oily. Cysts painful, burning, pruritus possible. **HS**: Soreness, pain, tenderness, restriction of movement; general malaise with flaring; decreased or absent apocrine sweating.

Investigations

A: Hormonal evaluation in adolescent girls with severe acne, women with signs of virilization, irregular menses, or normal menses but sudden onset or severe unexplained worsening of acne; no exogenous hormones 2–3 months before testing. Dehydroepiandrostenedione sulfate serum levels 400–700 ng/dL suggests adult-onset adrenal enzyme deficiency; > 800 ng/dL, adrenal neoplasm; > 1500 ng/dL, ovarian tumor. Total testosterone serum levels > 150 ng/dL, adrenal or ovarian neoplasm, hyperthecosis. Morning fasting glucose:insulin level ratio: if < 4.5, evaluate for insulin resistance or polycystic ovarian syndrome with glucose tolerance test. Other tests: thyroid function, prolactin level, midcycle follicle-stimulating hormone:luteinizing hormone ratio (> 3:1 indicates polycystic ovarian syndrome). **Bacterial culture and sensitivity**: If *Staphylococcus aureus* or gram-negative superinfection suspected. **HS**: Diagnosis clinical; can be confirmed histopathologically. Bacteria cultures positive in only 50% of all active cases. Erythrocyte sedimentation rate elevated; leukocytosis present.

Complications

A: *S. aureus* infection; gram-negative bacterial infection. **HS**: Scarring; local and systemic infections, rarely septicemia; restricted mobility of limbs secondary to scarring and pain; anal, rectal, and urethral fistulas; normocytic, normochromic anemia; asymmetrical pauciarticular arthritis or symmetrical polyarthritis/polyarthralgia syndrome; improves after surgical removal; rarely squamous-cell carcinoma. **Both**: Decreased self-esteem, social isolation, depression.

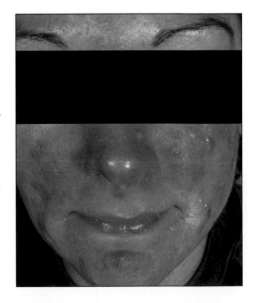

Comedones, inflammatory papules and cysts in a young woman with cystic acne.

Wendy Epstein

Treatment

Diet and lifestyle

• Diet and exercise consistent with normal menses for women; avoid foods high in iodides, supplemental Vitamin E, wheat germ; educate about not picking, no friction, avoidance of potentially comedogenic cosmetics and suncreens

Pharmacological treatment

Topical for acne

Cleansers: Benzoyl peroxide 2.5%, 5.0%, 10%. Salicylic acid 2%, glycolic acid washes. Benzethanium chloride 0.5%, for sensitive skin. Sulfur soap. Oil-control cleansers. some with acetone or surfactants. **Astrigents**: May contain glycolic acid, salicylic acid, other. Witch hazel for sensitive skin. **Masks**: Some contain anti-acne agents. **Polyacrylic acid strips**: Generally ineffective on smaller comedones. **Benzoyl peroxide**: Best agent against *P. acnes*; use with other antibiotics to prevent resistance. Wash, gel, lotion, usually 2.5%, 5.0%, 10%. **Benzamycin** gel, 3% erythromycin and 5% benzoyl peroxide, b.i.d., for antibiotic-resistant A. **Clindamycin** 1%; solution, gel, pledgets. **Erythromycin** 2%; solution, gel, pledgets. **Sulfur-resorcinol lotion**. **Retinoids**: Tretinoin (0.025%, 0.05%, 0.1% cream or 0.01%, 0.025% gel, or 0.05% solution or 0.1% in microsphere gel; nonphoto-sensitizing tazarotene, 0.05%, 0.1% gel; adapalene, 0.01% gel, 0.1% solution. Tazarotene, 0.05%, 0.1% gel, applied 2–5 minutes, b.i.d. **Azelex cream**: 20% azelaic.

Topical for hidradenitis suppurativa

Antibiotics: Clindamycin 1% or erythromycin 2% solution. **Silver-sulfadiazene or bactroban cream** for bacterial superinfection. **Intralesional triamcinolone acetonide**, 1.0-2.5mg/cc (0.01-0.03cc/cyst).

Systemic for acne

Antibiotics: Tetracyline, 250–500mg, b.i.d. to q.i.d.; minocycline, 50–100mg, b.i.d.; 5% develop dizziness/vertigo; rarely hepatic dysfunction, mononucleosis-like syndrome, dose-dependent bluish cutaneous hyperpigmentation; doxycycline, 50–100 mg, b.i.d.; increased phototoxicity. Erythromycin, 250–500 mg, b.i.d. to q.i.d.; not contraindicated during pregnancy, except for the erythromycin estolate preparation. Azithromycin, 250 mg, daily or every other day. Trimethoprin-sulfamethoxazole, one tablet, b.i.d.; against gram-negative acne. Clindomycin, ampicillin, cefradoxil. Isotretinoin: Choice for severe cystic acne, acne that causes scarring and recalcitrant acne unresponsive to other treatments. Usual dose is 1mg/kg/d (facial); 1.5mg/kg/d (chest, back) for 20 weeks. **Oral contraceptives**: Low estrogen contraceptives with less androgenic progestins such as norgestimate, desogestrel preferable; avoid androgenic 19-nortestosterone progestins; cyproterone acetate antian-drogen in combination with ethinylestradiol (available in Europe) effective. **Prednisone**, 5.0-7.5mg, at or before bedtime, to suppress ACTH and adrenal androgens, if adrenal hyperactivity suspected. At 0.5 to 1.0 mg/kg concommittantly or before treatment with isotretinoin in acne conglobata, and before treatment with isotretinoin in acne fulminans; taper dose as soon as possible. **Spironolactone**, DHT androgen receptor partial agonist, alone or in combination with oral contraceptives, starting with 50 mg/d, increasing to 100 mg, b.i.d.; adverse effects: menstrual irregularities, mastodynia, reduced libido and hyperkalemia, if preexisting renal disease.

Systemic for hidradenitis suppurativa

Antibiotics: According to results of cultures, sensitivities. If no pathogenic bacteria grows, oral tetracyclines in doses equivalent to those for acne. **Isotretinoin**, 1 mg/kg/d to 2 mg/kg/d.

Nonpharmacological treatment

A: Peels: 20% to 30% salicylic acid or 20% to 70% glycolic acid or 10% to 20% trichloroacetic acid. Triancinolone acetonide, 2.5 to 3.0 mg/cc diluted in saline, injected into inflammatory lesions; higher concentrations increase risk of atrophy. Cryotherapy. Augmentation for atrophic scars. Comedone extraction. Excision of scars, then dermabrasion or laser resurfacing. Mini-punch grafts from retroauricular area then laser resurfacing. Pulsed CO_2 or erbium laser resurfacing. Dermabrasion. **HS**: Incision and drainage of cysts. Unroofing and marsupialization of sinus tracts. CO_2 laser stripping with healing by secondary intention. Wide surgical excision beyond clinical borders with healing by secondary intention or grafting.

Treatment aims

A: To reduce or cure acne and prevent scarring.

HS: To reduce purulent, foul-smelling drainage; prevent infection and disability.

Prognosis

A: In women, sharp decline in incidence after age of 44 years.

HS: Chronic recurrent, often premenstrual flares. If untreated, spontaneous remission is rare and progressive disability common. Severity declines after menopause.

General references

Brown TJ, Rosen T, Orengo I: Hidradenitis Suppuritiva. *South Med J* 1998, **91**:1107–1114.

Jemec GB, Faber M, Gutschik E, Wendelboe P: The Bacteriology of Hidradenitis Suppurativa. *Dermatol* 1996, **193**:203–206.

Finley EM, Ratz JL: Treatment of hidradenitis suppurativa with carbon dioxide laser excision and second-intention healing. *J Am Acad Dermatol* 1996, **34**:465–469.

Boer J, Van Germert MJ: Long-term results of isotretinoin in the treatment of 68 patients with hidradenitis suppurativa. *J Am Acad Dermatol* 1999, **40**:73–76.

Jemec GBE, Wendelboe P: Topical clindamycin versus systemic tetracycline in the treatment of hidradenitis suppurativa. *J Am Acad Dermatol* 1998, **39**:971–974.

Diagnosis

Signs

Erythromelalgia (E): Symmetric warmth and redness of extremities with normal pulses. Distribution: legs (primary syndrome); arms and legs (secondary syndrome).
Acrocyanosis (A): Symmetric, prolonged but reversible, bluish, cyanotic discoloration of digits, hands, feet. Involved acral areas cool, moist. Pulses normal. Digits may be puffy.
Livedo reticularis (L): Reddish-blue, mottled, recticular, "fish-net" pattern of skin. Purpuric macules or nodules may develop, become ulcerated. Ulcers most often on lower legs, ankles, feet; heal as smooth or depressed ivory-to-white plaques with hyperpigmented borders with telangiectatic vessels.

Symptoms

E: Burning pain in extremities; attacks are paroxysmal, localized.
A: No pain; digits may be numb.
L: Subjective coldness of skin, numbness or pain (rare); pain, tenderness in ulcerated form. Secondary forms: symptoms of underlying disease.

Investigations

E: Secondary: erythrocyte, leukocyte, platelet counts, uric acid levels, antinuclear antibodies, blood pressure.
A: Cold agglutinins, anticardiolipin antibodies, cryoglobulins, platelet count.
L: Test for suspected underlying disease(s) (anti-nuclear antibodies, anti-cardiolipin antibodies, anti-2–GP1 antibodies; serum amylase; viral serologies and cultures.

Complications

A: Cosmetic appearance. Ulcerations when associated with combined cryoglobulins and cryoagglutinins.
L: Ulceration of purpuric macular or nodular lesions.

Differential diagnosis

E: Raynaud's phenomenon (hyperemic phase), ischemic vascular disease, arteriosclerosis obliterans, thromboangiitis obliterans, gout, fasciitis, neuropathies.
A: Raynaud's (blue phase). No sequential color changes; similar changes may occur with cold agglutinins, after inhalation of butyl nitrate, in fucosidosis or ethylmalonic aciduria, after treatment with bromocryptine or interferon α-2a, in presence of anti-cardiolipin antibodies, and with thrombocythemia.
L: Secondary form may accompany Raynaud's, vasculitis, lupus erythematosus, atheromatous embolization, drug reactions (amantidine), lymphomas, neurogenic diseases, hypertension, obstructive arterial diseases, Sneddon's syndrome (Livedo reticularis with cerebrovascular lesions), pancreatitis (Walzel's sign).

Etiology

E: Onset may be elicited by exposure to increased temperatures, limb dependency, exercise, occlusion of circulation. Abnormality in prostaglandin metabolism proposed. Primary syndrome: Etiology unknown. Secondary syndrome may be associated with thrombocythemia, polycythemia vera, hypertension, myeloproliferative diseases, lupus erythematosus, vasculitis, malignancy, hepatitis B vaccination, drugs (ticlopidine, nifedipine).
A: Vasoconstriction of small cutaneous arteries, arterioles; decreased blood flow on exposure to cold. Secondary dilation of capillaries, subpapillary venous plexus. Increased arteriolar tone (at room temperature), sympathetic vasomotor activity.
L: Accompanies vasospasm, obstruction of small perpendicular arterioles in dermis. Causes: increased sympathetic nerve activity; immune complex deposition in vasculitis; defects in fibrinolysis and platelet adhesiveness; infectious diseases; obstruction of arteries by vasculitis, embolization, hyperviscosity; drug induced localized vasoconstrictor release.

Epidemiology

E: Primary: Male predilection. Secondary: Usually after age 30. Rare familial cases.
A: Usually in third to fifth decade. **L:** Most common in women over 40. Ulcers may form in winter or summer.

Treatment

Diet and lifestyle

E: Avoidance of prolonged standing, overheating of extremities, excessive exercise; elevation or cooling of extremities
A: Avoidance of cooling of extremities, cold environment. Warm affected acral parts.
L: Cosmetic covering of affected skin areas: maintenance of body and extremity warmth.

Pharmacological treatment

Topical

L: Analgesic ointments, occlusive dressings for ulcerations.

Systemic

E: Piroxicam for primary syndrome. Treatment of underlying disease in secondary syndrome. Serotonin reuptake inhibitors (methysegide, pizotifen, fluoxetine, venlafaxine, sertraline). Sodium nitroprusside, intravenously. Sodium channel blockers: Intravenous lidocaine followed by oral mexiletine Aspirin or indomethacin in secondary syndrome due to polycythemia vera or thrombocytosis.

A: Inhibitors of sympathetic nerve activity, reserpine. Low-dose aspirin in thrombocythemia.

L: Sympatholytic drugs: Anticoagulants if thrombosis or anticardiolipin antibodies. Antiplatelet and fibrinolytic agents (aspirin, tissue plasminogen activator, stanozolol) Low molecular weight dextran infusions. Pentoxifylline. Nicotinic acid. Nifedipine. Immunosuppressives (Methotrexate, cytoxan). Prostacyclin or prostaglandin E infusions.

Nonpharmacological treatment

Surgery

E: Sympathectomy.

Physical modalities.

L: Psoralen and UVA photochemotherapy (PUVA).

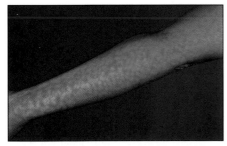

Livedo reticularis presents as a mottled red to bluish discoloration occurring in a net-like pattern.

Treatment aims

E: To decrease frequency of attacks.
A: To reduce frequency of episodes.
L: To improve appearance, treat underlying disease(s)

Follow-up and management

E: Attention to underlying diseases.
A: Treat underlying disease; remove causative drug(s).
L: Local treatment for ulcerations. Treatment of underlying disease in secondary forms.

Prognosis

E: Primary: partial control by avoidance of precipitating causes. Secondary: good control in polycythemia vera, thrombocytosis; other: depends on control of underlying disease(s).
A: Persistent, recurrent. No trophic changes. :: Benign form: excellent. With ulcers: may persist or recur with pain, disability, scarring. Secondary forms: depends on underlying disease(s).

General references

Rudikoff D, Jaffee IA: Erythromelalgia: Response to serotonin reuptake inhibitors. *J Am Acad Dermatol* 1997, 37:281–283.

Calderone DC, Finzi E: Treatment of primary erythromelalgia with piroxicam. *J Am Acad Dermatol* 1991, 24:145–146.

Kalgaard OM, Seem E, Kvernbo K: Erythromelalgia: A clinical study of 87 cases. *J Intern Med* 1997, 242:191–197.

Choi HJ, Hamm SK: Livedo reticularis and livedoid vasculitis responding to PUVA therapy. *J Am Acad Dermatol* 1999, 40:204–207.

Sams WM Jr: Livedo reticularis therapy with pentoxyfylline. *Arch Dermatol* 1988, 124:684–687.

Diagnosis

Signs

Addison's disease: Generalized bronze color of the skin. Brown pigmentation enhanced in areas around the eyes, gingival and buccal mucous membrane, tongue, nipples, palmar creases, and new scars. Linear streaks of pigmentation in nail plate. Gray scalp-hair may darken. Axillary hair may decrease. Brown or blue-black spotty pigmentation of the gingival or buccal mucosa.

Hypercorticism: Moon facies. Obesity, with redistribution of fat creating "buffalo hump," truncal obesity, and thin arms; purple striae on abdomen; hirsutism; ecchymoses; acne; hypertension.

Symptoms

Addison's disease: Nausea, vomiting, diarrhea and orthostatic hypotension, with dizziness and syncope.

Hypercorticism (Cushing's syndrome): Urinary frequency, thirst, fatigue, muscle weakness, psychiatric abnormalities.

Investigations

Addison's disease: Short cosyntropin stimulation test.

Hypercorticism: Overnight dexamethasone suppression test; 8:00 AM plasma cortisol; 24-hour urine cortisol. CT scan of the abdomen and the pituitary.

Complications

Addison's disease: Supine hypotension and death.

Hypercorticism: Hypertension, diabetes.

Differential diagnosis

Addison's disease: Hemochromatosis, porphyria cutanea tarda, chronic renal failure, hepatic cirrhosis, chemotherapy, carcinoid.

Hypercorticism: Obesity, sleep apnea.

Etiology

Addison's disease: Primary and secondary adrenal failure.

Hypercorticism: Adrenal hyperplasia resulting from pituitary hypersecretion, adrenocorticotropic hormone production from nonendocrine tumors or corticosteroid administration.

Epidemiology

Both: Affects all ages; no gender predilection.

Dina Began

Treatment

Pharmacological treatment

Addison's disease: Hydrocortisone, 100 mg, intravenously, every 8 hours.

Supportive methods

Addison's disease: Intravenous fluids for blood pressure support.

Special considerations

Addison's disease: Hospital admission, with endocrinologic consultation.

Hypercorticism: Consult an endocrinologist.

Treatment aims

Addison's disease: Correct cortisol deficiency; maintain blood pressure.

Hypercorticism: Decrease serum cortisol and control blood pressure and blood glucose.

Prognosis

Both: Varies with etiology.

General references

Williams GH, Duffy RG: Diseases of the adrenal cortex. In: *Harrison's Principles of Internal Medicine,* edn. 14, vol 2. Edited by Fauci AS, Braunwald E, Isselbacher KJ, *et al.* New York: McGraw-Hill Health Professions Division; 1998:2053–2054.

Freinkel RK: Other endocrine diseases. In: *Fitzpatrick's Dermatology in General Medicine.* Edited by Freedberg IM, Eisen AZ, Wolff K, *et al.* New York: McGraw-Hill Health Professions Division; 1999:1979–1982.

Diagnosis

Signs

- Age-related skin changes inevitably involve the entire integument.
- Photoaging superimposed on intrinsically aging skin in sun-exposed areas causes features typical of actinic damage.
- Clinical features: coarse textural changes and irregular pigmentation (*eg*, lentigines, macular hypomelanosis, persistent hyperpigmentation).
- Other signs: Wrinkling (fine surface lines, deep furrows); miniaturization and depigmentation of hair follicles; loss of translucency, elasticity, skin laxity; sallow color; telangiectasias; easy bruisability; associated benign, malignant neoplasms.

Symptoms

- Skin feels looser, less resilient, dry, and sensitive.

Investigations

- Ultraviolet lamp examination: Enhances visualization of photodamage.
- Biopsy: Histologic features: atrophy of epidermis, nuclear atypia, decreased dermal thickness, solar elastosis, fewer adnexal structures.

Complications

- Solar lentigos, actinic keratosis, malignancies (basal cell carcinoma, squamous cell carcinoma, melanoma) correlate primarily with sun exposure.
- Impaired barrier function, moisture retention; diminished wound healing, mechanical protection; loss of sensory perception, chemical clearance; decreased ability to sweat and thermoregulate; inadequate production of sebum, vitamin D.

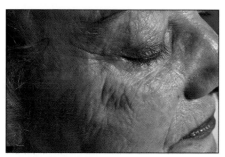

Advanced photoaging with atrophic skin, irregular pigmentation, telangiectasias, skin sagging, criss-crossed lines and periorbital and perioral rhytides.

Differential diagnosis

Premature aging syndromes (progeria, metageria, pangeria, acrogeria); diseases associated with poor nutrition, tissue breakdown (metastatic cancer); phototoxicity (porphyria cutanea tarda), HIV-associated wasting syndrome.

Etiology

Intrinsic aging changes: Genetically predetermined, gradual, and inevitable.

Physiologic organic changes: Particularly hormonal ones (specially estrogen deficiency), have a significant effect on skin senescence.

Extrinsic changes: Represent the cumulative effect of environmental factors on the skin. Ultraviolet (UV) radiation is the overwhelmingly predominant cause; by age 18, 50% of UV light (UVL) exposure has occurred. UVL radiation elevates matrix metalloproteinases, which degrade skin collagen. Susceptibility to environmental factors varies among individuals, based on intrinsic factors, such as skin type. Cigarette smoking and poor nutrition accelerate aging.

Epidemiology

Photoaging most pronounced if fair coloring, significant sun exposure.

Paul Frank and Ellen Gendler

Treatment

Pharmacological treatment

Topical

• All-trans-retinoic acid (tretinoin): Dose dependent effects; increase with long-term usage. Tretinoin .05% cream (used sparingly nightly or every other night) specifically marketed for this indication; other preparations, other retinoids (*eg*, adapalene, tazaratene), may be as effective. Dryness, erythema, desquamation improve with time. Treatment for at least 3–6 months is needed to detect improvement (*eg*, smoother skin texture, decreased pigmentation, reduction of fine lines, wrinkles). Perpetual treatment is needed to maintain beneficial effects.

• N-furfuryladenine 0.1% cream; nonprescription, derived from plant-growth hormone: effects poorly studied, but thought to be similar to topical retinoids, without irritation, photosensitivity.

• α-hydroxy (glycolic, lactic, citric) acids (AHAs) used daily in low concentrations (also in superficial chemical peels, at higher concentrations). Glycolic acid penetrates skin more easily than other AHAs. AHAs exfoliate upper layers of skin, stimulate collagen production to improve textural, pigmentary imperfections. β-hydroxy acids (salicylic acid) are keratolytic; similar effect, supposedly greater tolerability.

• Antioxidants (vitamin C [ascorbic acid], vitamin E [tocopherols], beta-carotene, CoQ10, bioflavinoids): efficacy as topical agents controversial. Vitamin C may improve protective effect of sunscreens, but rapidly deactivated by light, oxygen; instability in compounds a big obstacle.

• Estrogen replacement: When used in postmenopausal women, could help maintain total skin thickness and collagen content.

Nonpharmacological treatment

Microdermabrasion: Chemical peels (superficial: glycolic, 15% to 35%, or salicylic acid, 20% to 30%; medium: glycolic acid, 50% to 70% or TCA, 15% to 35%) provide gradual improvement. Skin resurfacing with dermabrasion or laser (crbium, pulsed CO2) stimulates new collagen production and revivifies skin. With deeper destruction, efficacy increases, but longer recovery period, increased risk of side effects (persistent erythema, hyperpigmentation, scarring). **Soft tissue augmentation.** Several filling agents can soften rhytides, age lines. Bovine-derived collagen, alone or mixed with patient's serum; requires prior allergy testing; lasts 4 to 9 months, depending on injection site. Collagen derived from human cadaver or patient's skin: nonallergenic; may last up to 2 years. Transplanted human dermis, burrowed under lines, scars: provides long-term results without risk of rejection. Hylaform gel (cross-linked chains of hyaluronic acid derived from rooster combs) is nonallergenic. Autologous fat injected into wrinkles, fallen areas (cheeks, chin) may last months to years. Polytetrafluoroethelene enhances lip-lines, nasolabial folds permanently.

Botulinum toxin (1 IU/0.1 mL): Temporarily paralyzes injected muscles; eliminates frown lines, wrinkles for approximately 3 to 6 months; in addition to glabellar creases (0.4 to 0.08 mL/corrugator), frown lines or periorbital lines (0.4 to 0.6 mL/corrugator), platysmal bands, and perioroficial lines can also be improved.

Surgery: Rejuvenation, reconstructive surgery; liposculpture; hair transplantation.

Supportive methods: Photoprotection with broad spectrum sunscreens (UVA, UVB), protective clothing essential to maintain improvement, prevent further acute UVL damage. Moisturizers help protect skin from environmental detriments. Oral antioxidants may retard aging; no evidence confirms Gingko bilboa, dihydroethylstilbesterol, other supplements are beneficial.

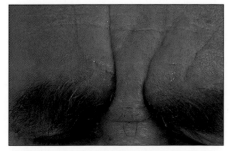

Deep glabellar lines that may improve with injections of botulinum toxin.

Paul Frank and Ellen Gendler

Treatment aims

Reverse actinic damage, to prevent skin cancer, restore integrity of skin, cosmetically and functionally.

Follow-up and management

Patients with significant photodamage need yearly screening for skin cancer. Cosmetic interventions (*eg*, soft tissue augmentation, chemical peels), must be maintained at varying intervals to maximize their effects.

General references

Uitto J. Understanding premature skin aging. *N Engl J Med* 1997, **337**:1463–1465.

Drake LA, Dinehart SM, Farmer ER, *et al.*: Guidelines of care for photoaging/ photodamage. *J Am Acad Dermatol* 1996, **5**:462–464.

Gendler EC: A practical approach to the use of retinoids in aging skin. *J Am Acad Dermatol* 1998, **39**:S114–S117.

Krauss MC: Recent advances in soft tissue augmentation. *Semin Cutan Med Surg* 1999, **18**:119–128.

Diagnosis

Signs

- Acute: Well-demarcated, erythematous, edematous papules and plaques with vesicles, bullae, and erosions at the site of exposure. The lesions may become crusted. The eruption is usually symmetrical, but atypical patterns develop, and localized or generalized spread may occur. The distribution is determined by site of contact with the external agent. Areas distant from application of offending agent may develop so-called ectopic contact dermatitis (*eg*, eyelid involvement from nail polish). Linear distribution is the hallmark of toxicodendron ("poison ivy") dermatitis. Airborne and photo contact dermatitis affect exposed areas of face, neck, arms, and hands.

- Subacute: Erythematous papules and plaques with fine, dry scale.

- Chronic: Lichenified, slightly erythematous, scaly (even hyperkeratotic) papules and plaques, with excoriations, hyperpigmentation, vesiculation, or fissures.

Symptoms

- Pruritus, fissuring with pain, dryness, scaling.

Investigations

- Patient history and distribution of dermatitis may suggest cause, but is often insufficient to identify the causative agent.

- Skin biopsy: Shows epidermal spongiosis and a superficial, perivascular, lymphohistiocytic dermal infiltrate, occasionally with eosinophils. Acanthosis and hyperkeratosis with areas of parakeratosis are present in chronic cases. Histopathologic evaluation does not reliably differentiate between allergic and irritant contact dermatitis.

- Patch testing: The mainstay of diagnosis for allergic contact dermatitis. Starts with the T.R.U.E. Test (Thin-layer Rapid Use Epicutaneous Test; Glaxo Wellcome, Research Triangle Park, NC, USA; http://www.truetest.com) and progresses to testing for other suspected standardized allergens. Increasing the number of allergens tested increases the yield of patch testing. Only standardized allergens should be tested; compounds of unknown composition should not be used. Patch tests are applied to the upper back, but the inner arms may also be used. Patches are removed and interpreted after 48 hours and interpreted again 72 or 96 hours after placement. Determining relevance of positive patch tests is vital to successful diagnosis. Patients should not use systemic or topical corticosteroids for 1 week before patch testing. No standardized tests exist for irritant contact dermatitis, but patch testing may be necessary to exclude a concomitant allergy.

- Repeated open application testing (ROAT): Patients self-test with nonoccluded application of own suspected products on the volar forearm twice daily for 7 days. Only test with products designed for skin application (avoid soaps and detergents, etc.).

Complications

- Exfoliative erythroderma, lichen simplex chronicus, postinflammatory hypopigmentation, hyperpigmentation, impetiginization.

Differential diagnosis

Dyshidrosis, atopic dermatitis, nummular eczema, autoeczematization dermatitis (id reaction), stasis dermatitis, seborrheic dermatitis, psoriasis, dermatophytosis.

Etiology

Allergic contact dermatitis: Occurs only in sensitized individuals and represents a type IV, cell-mediated, delayed hypersensitivity reaction against the allergen. Langerhans cells carry the antigen via the lymphatics to the regional lymph nodes and sensitized CD4+ T lymphocytes migrate to all areas of the skin. Persons may be exposed to allergens for years before developing hypersensitivity. The most frequent allergens in the United States are nickel sulfate, fragrance mix, thimerosal, quaternium-15, neomycin sulfate, formaldehyde, bacitracin, thiuram mix, balsam of Peru, cobalt chloride, para-phenylenediamine, and carba mix.

Irritant contact dermatitis: Occurs via a nonimmune mechanism and may occur in any exposed person. Common irritants include alkalis (*ie*, soaps, detergents, lye, ammonia-containing compounds), acids, and solvents.

Important factors in the development of irritant contact dermatitis include the nature of the chemical, its concentration, the duration of contact, and the permeability of the stratum corneum.

Epidemiology

Contact dermatitis accounts for 4% to 7% of all dermatologic consultations. Irritant contact dermatitis is more common than allergic contact dermatitis.

Irritant contact dermatitis: The most common form of occupational skin disease. Increased incidence of contact dermatitis occurs in certain occupational groups exposed to "wet work" (eg, hairdressers, nurses, metal and chemical industry workers).

Certain allergens have a marked sex predilection (eg, nickel allergy is more common in women, and allergy to potassium dichromate is more common in men). Periorbital contact dermatitis occurs more commonly in women.

Joshua P. Fogelman and Ronald R. Brancaccio

Treatment

Diet and lifestyle

•Contact dermatitis due to occupational exposure may require alteration of workplace conditions. The Americans with Disabilities Act of 1990 protects workers.

•Allergen avoidance may necessitate changes in skin-care products, clothing, and hobbies.

•Medicaments and allergens present in certain foods, such as flavoring agents, preservatives, and nickel, may cause systemic contact dermatitis in patients sensitized topically. Specific dietary restrictions may be indicated in these patients.

•Bentoquatam 5% lotion is useful as a barrier against Rhus dermatitis.

Pharmacological treatment

Topical

•Simple emollients (*eg*, petrolatum); avoid sensitizing agents.

•Antipruritic agents such as pramoxine may be useful, but avoid topical antihistamines and benzocaine-related topical anesthetics.

•Topical corticosteroids, preferably ointment-based (*eg*, fluocinolone 0.025% ointment contains petrolatum only in its base).

•For areas with vesiculation and weeping: open wet compresses with saline or aluminum sulfate/calcium acetate.

•Topical tacrolimus 0.1% ointment.

Systemic

•Severe acute or generalized contact dermatitis: oral corticosteroid therapy (prednisone at 1 mg/kg of body weight, as a single dose in the morning, with food, tapered over 2–3 weeks.

•Cyclosporine, 3–5 mg/kg divided into two doses daily for chronic contact dermatitis; given for a limited interval with careful monitoring of the patient's blood pressure, electrolytes, and renal function.

•Sedating antihistamines, (*eg*, diphenhydramine and hydroxyzine), for pruritus.

Nonpharmacological treatment

•Ultraviolet B phototherapy

•Topical or systemic psoralen plus ultraviolet A photochemotherapy

•Grenz ray radiation therapy

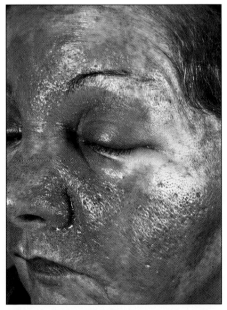

Allergic contact dermatitis from facial products: diffuse erythema, edema, vesicles, weeping.

Treatment aims

Ameliorate inflammation and pruritus. Identify and avoid the allergen or irritant. Treat secondary infection, if present. Educate patients to avoid offending agent(s) and suggest available substitutes.

Prognosis

Contact dermatitis may resolve with proper treatment or avoidance of the causative allergen or irritant, or it may progress to a chronic dermatitis.

Prognosis is good with proper treatment and avoidance of offending allergens or irritants.

Follow-up and management

Avoidance of offending allergens or irritants; use of physical modalities, if complete avoidance cannot be achieved. Induction of desensitization/hyposensitization has not been shown to be efficacious.

Allergic and irritant contact dermatitides often coexist. Contact dermatitis may complicate an underlying dermatosis because of a compromised epidermal barrier and exposure to topical medications.

Contact allergy to the topical corticosteroid itself, rather than to the base ingredients, is increasingly common and may complicate or be the underlying cause of recalcitrant contact dermatitis. Patch testing or ROAT with the corticosteroid used by the patient or two screening agents (tixocortol pivalate 1% in petrolatum and budesonide 0.1% in petrolatum) should be performed in resistant cases.

Sedating antihistamines should be used with caution in the elderly because of anticholinergic side effects (*eg*, urinary retention) and should be avoided in patients operating vehicles or potentially dangerous equipment.

Unscented products contain a masking fragrance.

Support Organizations

American Contact Dermatitis Society, 930 North Meacham Road, Schaumburg, IL 60173-6016, tel: 847-330-9830.

General references

Rietschel RL, Fowler JF: *Fisher's Contact Dermatitis.* Baltimore: Williams & Wilkins; 1995.

Marks JG, Belsito DV, DeLeo VA, *et al.*: North American Contact Dermatitis Group patch test results for the detection of delayed-type hypersensitivity to topical allergens. *J Am Acad Dermatol* 1998, **38**:911–918.

Joshua P. Fogelman and Ronald R. Brancaccio

Diagnosis

Signs

Acquired systemic amyloidosis (primary; ASA): Petechiae, purpura, ecchymoses on eyelids, axilla, umbilicus and anogenital regions; waxy translucent or purpuric papules, nodules, plaques; tumefactive lesions; less common pigmentary changes; scleroderma-like bullous lesions. Alopecia, cutis laxa, nail dystrophy, macroglossia.

Lichen amyloidosis (LA): Discrete, intensely pruritic, often scaly brownish red papules; most common on shins.

Macular amyloidosis (MA): Pruritic, gray-brown reticulated macules with reticulated or rippled pattern; most common on back.

Nodular amyloidosis (NA): One or several, 1–3 mm nodules (occasionally plaques), atrophic epidermis in center of lesion; usually on legs or face.

Symptoms

• Chronic constitutional symptoms (fatigue, weakness, anorexia, weight loss, malaise), dyspnea, paresthesia related to carpal tunnel syndrome.

Investigations

Skin biopsy for histopathologic diagnosis is test of choice.

ASA: Amorphous, eosinophilic masses in dermis, around fat cells, in walls of blood vessels; Congo red stain: "apple-green" birefringence.

MA, LA: Amyloid deposits limited to subpapillary plexus; in lichenoid lesions, epidermis shows acanthosis, hyperkeratosis.

NA: Large amyloid accumulations throughout dermis, involving subcutaneous fat. Amyloid also in blood vessel walls, sweat glands, around fat cells.

Complications

ASA: Cardiac (congestive heart failure, partial heart block, arrhythmias); renal (nephrosis); neurologic (neuropathy); coagulopathies; urinary losses of clotting factors and acquired deficientcy of factors IX and X; gastrointestinal bleeding.

NA: Sjögren's syndrome.

Differential diagnosis

ASA: Lipoid proteinosis, senile purpura.
Secondary amyloid: Lichen simplex chronicus, ashy dermatosis, post-inflammatory pigmentation.

Etiology

Amyloid accumulates due to various pathogenic mechanisms; biochemical composition of amyloid fibrils varies with clinicopathologic type of amyloidosis.

ASA: In primary systemic (occult dyscrasia) and myeloma-associated ASA, amyloid fibril protein is AL; secondary: AA; nodular: A1; macular, lichen, nodular: altered keratin.

Systemic amyloidosis may be caused by several diseases, especially rheumatoid arthritis, osteomyelitis, familial Mediterranean fever; rare causes: psoriatic arthritis, lepromatous leprosy, tuberculosis; skin-disease causes: hidradenitis suppurativa, dystrophic epidermolysis bullosa, stasis ulcers.

Epidemiology

LA: Most common in Chinese ancestry.
MA: Central, South American; Asian; Middle Eastern populations.
NA: in association with Sjögren's syndrome; 2:1 female predilection; usually in sixth, seventh decades of life.

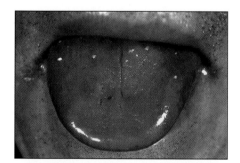

Macroglossia, with pale, smooth surface due to infiltration of amyloid, occurs in 10% of cases with primary amyloidosis.

Dina Begany

Treatment

Pharmacological treatment

Topical
MA, LA: Topical dimethyl sulfoxide (DMSO), 50% in water, with treatment continued for 6–20 weeks. Intralesional corticosteroids: 5–10 mg/mL of triancinolone acetonide.

Systemic
Primary and myeloma-associated amyloidosis: Investigational therapies: melphalan plus prednisone, thalidomide, stem cell transplant and high-dose chemoptherapy, dendritic cell therapy, 4'-iodo-4'-deoxydoxorubicin, chemotherapy, interferon-γ. Colchicine preferred for familial Mediterranean fever.

MA, LA:

• Antihistamines for itching.

• Acitretin, 25–50 mg, daily.

• Thalidomide.

Nonpharmacological treatment

Physical modalities
• UVB phototherapy for **MA, LA**.

Surgery
• Dermabrasion for MA, LA.

• Excision of nodular lesions of primary localized cutaneous amyloidosis.

• CO_2 laser ablation for MA, LA.

• Electrodesiccation and curettage for MA, LA.

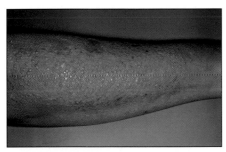

Lichen amyloisosis presents as firm, papular lesions that are commonly in areas where the skin has been traumatized by rubbing or scratching.

Treatment aims
Primary: To correct the underlying immunocyte dyscrasia.
Secondary: To relieve itching and promote resolution of all lesions.

Prognosis
ASA: Disease regression and prolonged survival in few patients treated with alkalating agents. Poor prognosis with renal involvement.

Follow-up and management
ASA: Oncology consultation is recommended.

Support organizations
Amyloidosis support network. www.amyloidosis.org

General references
Tourat DM, Sau P: Cutaneous deposition diseases. Part I. J *Am Acad Dermatol* 1998, 39:149–156.

Breathnach SM. Amyloidosis of the skin. In *Fitzpatrick's Dermatology in General Medicine*. Edited by Freedberg IM, Eisen AZ, Wolff K, *et al*. New York: McGraw-Hill Health Professions Division; 1999: 1756–1763.

Diagnosis

Signs

Swimmer's ear (otitis externa; OE): Erythema, fissuring in external ear canal visible with otoscope. Later, thin white discharge

Stings by Jellyfish, Portuguese Man-of War (S): Erythematous papules or wheals in a linear pattern corresponding to the areas where the tentacle contacted the skin. Long term toxicities include scarring, keloids and fat atrophy.

Seabather's eruption (SE): Inflammatory papules; distribution concentrated in the parts of the body covered by swimsuit and in hairy areas.

Swimmer's itch (SI): Erythematous macules and papules present on areas of the skin that were exposed to the water and not covered by swimware.

Sea urchin injuries (SU): Usually, the victim is well-aware of having been in contact with a sea urchin. The imbedded spines give off a purple dye that causes a stain to appear at the puncture site. There are also multiple black macules in a cluster.

Symptoms

OE: Initially, ear pruritus; pain, increasing with pressure on tragus or pulling of lobe. Pain can be severe.

S: Localized toxic reaction: immediate pain, mild or severe, in distribution of nematocysts. Initial prickly or stinging sensation. Intensity increases over about 10 minutes. Systemic toxic reactions range from mild to severe and may include headache, nausea, vomiting, weakness and delerium. Cardiac arrest and respiratory arrest have been reported, particularly in the case of box jellyfish envenomation. Species that are associated with the most toxic and potentially lethal stings include the Portuguese man-of-war and box jellyfish.

SE: Pruritis and burning in the distribution of the rash.

SI: Pruritis and burning that can be severe in the area of the rash.

SU: The puncture wound is very painful. Paresthesias may develop at the wound site. Systemic symptoms are rare, but include nausea, paresthesias, ataxia, muscle cramps, syncope, paralysis and respiratory distress.

Complications

OE: Rarely, can lead to cellulitis, especially in patients with diabetes.

SU: Delayed foreign-body reaction to sea urchin spines possible. Wounds can be nodular or diffuse. The nodular reaction consists of pink papules. The diffuse form is usually on the fingers or toes with fusiform swelling and pain and loss of function.

Differential diagnosis

OE: Otitis media; in OE, pain increases with pressure on tragus or pulling of lobe; in otitis media, it does not.

SE, SI: Should be differentiated from each other. SE occurs in covered areas; SI in uncovered areas.

Etiology

S: Injury is caused by stinging capsules or nematocysts on tentacles. Each nematocyst contains a toxin or toxins that is discharged into the skin when the victim is stung.

SU: Sea urchins are encased in a shell, which has multiple mobile spines that are responsible for the injury. Generally the injury is a puncture wound that occurs when a person steps on a sea urchin or falls and impales a hand on a sea urchin. After piercing the skin, the spines break off and become imbedded.

SE: The eruption is caused by the larval forms of marine colenterates, thimble jellyfish and a sea anemone. The eruption is due to stings from the nematocysts of the larvae, which become trapped underneath swimware or may adhere to body hair. The nematocysts are triggered to fire by processes including mechanical pressure, changes in osmotic pressure as the swim suit dries or contact with freshwater while wearing the swimware.

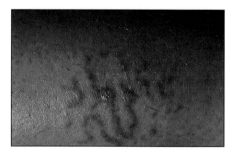

Linear, whip-like, erythematous welts due to jellyfish stings.

Treatment

Pharmacological treatment

Topical

OE: Cleanse the ear canal with lukewarm tap water or 1.5% hydrogen peroxide and dry the canal with a hair dryer. If there is a tympanic membrane perforation, irrigation should be avoided. Ear drops that contain an antibiotic as well as a corticosteroid (*eg*, Cipro HC, Tobradex or Corticosporin) should be used t.i.d or q.i.d.

S: After victim is removed from water, area must be washed with an appropriate solution to disarm the nematocysts. Vinegar is generally effective. If no denaturing agent is available, seawater can be used to wash the skin. The tentacles should be removed gently using gloves to prevent further stings. Washing with fresh water or alcohol may cause remaining nematocyts to fire. Ulcerated or open wounds should be given routine wound care.

SE, SI: Treatment is generally symptomatic; antipruritic lotions and topical steroids are generally effective.

SU: The affected area should be immersed in hot water (about 45°C,113°F) for 30–90 minutes, until the pain is relieved. Infiltration with lidocaine without epinephrine may be required. For nodular delayed reaction, intralesional corticosteroids.

Systemic

OE: Systemic antibiotics can be used in severe cases. Appropriate cultures should be obtained from the ear canal.

SU: Systemic antibiotics may be required, and the patient should receive tetanus prophylaxis if indicated.

Nonpharmacological treatment

SU: Spines that are protruding should be gently removed, however they are likely to break. For the diffuse reaction, the spines may need to be surgically removed. Prior to removal, an X-ray should be obtained to confirm the position of the spines.

Special therapeutic considerations

OE: Best treatment is prevention. Otic Domeboro solution should be instilled into the external ear canal after every swim or dive. All swimming and diving should cease until OE has cleared, usually in 5 to 7 days.

SE: Swimmers should remove their swimware and shower as soon as they exit the water. The swimsuit should be removed prior to showering; if possible, the individual should rinse with salt water. Bathing suits should be rinsed out with soap and water and heat-dried.

SI: Whole-body Lycra swimsuits or wet suits give some protection. Toweling off vigorously after swimming in waters where swimmer's itch is endemic.

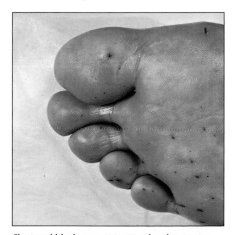

Clustered black, punctate macules due to sea urchin spines.

Prognosis

SE: The eruption generally lasts 7–10 days.

General references

Bove AA, Davis JC: *Diving Medicine*, edn 2. Philadelphia: W.B. Saunders; 1990.

Fisher AA: *Atlas of Aquatic Dermatology*. New York: Grune and Stratton; 1978.

Diagnosis

Signs

Brown recluse spider (BRS): Within 8 hours, urticaria, erythematous/violaceous discoloration, subsequent full-thickness necrosis in < 10%. Central blister, surrounding gray to purple discoloration, blanched ring followed by a ring of symmetric erythema.

Black widow spider (BWS): Usually, two fang marks at site; progression from slight erythema to piloerection to mild edema or urticaria to local perspiration to lymphangitis.

Mosquito (M): No response to first bite. Subsequent bites: Wheals 24 hours later, persists days. Further bites: Immediate wheal then delayed wheal. More bites: Delayed wheal disappears. Ultimately: Tolerance, no response.

Tick (T): Potentially painful, red papule; may progress to local swelling, erythema, blistering, ecchymosis, necrosis.

Chigger (C): May be intense pruritus on ankles, legs, belt line; erythematous macules may develop at bite site, also on feet, groin, genitalia, axillae, wrist, antecubital fossa.

Flea (F): Linear or clustered urticarial papules, usually on legs, below knees, occasionally forearms. Lesions more severe in allergic individuals.

Bedbug (B): Linear asymptomatic purpuric macules on face, neck, hands, arms. Sensitized individuals: intensely pruritic wheals, papules.

Hymenoptera (H): Bee, wasp: Erythematous papules, edema, urticaria. Honeybee leaves venom sac, stinger at site. Fire ant: Multiple stings; lesions often semicircular, develop into sterile pustules.

Symptoms

BRS: Bite painless. Site may become painful, with exanthem, fever, headache, malaise, arthralgias, nausea, vomiting.

BWS: Pinprick or sharp pinch; dull, aching pain or numbness 1 hour later.

M, T, C, F, B: Depends on previous exposure, sensitization to antigens in saliva, venom; immune status.

H: Extreme pain.

Investigations

BRS, BWS: Capture of spider allows definitive diagnosis. Histology can be suggestive but not specific.

Complications

• Papular urticaria may appear in batches after arthropod bites

BRS: Rarely, mild hemolysis, coagulopathy; more rarely, viscerocutaneous loxoscelism.

BWS: From 10 minutes to 24 hours after bite, regional muscle spasms (usually near bite), sometimes accompanied by dizziness, headache, sweating, nausea, vomiting; later, tachypnea, hypertension, restlessness. Mortality: less than 1%.

T: Tick-borne diseases. **F**: Tunga penetrans (sand flea); possible secondary infection.

M: Mosquito-borne diseases; anaphylactic reactions rare; bullae, cellulitis not uncommon sequelae.

H: Angioedema, generalized urticaria in < 5%; anaphylaxis in < 1%, within 20 minutes; serum sickness. Systemic reactions most common from yellow-jacket stings.

Etiology

BRS: Most in Midwest, south central US. Venom generates leukocyte chemoattractants, liberates thromboxane B2 in vitro. Bites most often March to October in closets, attics, outbuildings.

BWS: In all 48 contiguous US states, usually in warm climates. Venom destabilizes nerve cell membranes by opening ionic channels at synapses.

M: Female injects salivary secretions that anticoagulate blood, induce local skin reaction.

B: Blood-sucking ectoparasites; feed nocturnally, injecting saliva containing anticoagulant, anesthetic; feeding duration: a few minutes.

F: Can jump 18 cm; all species bite humans.

C: Humans infested while walking through vegetation or tall grass.

T: *Ixodidae* (hard tick) responsible for most diseases. Insert barbed hypostome through skin, secrete cement-like substance that firmly anchors hypostome to skin; feed for approximately 7 days, then fall off. All stages require blood meal.

H: Bee, wasp: Honeybee venom contains phospholipase A and various biogenic amines. Fire ant; Venom contains solenopsin D, a piperidine derivative causing release of histamine and vasoactive amines from mast cells.

Epidemiology

Arthropod bites common during summer.
M: Preference for black, young, cool, and scented skin; attracted to bright colors, elevated carbon dioxide concentrations.
F: Worldwide. Domestic animals.
C: Rural areas, agricultural workers.
T: Spring, summer.
B: Impoverished living conditions.
H: Bee, wasp, hornet stings peak in August. Fire ants attack those who disturb their nests and bed-ridden individuals; attacks can occur within homes and institutions.

Preventive Measures
Protective clothing, repellants (DEET against mosquitoes, fleas, gnats, chiggers; permethrin against ticks). No perfumes, bright colors. Antibiotics for secondary infection.

Bruce E. Strober and Doris J. Day

Treatment

Pharmacological treatment

Topical

M, T, C, F, B: Local cleansing, cold packs. Lotions/creams containing menthol, pramoxine, doxepin, lidocaine, for temporary relief. Corticosteroids (relief is delayed, more potent agents cause faster improvement).

H: Cutaneous reactions managed by ice, topical or local lidocaine injection, analgesics. Efficacy of antihistamines, baking soda, papain, and corticosteroids unproven.

Systemic

BRS: Corticosteroids for hemolysis and viscerocutaneous loxoscelism. Dapsone, 50–100 mg, qd. Antibiotics only for secondary infection.

BWS: Muscle spasms: calcium gluconate 10% solution (10 mL i.v. push over 5 minutes, repeat every 2 hours, as needed). Narcotics for persistent pain; muscle relaxants. Antivenin to prevent latrodectism; reserved for those under age 16, elderly, pregnant, hypertensive, symptomatic within 3 hours of bite, or no improvement after symptomatic treatment.

M, T, C, F, B: Oral antihistamines. Tapering course of prednisone in very severe cases.

H: Mild anaphylactic symptoms: Pruritus, itchy nose/eyes, sneezing, urticaria and localized angioedema: observation or intramuscular/intravenous H_1 and H_2 antihistamines. Moderate/severe anaphylactic symptoms: Epinephrine (1:1,000) subcutaneously, with additional doses every 20–30 minutes if no resolution; antihistamines alleviate urticaria, headache and flushing, i.v. or i.m; if systolic blood pressure < 60, i.v. epinephrine (1:10,000); airway maintenance, O_2 therapy, volume expansion with i.v. fluids. Patients taking beta-blockers may not respond to epinephrine; give glucagon, i.m., i.v., or s.c. Serum sickness: treat with brief course of corticosteroids, with or without antihistamines.

Nonpharmacological treatment

BRS, BWS: Treat symptoms with ice, analgesics, elevation.

BWS: Delay surgical debridement until wound is stabilized with medical management. **H**: Honeybee: Remove stinger unit, which continues to operate after separation from insect. Hold sharp-edged object (for example, credit card, knife blade) at right angle to skin, and scrape horizontally to extract stinger without compression of venom sac.

Special therapeutic considerations

• Tick paralysis: Likely due to toxin secreted in saliva of tick; lower motor neuron paralysis that is rapidly treated by removal of tick; treatment may involve respiratory support.

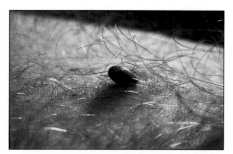

Local erythema and edema at the site of a tick bite. The engorged tick remains attached to the skin.

General references

Kemp ED: Bites and stings of the arthropod kind. *Postgrad Med* 1998, **103**:88–106.
Reisman RE: Insect Stings. *New Eng J Med* 1994, **331**:523-27.
Jerrard DA: Management of Insect Stings. *Amer J Emer Med* 1996, **14**:429–33.

Diagnosis

Signs

Structure

Nonbullous impetigo (NI): Vesicles or pustules on erythematous base that rupture to form honey-colored crusted or weeping plaques.

Bullous impetego (BI): Vesicles and bullae containing serous fluid that rupture to leave moist erosions covered with thin crust.

Ecthyma (E): Vesicles or pustules on an erythematous base that enlarge and develop into a shallow ulcer covered with central yellow-green crust and surrounded by a violaceous halo.

Superficial folliculitis (SF): Erythematous papules and pustules at openings of hair follicles.

Deep folliculitis (DF): Furuncles are deep, erythematous nodules involving hair follicles. Carbuncles are grouped, coalescing furnuncles.

Erysipelas: Well-demarcated, raised erythematous, indurated plaque.

Cellulitis: Patients may have erythematous streaking, spreading erythematous, hot area of skin (lymphangitis) and regional lymphadenopathy.

Distribution

Impetigo: Face (especially perinasal), scalp, extremities. **Ecthyma**: Lower extremities. **Folliculitis, furuncles**, and **carbuncles**: Any hair-bearing site, but commonly on scalp, beard, axillae, extremities, and buttocks. ***Pseudomonas* ("hot-tub") folliculitis**: Buttocks, trunk, axillae. **Gram-negative folliculitis**: Perioral regions. **Erysipelas**: Face, scalp, lower extremities, hands, genitalia. **Cellulitis**: Usually lower extremities.

Symptoms

• Common symptoms include pruritus (impetigo or folliculitis); skin tenderness (ecthyma, cellulitis, erysipelas); fever, chills, and malaise (cellulitis, erysipelas).

Investigations

• In most cases, a specific clinical diagnosis can be made.

Microbiology: Swab areas of impetigo for Gram stain and culture. **Culture of nares**: In recurrent infections, to detect *Staphylococcus* carriage. **Blood culture**: If skin is intact over areas of cellulitis. **Biopsy**: Usually unnecessary.

Complications

• Glomerulonephritis, due to group-B streptococcal infection. Bacteremia and septicemia, allowing spread to internal organs. (pneumonia, endocarditis, visceral abscesses). Absecces, osteomyelitis, septic arthritis, gangrene. Multiple systems organ failure. Death.

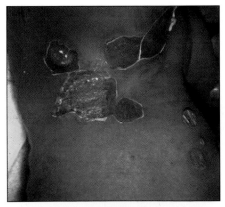

Bullous impetigo: superficial bullae leave erythematous erosions that heal without scarring.

Differential diagnosis

NI: Allergic contact dermatitis (ACD), atopic dermatitis, dermatophytosis, herpes or varicella infection, seborrheic dermatitis. **BI**: ACD, pemphigus vulgaris, bullous pemphigoid, erythema multiforme, dermatitis herpetiformis, thermal burns, bullous fixed drug eruption, staphylococcal scalded skin syndrome, bullous dermatophytosis, bullous insect bite reaction. **Ecthyma**: Chronic herpes, excoriated insect bites, neurotic excoriations, arterial ulcers. **SF**: Pseudofolliculitis barbae, acne vulgaris, rosacea, drug-induced acneiform eruption, hidradenitis suppurativa, eosinophilic pustular folliculitis, *Pityrosporum* folliculitis. **DF**: Kerion (dermatophytic folliculitis), cystic acne, hidradenitis suppurativa, ruptured inclusion cyst.

Etiology

Staphylococcus aureus is the most common agent causing folliculitis, furuncles, carbuncles, and cellulitis. Group A β-hemolytic *Streptococcus* species in ecthyma and erysipelas. *S. aureus* phage group II is responsible for BI. *Klebsiella*, *Enterobacter*, and *Proteus* species: Gram-negative folliculitis. *Pseudomonas aeruginosa*: "Hot tub" folliculitis, ecthyma gangrenosum.

Epidemiology

Impetigo: Late summer and early autumn. Predispositions: preschool children, crowding, poor hygiene, contact sports, neglected minor skin trauma, certain skin diseases (atopic dermatitis, scabies, varicella, Darier's disease). **Ecthyma**: Immunocompromised patients. **SF**: Usually seen in healthy persons, especially athletes. **DF** predispositions: Nasal colonization with *S. aureus*, infestations (pediculosis, scabies), diseases (diabetes, hematologic disorders, immunoglobulin deficiency states, obesity), medications (cytotoxic agents, corticosteroids). **Erysipelas**: Infants, children, older adults. Predispositions: Diabetes, alcoholism, nephrotic syndrome, immunosuppression, venous or lymphatic obstruction. **Cellulitis** predispositions: Dermatophytosis, eczema, ulcerations, skin trauma, burns, diabetes, edema, peripheral vascular disease.

Narayan S. Naik and Doris J. Day

Treatment

Diet and lifestyle

•Important in patients with diabetes, hypertension, lymphedema, or neuropathy. Improved blood sugar control in diabetic patients. Regular inspection and protection of extremities from trauma, temperature extremes, dryness.

Pharmacological treatment

Topical

•Antibiotics, including bacitracin, mupirocin, clindamycin, erythromycin, benzoyl peroxide for localized impetigo or folliculitis.

Systemic

•When possible, choose antibiotic on the basis of culture results.

•Oral antibiotics effective mainly against *S. aureus* and group A streptococci can be empirically used. **Penicillinase-resistant penicillin**: Dicloxacillin, 250–500 mg, p.o., q.i.d. **First-generation cephalosporins**: Cephalexin, 250–500 mg, p.o., q.i.d. **Penicillin-allergic patients**: Erythromycin, 250–500 mg, p.o., q.i.d.; clindamycin, 300 mg, p.o., q.i.d.

•Gram-negative folliculitis: Ampicillin, 250–500 mg, q.i.d. or trimethoprim-sulfamethoxazole, one double-strenght tablet, b.i.d.

•Most infections are treated with 10–14 days; ecthyma often needs several weeks. More serious infections require parenteral therapy: nafcillin, 1–1.5 g i.v./i.m. every 6 hours, or cefazolin, 1g i.v./i.m. every 8 hours; for penicillin-allergic patients, vancomycin, 1–2 g i.v. every 12 hours, or clindamycin, 600 mg i.v. every 6 hours.

Nonpharmacological treatment

•Supportive: Crust debridement; antibacterial soap, antiseptics (povidone, chlorhexidine), aluminum acetate soaks, warm compresses. Handwashing is vital to prevent infection transmission. Water chlorination usually prevents pseudomonas folliculitis.

•Physical modalities: Leg elevation, immobilization (cellulitis); moist compresses for deep folliculitis (furuncles, carbuncles).

•Surgery: Incision and drainage (abscesses, furuncles and carbuncles); debridement of necrotic tissue.

Special considerations

•Eliminate nasal *Staphylococcus* carriage with rifampin, 600 mg orally daily for 10 days, together with dicloxacillin or trimethoprim-sulfamethoxazole, or with topical mupirocin, intranasally twice daily for 5–10 days. Obtain radiographs or MRI scans of patients with recurrent cellulitis, to rule out osteomyelitis, which requires longer parenteral antibiotic regimens.

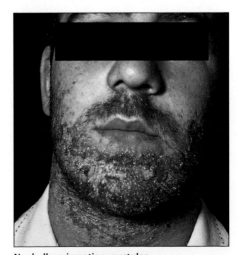

Nonbullous impetigo: pustules arising from erythematous skin; weeping, crusted erosions.

Narayan S. Naik and Doris J. Day

Treatment aims

To eradicate pathogenetic bacteria; drain purulent fluid; debride crust, necrotic tissue; prevent spread and recurrence of infection.

Prognosis

With appropriate treatment, prompt resolution is usual. *Pseudomonas* folliculitis is often self-resolving.

Follow-up and management

Necessary because causative organisms may be resistant to initial antibiotic regimens or require prolonged courses of therapy.

Patient education on proper hygiene is very important in preventing future episodes.

General references

Lee PK, Weinberg AN, Swartz MN, *et al.*: Pyodermas: *Staphylococcus aureus*, *Streptococcus*, and other gram-positive bacteria. In *Dermatology in General Medicine*, edn 5. Edited by Freedberg IM, *et al.* New York: McGraw-Hill; 1999:2182–2205.

Diagnosis

Signs

Balanoposthitis erosiva: Smegma, subpreputial smegmatic stones possible. **Pseudoepitheliomatous keratotic and micaceous balanitis (PKMB)**: Hyperkeratotic, white laminated plaques; may involve whole glans penis. **Desquamative balanitis (DB)**: Desquamation, redness, erosions of glans penis. **Balanitis xerotica obliterans (lichen sclerosus; BX)**: Erythematous papules, macules; glans, foreskin, meatus. Slowly progress to atrophic, ivory-white, sclerotic plaques. May present with diffuse or localized blue-white or yellow-white atrophic mottled plaques of glans; friable fissures, erosions, constricting bands, bullae, telangiectasia, hemorrhage of affected skin; stenosis or obliteration of meatus, anterior urethra. **Balanitis plasmacellularis (plasma cell balanitis; BP)**: Solitary, velvety red-orange patch or plaque of glans or prepuce; only in uncircumcised. Petechial "cayenne pepper" macules may dot lesion. **Balanitis circinata (BCi)**: Well-demarcated, serpiginous erythematous plaque, irregular scaly border. Superficial erosions possible. If circumcised, plaques dry, scaly; if uncircumcised, moist. **Balanitis candidomycetica (BCa)**: Early lesions: red, pinpoint papules on glans, prepuce; become eroded. Prepuce may develop dry glazed appearance. Eventually, beefy red erythematous patches; satellite pustules, erosions. White discharge usual. **Bacterial balanitis (BB)**: Red, tender, warm, edematous foreskin, glans penis; purulent discharge; inguinal adenitis. Gonococcal: tender ulcers, pustules, furuncles on penile shaft. *Bacteroides* strains: anaerobic balanitis, superficial erosions, malodorous subpreputial discharge, preputial edema. *Gardnerella vaginalis*: Usually redness, edema of prepuce, glans penis; malodorous, fishy subpreputial discharge. *Streptococcus* group B: Nonspecific erythema with or without exudate; may progress to penile cellulitis, especially if abrasions. **Human papillomavirus balanitis (HPB)**: Flat or cauliflower-like condylomata, may result in patchy or complete involvement of glans penis, mucosal foreskin. *Trichomonas* balanitis: Sexually acquired, superficial erosive balanitis; may lead to phimosis.

Symptoms

BE: Foreskin red, painful, swollen, often weeping. **BX**: Soreness, itching, loss of glans penis sensation, erectile dysfunction, dyspareunia, dysuria, phimosis, irritative and obstructive micturition. **BP**: Mild itching, tenderness. **BCi**: Usually asymptomatic. **BCa**: Mild itching, burning.

Investigations

BX: Histopathologic examination.
BP, **BCi**: 3-mm punch biopsy; heals in days.
Potassium hydroxide or fungal culture for confirmation, culture of purulent discharge, gram stain of exudate, serologic tests for syphilis, darkfield examination. Viral culture if herpes simplex virus suspected (60% to 90% sensitive); Tzanck smear. Patch testing if allergic hypersensitivity suspected; consider antiseptics, anesthetics; substances in prophylactic products, lubricants, hygiene products; topical medications, vaginal products used by sexual partner; chemicals transmitted from hand to penile skin.

Complications

• Usually, no serious complications, but cellulitis can lead to gangrene, penectomy. Lichen sclerosis (LS): Meatal stenosis may lead to urinary retention, bladder, kidney damage. Rarely, nonmelanoma skin cancer in LS lesions.

Differential diagnosis

Penis, foreskin: Most commonly lichen planus, psoriasis; other: fixed drug eruption, lichen nitidus, seborrheic dermatitis, sarcoidosis, erythema multiforme, morphea, scabies, foscarnet-related ulcerations, inflammatory bowel disease. **Extramammary Paget's disease**: Rare on penis; consider if underlying genitourinary malignancy. **Erythroplasia of Queyrat (EQ)**: Slightly elevated erythematous plaques; may be confused with balanitis. Usually asymptomatic, but itching, pain, bleeding, difficulty retracting foreskin. **Squamous cell carcinoma** of glans may appear as ulcer with indurated edges.

Etiology

BE: Retention of moisture, smegma; growth of pathogens. Risk factors: excessively long foreskin, partial or complete phimosis, poor hygiene, sexually transmitted diseases, trauma, incontinence, diabetes mellitus. **DB**: Most common: Pemphigus, linear IgA disease, cicatricial pemphigoid. Ulcerative balanoposthitis may be manifestation of acute promyelocytic leukemia. **BCa**: Generally sexually acquired through carriage of yeasts. Colonization rate of yeast 14% to 18%; no circumcision predeliction. **BB**: Group A hemolytic streptococci contracted through fellatio. *Staphylococcus aureus* balanitis rare. **Fourth venereal disease of Corbus**: Severe erosive, gangrenous form of anaerobic balanitis; caused by anaerobes, *Fusobacterium*. Anaerobes may be isolated from genital ulcers but do not appear to cause ulceration. **BX**: Probably multifactorial. Risk factors: circumcision after age 13, autoimmune disease. **BP**: Unknown; middle-aged, uncircumcised men. **BCa**: About 40% with Reiter's syndrome; usually in third decade. Higher incidence among Native Americans. Up to 90% positive for HLA-B27. Likely related to previous gastrointestinal, venereal infection, especially *Chlamydia trachomatis*. **BCi**: *Candida albicans* about a third of balanitis cases. Disposing factors: occlusion; skin moisture, maceration; Down's syndrome; diabetes mellitus; immunodeficiency; broad-spectrum antibiotics; corticosteroids; other immunosuppressive medications.

Casey Gallagher and Miguel Sanchez

Treatment

Pharmacological treatment

Topical

BE: Wet dressings: 0.25% silver nitrate; Burrow's solution. Low potency topical corticosteroids with imidazole cream, b.i.d.. Mycostatin cream, with or without Vioform, b.i.d. Aqueous gentian violet or carbol-fuchsin, diluted 1:1 with water. Phisoderm or similar, according to tolerance.

BX: Clobetasol cream (carefully monitor for atrophy). Intralesional triamcinolone, 3–5 mg/mL, every 3–4 weeks. Retinoids may help.

BCi: Low potency corticosteroids.

BCa: Topical imidazole creams (Nizoral, oxiconazole) or mycostatin powder for limited disease.

EQ: Topical 5-fluorouracil 5% or 1% for early, superficial lesions.

Systemic

BX: Testosterone: disappointing results. Penicillin: anecdotal cures. Oral vitamin E ineffective.

BCa: Widespread infection, or failure to improve: fluconazole or itaconazole, 200 mg daily.

PKMB: 5-fluorouracil results in high recurrence rate.

Nonpharmacological treatment

BX: Circumcision for lesions confined to prepuce; variable success if more extensive. CO_2 laser ablation. Excision with skin grafting. Sequential urethral dilation , electrosurgical meatotomy, urethroplasty, meatoplasty, proximal diverting meatostomy for urethral involvement. Radiotherapy: increased cancer risk.

PKMB: Surgical excision of lesion; Mohs' micrographic surgery may be optimal, but experience limited.

BP: Circumcision; CO_2 laser ablation.

EQ: Mohs' micrographic surgery. Excision with histologic examination of margins. Early circumcision drastically reduces incidence.

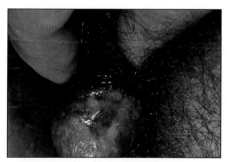

Eroded erythematous patch on glans penis. Erosive balanitis nonspecific; may be due to infectious (syphilis), neoplastic (SCC), inflammatory (cicatriceal pemphigoid) cause. Biopsy indicated.

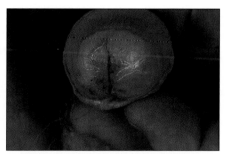

Well demarcated, depigmented, atrophic, periurethral patch due to balanitis xerotica obliterans (lichen sclerosus). Note excoriations, petechiae due to scratching, rubbing.

Treatment aims

To relieve symptoms and cure or arrest progression of disease.

Prognosis

LS: Chronic; poor response to treatment.
BP: Chronic; appropriate treatment curative.
BCi: Readily responds to appropriate therapy.
BB: In *Candida* infection, 90% respond to topical treatment; most others to oral medication. Clearing takes 1–3 weeks, depending on immune status.
PKMB: May represent premalignant condition leading to verrucous or invasive squamous cell carcinoma.

Follow-up and management

Observe until resolution. Rule out diabetes if *Candida* infection. Evaluate sexual partner(s) for candidal vaginitis; treat, as necessary. Promptly evaluate recurrent infection immunosuppression.

General references

English JC III; Laws RA; Keough GC, *et al.*: Dermatoses of the glans penis and prepuce. *J Am Acad Dermatol* 1997, 37:1–24.

Clinical Effectiveness Group (Association of Genitourinary Medicine and the Medical Society for the Study of Venereal Diseases): National guideline for the management of balanitis. *Sex Transm Infect* 1999, 75(Suppl. 1):S85–S88.

Waugh MA. Balanitis. *Dermatol Clin* 1998, 16:757–762.

Diagnosis

Signs

Nodular (most common type): Skin-colored, dome-shaped papule with telangiectasias and a "pearly" border. The surface may be ulcerated and crusted. Cystic lesions may occur.

Pigmented: Features of nodular type of basal-cell carcinoma (BCC) associated with black or brown pigmentation. It is more common in darker-skinned individuals.

Superficial, multicentric: Erythematous, scaly plaque with slightly raised border. It may be eroded or covered with crust. Most commonly seen on the trunk.

Morpheaform (sclerosing): Indurated, white to waxy plaque with ill-defined margins resembling a scar. Most commonly seen in the head and neck area.

Fibroepithelioma of Pinkus: One or several raised, firm, slightly pedunculated pink papules. Most commonly seen on the lower trunk.

Nevoid basal-cell carcinoma syndrome (NBCCS or Gorlin syndrome): Autosomal dominant syndrome characterized by multiple BCCs, palmar and plantar pits (50% of patients), odontogenic keratocyst of the jaws, calcification of the falx cerebri, bifid ribs, hypertelorism, and partial agenesis of corpus callosum. The lesions tend to present between puberty and age 35 years as smooth, skin-colored papules resembling nevi. The syndrome may be associated with medulloblastomas, ovarian fibromas, and fibrosarcoma (jaw).

Symptoms

• Asymptomatic. Lesions may ulcerate and bleed.

Investigations

• Diagnosis should be confirmed by skin biopsy. Histopathologic testing shows nests of proliferating atypical basal cells, which at the periphery tend to be arranged in palisades and are surrounded by connective tissue stroma.

Complications

• Disfigurement, ulceration (rodent ulcer), bleeding, and progressive destruction of vital organs (eyes, lips, nose, ears). Recurrent tumors have a more aggressive behavior. Direct invasion into sinuses and brain and, rarely, metastasis cause death.

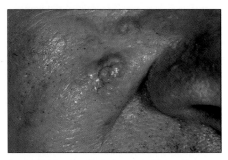

A nodular basal cell carcinoma with pearly, rolled borders and telangiectasias

Differential diagnosis

Fibrous papule, sebaceous hyperplasia, nevus, seborrheic keratosis, amelanotic melanoma (nodular BCC); malignant melanoma, pigmented seborrheic keratosis, angiokeratoma, traumatized nevus (pigmented BCC); nummular eczema, psoriasis, extramammary Paget's disease, Bowen's disease (superficial BCC), scar, localized scleroderma (morpheaform BCC).

Etiology

The etiology of BCC is unknown. Predisposing factors include exposure to ultraviolet radiation; radiation therapy; long-term arsenic exposure; immunosuppression (from drugs or HIV); chronic ulcers, scars, or burns; genodermatoses (NBCCS, xeroderma pigmentosum, albinism, Basex syndrome); nevus sebaceous, porokeratosis, and linear epidermal nevi.

In NBCCS, mutations in the *PATCHED* gene located on chromosome 9 appear to be responsible for tumor growth.

Ultraviolet light may cause carcinogenesis through injury to the tumor suppressor *p53* gene.

Epidemiology

BCC is the most common cancer in white populations, with an estimated incidence of 900,000 cases per year in the United States. Most frequent in light-skinned, older patients with a history of exposure to ultraviolet light. NBCCS has a prevalence of 1/56,000.

Brian Jiang and Perry Robins

Treatment

Diet and lifestyle

• Sun avoidance, sun protection using broad-spectrum sunblock (ultraviolet A and B) with sun protection factor greater than 15, and protective clothing.

Pharmacological treatment

Topical

• Intralesional interferon-α 1.5×10^6 IU three times weekly for 3 weeks, for a total dose of 13.5×10^6 IU (70%–100% cure rates reported in studies with suboptimal follow-up).

• 5% 5-fluorouracil cream applied at bedtime for months (for surgery-inaccessible cases): at least 20% recurrence rate for nodular BCC.

• Imiquimod cream is under investigation: small studies suggest good response with thrice-weekly application, but no long-term follow-up data are available.

Nonpharmacological treatment

Surgery

• Small, low-risk BCCs can be treated by electrodesiccation and curettage, CO_2 laser ablation, excision, and cryosurgery. For patients who are poor surgical candidates or have lesions in difficult-to-reach areas, the use of radiation may be indicated.

• High-risk BCCs should undergo Mohs micrographic surgery because this technique offers the highest cure rate (98%–99%) with maximal conservation of normal tissue. High-risk BCCs include recurrent tumors, tumors > 2 cm, locations with high recurrence rates (periorbital, nasolabial, perioral, and nasal ala), aggressive histologic pattern, ill-defined clinical borders, multicentricity, previous radiation exposure to the site, perineural invasion of tumor, areas where tissue conservation is important, and incompletely excised tumor.

• With photodynamic therapy using 5-aminolevulinic acid cream (under occlusion for several hours) and photoactivating light for about 30 minutes, 86% of superficial BCCs have complete response; recurrence rate at 48 months is 28%.

Physical modalities

• Fractionated superficial radiation therapy (especially for BCC in eyelids, nose, and ears in elderly patients).

• Gold-grain brachytherapy. Elastoplast mould (EPM).

Treatment aims

To eradicate the tumor while maintaining the best cosmetic and functional results.

Prognosis

Recurrences usually occur 4–12 months after the initial treatment, and the risk of acquiring a second lesion is about 40%. BCC rarely metastasizes (fewer than 300 reported cases). If this does occur, survival is approximately 8 months. Chemotherapy with cisplatin and bleomycin given 4 days a week for 3 weeks before surgery may improve prognosis in patients with advanced, unresectable tumors.

5-year recurrence rate for primary BCCs: surgical excision, 10.1%; radiation therapy, 8.7%; curettage and electrodesiccation, 7.7%; cryosurgery, 7.5%; all non-Mohs surgical modalities 8.7%; Mohs micrographic surgery, 1.0%.

Follow-up and management

Patients should have follow-up visits 3 months after therapy and every 6 months to 1 year thereafter over the patient's lifetime. For NBCCS, a multidisciplinary approach is recommended. Skin cancer screening every 3 months is recommended for early diagnosis and treatment of tumors. Patients should be evaluated annually for associated tumors, with imaging studies of the jaws, head, heart, and bones. Genetic counseling is strongly recommended given the autosomal dominant mode of inheritance. Therapy with isotretinoin, 1.0–2.0 mg/kg of body weight per day, or acitretin, 0.6–1.2 mg/kg per day, reduces the appearance of new BCCs and decreases growth of present BCCs, but must be continued indefinitely. Radiation therapy is contraindicated in patients with NBCCS.

General references

Randle HW: Basal cell carcinoma. Identification and treatment of the high-risk patient. *Dermatol Surg* 1996, **22**:255–261.

Lawrence CM: Mohs' micrographic surgery for basal cell carcinoma. *Clin Exp Dermatol* 1999, **24**:130–133.

Kopera D, Cerroni L, *et al.*: Different treatment modalities for the management of a patient with the nevoid basal cell carcinoma syndrome. *J Am Acad Dermatol* 1996, **34**:937–939.

Diagnosis

Signs

Skin: Usually painful oral or genital aphthous ulcers (round ulcers with sharp, erythematous border, covered with yellow pseudomembrane); erythema nodosum–like lesions; papulopustular lesions; follicular acneiform lesions; pyoderma gangrenosum–like lesions; cutaneous necrotizing vasculitis; Sweet's syndrome–like lesions.

Ophthalmologic: Posterior uveitis, conjunctivitis, corneal ulcers, papilledema, retinal vasculitis, hypopyon, blurred vision, eye pain, photophobia, floaters, lacrimation.

Neurologic: Meningoencephalitis, seizures, cerebral venous thrombosis, cranial nerve palsies, cerebellar ataxia, hemiplegia, benign intracranial hypertension, headaches, dementia.

Musculoskeletal: Oligoarthritis.

Gastrointestinal: Terminal ileal and cecal ulcers, abdominal pain, diarrhea.

Cardiovascular: Angina, pericarditis, endocarditis, valvular abnormalities, aortic pseudoaneurysms, venous thrombosis.

Pulmonary: Tracheobronchial ulcers, pulmonary embolism, pulmonary artery aneurysms, pneumonitis.

Renal: Glomerulonephritis.

Investigations

• Viral and fungal cultures of aphthae.

• Complete blood count, serum B12, folate, iron studies.

• Urinalysis.

• Skin or mucosal biopsy.

• Pathergy testing (pustular lesion develops 24 hours after cutaneous trauma).

• HLA-B27 testing and gastrointestinal evaluation for inflammatory bowel disease (in patients with family history).

• Radiologic evaluation of joints.

• Magnetic resonance imaging (MRI) evaluation of central nervous system.

• Computed tomography, MRI, angiography, and ventilation–perfusion scanning for cardiovascular and pulmonary evaluation.

Complications

• Blindness, glaucoma, intracranial hemorrhage, cerebral aneurysms, cerebral thrombosis.

• Hearing and vestibular defects, deforming arthritis, bowel perforation, Budd-Chiari syndrome, myocardial infarction, arterial aneurysms, venous thrombosis, pulmonary embolism, pneumonitis, renal failure.

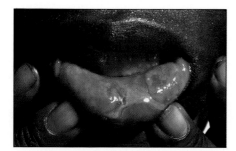

Aphthous-like lesions on the inner lower lip due to Behçet's disease.

Differential diagnosis

Viral and candidal ulcerations; deficiency of vitamins B_1, B_2, B_6, and B_{12}, folate, iron, and zinc; inflammatory bowel disease; Sweet's syndrome; Reiter's syndrome; genitoulcerative sexually transmitted diseases.

Etiology

Genetic factors: HLA-B51 association (particularly among persons from the Middle East and Asia).

Infectious triggers: possible association with *Streptococcus* species and herpes simplex virus.

Immunologic factors: circulating immune complex deposition, vascular injury and enhanced neutrophil migration; elevated cytokine levels; autoreactive anti-heat shock protein, T-cell and B-cell autoantibodies.

Epidemiology

Highest prevalence in Turkey (80–370 cases per 100 000). Prevalence in East Asia and the Middle East, 13.5–20 per 100,000. In the United States and United Kingdom, prevalence ranges from 0.12 to 0.64 per 100,000. Mean age at onset is third to fourth decade (slightly higher among East Asian women and Middle Eastern men). Rare among blacks.

O'Duffy criteria

Aphthous genital ulceration.

Uveitis.

Cutaneous "pustular" vasculitis.

Synovitis.

Meningoencephalitis.

Diagnosis: Recurrent oral aphthous ulceration and 2 or more of above criteria present.

Incomplete form: Recurrent aphthous ulceration and 1 or more criteria present.

Exclusions: Inflammatory bowel disease, systemic lupus erythematosus, Reiter disease, and herpes simplex.

International study group criteria

Recurrent oral ulceration: aphthous ulceration recurring at least 3 times in 12 months, plus 2 of the following criteria:

Recurrent genital ulceration.

Eye lesions (anterior uveitis, posterior uveitis, cells in vitreous on slit-lamp examination; or retinal vasculitis).

Skin lesions (erythema nodosum, pseudofolliculitis or papulopustular lesions; or acneiform nodules in postadolescent patient not receiving corticosteroids).

Positive pathergy test result.

Macrene Alexiades-Armenakas and Andrew Franks, Jr

Treatment

Diet and lifestyle
• Avoid implicated food allergens, such as cow's milk, gluten, food dyes, and preservatives; implicated drugs, such as nonsteroidal anti-inflammatory drugs; and implicated dentrifices, such as sodium lauryl sulfate.

Pharmacological treatment

Topical
• Class I and II corticosteroids in gel or ointment base to ulcers 3–10 times per day (for oral and genital ulcers).

• Intralesional triamcinolone acetonide, 5 mg/mL, to ulcers.

• Pain control measures include dyclonine hydrochloride, mixture of viscous lidocaine, pectin/kaolin, and diphenhydramine; viscous lidocaine, aloe vera gel extract (Carrington patch), and Zilactin gel.

• Chlorhexidine gluconate oral rinses (antiseptic).

• Amlexanox paste 5%, applied frequently to ulcers.

• Tetracycline, 250 mg dissolved in water rinses, four times daily. Sometimes nystatin and diphenhydramine are added to rinse.

Systemic
• Colchicine, 0.6 mg orally three times daily initially; decrease to 0.6 mg orally twice or once daily if nausea, vomiting, or diarrhea develop (use concomitantly with topical corticosteroids for skin and mucosal involvement).

• Dapsone, 100 mg orally daily initially; decrease to 50 mg orally daily if hematocrit drops or fatigue develops (for persistent aphthae and cutaneous manifestations).

• Thalidomide,100 mg orally daily initially, up to 300 mg orally per day maximum.

• Prednisone, 1 mg/kg per day, or prednisolone, 20–100 mg orally daily, or pulse therapy with methylprednisolone, 1000 mg i.v. daily, with close monitoring for 3 days (for acute severe flares and gastrointestinal, central nervous system or large-vessel involvement).

• Indomethacin, 25–50 mg orally 3 times daily (for arthritis).

• Sulfasalazine, 1.0 g 3–4 times daily.

• Cyclosporine, 2.5–5 mg/kg orally, in two divided doses (for retinal vasculitis or very severe systemic disease). It may be used in combination with corticosteroids.

• Methotrexate, 7.5–20 mg orally each week (for severe mucocutaneous involvement without liver disease).

• Interferon- α 2a, 3–12 million U subcutaneously 3 times per week (for severe mucocutaneous and articular involvement; has not been used in central nervous system or ocular disease).

• Pentoxyfylline, 400 mg orally 3 times daily (for recalcitrant mucocutaneous disease).

• Azathioprine, 1–2 mg/kg orally daily in 2 or 3 divided doses (for prevention of ocular complications).

• Tacrolimus, dose adjusted to maintain the whole blood trough level between 10 and 15 ng/mL; then decreased as soon as response occurs.

• Cyclophosphamide, 1–5 mg/kg per day orally or 700–1000 mg/month intravenously as pulse therapy (for vasculitis and aneurysms).

• Chlorambucil, 5 mg orally daily (for severe ocular, central nervous system, and large-vessel disease).

• Anticoagulants (warfarin, heparin, or low-molecular-weight dextran) (for venous thrombosis).

Treatment aims
To minimize systemic complications.

Most aggressive treatment reserved for gastrointestinal, central nervous system, and large-vessel involvement.

Less aggressive treatment is used for ocular disease, and conservative therapy is used for mucocutaneous disease.

Special therapeutic considerations
Betamethasone eye drops for anterior uveitis and retinal vasculitis, 1–2 drops three times daily, or tropicamide eye drops for anterior uveitis, 1–2 drops twice daily.

Prognosis
Mucocutaneous and ocular manifestations recur cyclically.

Oral ulcers typically ulcers heal in 10 days without scarring; genital ulcers heal with scarring.

Usually, initial manifestations are oral and genital ulcers, followed by cutaneous lesions and arthritis; and ocular and neurologic involvement occurs months to years later.

Mortality is low and usually due to pulmonary or central nervous system hemorrhage or bowel perforation.

Follow-up and management
Monitor patients who have complex aphthosis for development of systemic signs.

General references
Ghate JV, Jorizzo JL: Behçet's disease and complex aphthosis. *J Am Acad Dermatol* 1999, **40**:1–18.

O'Duffy JD, Goldstein NP: Neurologic involvement in seven patients with Behçet's disease. *Am J Med* 1976, **16**:17–18.

International study group for Behçet's disease: Criteria for diagnosis of Behçet's disease. *Lancet* 1990, **335**:1078–1080.

Sakane T, Takeno M, Suzuki N, et al.: Behçet's disease. *N Engl J Med* 1999, **341**:1284–1291.

Diagnosis

Signs

•Focal areas of hair loss (typically scalp); associated erythema; papules, plaques, nodules; scale; pustules; vesicles; scars; or hypopigmentation/ hyperpigmentation of skin; combination of signs.

Symptoms

•Range from asymptomatic to focal pruritus or pain.

Investigations

•Punch biopsy of lesion (vertical or horizontal sections); culture or microscopic examination of stained smear obtained from lesions of suspected infectious causes.

Complications

•Typically, permanent loss of hair in affected areas.

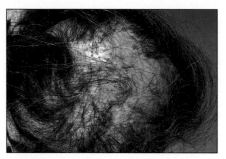

Late-stage scarring alopecia due to lichen planopilaris; perifollicular erythema is barely noticeable.

Differential diagnosis

Clinical syndromes and dermatoses of uncertain origin

1a, lichen planopilaris; 1b, folliculitis decalvans; 1c, pseudopelade of Brocq; 1d, scleroderma/morphea; 1e, discoid lupus erythematosus; 1f, sarcoidosis; 1g, acne keloidalis; 1h, dissecting perifolliculitis (perifolliculitis capitis abscedens et suffodiens); 1i, follicular degeneration syndrome; 1j, lichen sclerosus et atrophicus; 1k, cicatricial pemphigoid; 1l, necrobiosis lipoidica diabeticorum; 1m, dermato-myositis; 1n, follicular mucinosis; 1o, amyloidosis; 1p, erosive pustular dermatosis; 1q, lipedematous alopecia.

Infectious processes

2a, bacterial; 2b, fungal; 2c, viral; 2d, protozoan.

Hereditary disorders and developmental defects

3a, aplasia cutis congenita; 3b, epidermal nevi (eg, nevus sebaceous, syringocys-tadenoma papilliferum); 3c, facial hemiatrophy (Romberg's syndrome); 3d, Darier's disease; 3e, recessive x-linked ichthyosis; 3f, epidermolysis bullosa (recessive dystrophic type); 3g, inconti-nentia pigmenti; 3h, porokeratosis of Mibelli; 3i, scarring follicular keratosis; 3j, Conradi's syndrome; 3k, polyostotic fibrous dysplasia; 3l, Graham-Little syndrome.

Neoplasms

4a, basal-cell carcinoma; 4b, squamous-cell carcinoma; 4c, metastatic tumors; 4d, lymphomas; 4e, adnexal tumors.

Chemical/physical agents

5a, mechanical trauma (including factitial); 5b, burns; 5c, radiation; 5d, caustic agents; 5e, other chemicals/drugs.

Etiology

See classification in above section on differ-ential diagnosis.

Epidemiology

Childhood to adult: Hereditary disorders and developmental defects. **Adult:** Typically, neoplasms;,clinical syndromes, dermatoses of uncertain origin. **Any age:** Infectious processes; chemical/physical agents.

Arthur P. Bertolino

Treatment

Diet and lifestyle
•Condition can be emotionally devastating. Wigs or hair extensions are sometimes useful during treatment.

Pharmacological treatment
•Treatments for disorders are grouped by pharmacologic agent. Each disorder is specified by the number and letter designated in the differential diagnosis section (*eg*, 1a is lichen planopilaris). Specific doses are not listed because of questionable efficacy.

Topical
Corticosteroids (topical/ intralesional): 1a, 1b, 1c, 1d, 1e, 1f, 1g, 1h, 1i, 1j, 1k, 1l, 1m, 1p. **Retinoids (adapalene, tazarotene)**. 3d. **Calcipotriene**. 1d. **Local wound care**: 5a–c.

Systemic
Corticosteroids (systemic): 1d,1f, 1k, 1p. **Antibiotics, antifungal agents, anti-infective agents**: rifampicin/clindamycin (1b); tetracycline (1g, 1h, 1i, 1k); erythromycin (1h); drugs appropriate for infection (1p, 2a–d). **Retinoids (topical/oral)**: isotretinoin (1e, 1f, 1h, 1n, 1p, 3d); acitretin (1j, 3d), vitamin A (3d), acitretin (3e), etretinate, (3h). **Antimalarials**: hydroxychloroquine sulfate (1c, 1e, 1j, 1m), chloroquine phosphate (1f). **Azathioprine**: 1e, 1k. **Dapsone**: 1e, 1k, 1n. **Methotrexate**: 1e, 1m. **Penicillamine**: 1d. **Phenytoin**: 1e, 3f(?). **Sulfasalazine**: 1e. **Thalidomide**: 1e, 1f. **Immune modulators**: i.v. immunoglobulin (1d), interferon-α2a (1e), interferon-α2b, interferon-γ (1n). **Other pharmacologic agents**: chemotherapy for systemic cancer (4c, 4d); oral/topical fusidic acid:oral zinc sulfate (1b), zinc sulfate (1h), testosterone propionate (1j), cyclophosphamide, sulfamethoxypyridazine, tetracycline/nicotinamide (1k), zinc sulfate (1p),topical 5-fluorouracil (3d, 3h), topical camostat mesylate (3f). **No established pharmacologic treatment**: 1o, 1q, 3a–c, 3g, 3i, 3j, 3k, 3l, 4a, 4b, 4e.

Nonpharmacological treatment

Supportive methods
•Tar-containing shampoos for pruritus/scalp discomfort, as needed.

• Localized topical wound care for weeping or eroded lesions.

Physical modalities
•Psoralen and ultraviolet A photochemotherapy (PUVA): 1d, 1n. Ultraviolet A-1: 1d.

Surgery
•Excisional surgery is typically performed at the outset for focal malignant neoplasms or at any convenient time for nonmalignant neoplasms. Focal areas of cicatricial alopecia that have been inactive for 6 months without treatment may be considered for excision or hair transplantation.

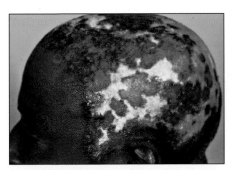

Complete scarring alopecia due to lupus erythematosus; note hypopigmented and hyperpigmented patches.

Treatment aims

To limit extent of permanent alopecia so that repair may eventually be realized through surgical intervention once process is inactive. In general, efficacy of treatment is limited and should not be expected to provide uniformly satisfactory results.

Prognosis

For progressive disorders, stabilization may take a few to many months.
Surgical options for repair of areas of alopecia are usually viable as long as extensive alopecia is prevented.

Follow-up and management

Patients receiving pharmacologic treatments are usually followed monthly until the alopecia process becomes inactive. Correctional surgery is usually considered once the process has been inactive for 6 months without treatment. For disorders treated surgically, lesions are removed on a timely basis; periodic follow-up is done to check for possible recurrence.

General references

Rook A, Dawber R: *Diseases of the Hair and Scalp*, edn 2. Boston: Blackwell Scientific Publications; 1991.

Newton RC, Hebert AA, Freese TW, Solomon AR: Scarring alopecia. *Dermatol Clin* 1987, **5**:603–618.

Headington JT: Cicatricial alopecia. *Dermatol Clin* 1996, **14**:773–782.

Sullivan JR, Kossard S: Acquired scalp alopecia. Part I: A review. *Australas J Dermatol* 1998, **39**:207–221.

Sullivan JR, Kossard S: Acquired scalp alopecia. Part II: A review. *Australas J Dermatol* 1999, **40**:61–72.

Arthur P. Bertolino

Diagnosis

Signs

Lentigines (lentigo simplex): 2–3 mm (rarely >5 mm) circular or polycyclic, brown to black-brown macules in non–sun-exposed areas. Solar lentigo is a small, circumscribed, tan to brown, 0.5- to 3-cm patch in sun-exposed areas.

Seborrheic keratosis: Single or multiple round to oval brown papules or plaques, 0.5 to 3 cm, that occur on any body site but predominate on the trunk, upper extremities, and face. Lesions can be aligned in skin folds (inframammary area). Sizes vary from 1 mm to several centimeters, and appearance is often greasy, warty, and "stuck-on." Follicular prominence increases as these lesions mature. Colors can be white-gray, yellow-pink, tan, brown, black ,or a mixture of colors. Stucco keratosis is a 1- 3-mm gray, "stuck-on" seborrheic keratosis, usually on the legs.

Dermatosis papulosa nigra: Brown to black, flattened, 1- 5-mm smooth papules, usually seen on the face (specially the malar region) but also on the neck and upper trunk. On the neck and trunk, the lesions are more pedunculated.

Symptoms

• Lentigines and dermatosis papulosa nigra lesions are usually asymptomatic. Seborrheic keratosis can rarely be pruritic and may become tender if inflamed by rubbing or picking, or if secondarily infected, causing swelling and bleeding.

Investigations

Seborrheic keratosis: Excisional biopsy if melanoma is suspected.

Lentigo: Biopsy should be performed if lentigo maligna melanoma is suspected. Pathology shows club-shaped elongated rete ridges with increased number of melanocytes in the basal layer and hypermelanosis.

Complications

Seborrheic keratosis: Lesions can become irritated or secondarily infected. Rarely, eruptive lesions have been associated with malignancy (sign of Leser-trelat).

Lentigo: If systemic abnormalities occur concomitantly with lentigines, then investigate for LEOPARD syndrome (multiple lentigines syndrome—lentigines, electrocardiographic conduction abnormalities, ocular hypertelorism, pulmonary stenosis, abnormal genitalia, retardation of growth, and sensorineural deafness) or NAME syndrome (Carney's syndrome–nevi, atrial myxoma, myxoid neurofibromas, ephelides). If Peutz-Jeghers syndrome is suspected, evaluate for gastrointestinal hematomatous polyps causing intussusception, bleeding, and obstruction. Adenocarcinoma can develop within polyps; increased risk for breast, ovarian, and pancreatic carcinoma.

Solar lentigos from exposure; common on whites older than 70, on face, hands.

Differential diagnosis

Seborrheic keratosis: Malignant melanoma, solar lentigo, pigmented actinic keratosis, pigmented basal cell carcinoma, and verruca vulgaris.

Dermatosis papulosa nigra: Acrochordons, pigmented flat warts.

Lentigo: Must be differentiated from a junctional nevus; cafêau lait macule; pigmented solar keratosis; early, seborrheic keratosis; lentigo maligna; and freckles.

Etiology

Seborrheic keratosis: Unknown etiology. May be familial with an autosomal dominant inheritance pattern. These lesions may occur earlier in tropical regions because of sun exposure. Because some lesions are verrucous, human papillomavirus has been suggested but not confirmed.

Dermatosis papulosa nigra: Probably genetically determined, with 45%–50% of patients having positive family histories. The lesions are nevoid developmental defects of the pilosebaceous follicles.

Lentigo: Can be acquired or congenital. Solar lentigo is induced by ultraviolet radiation. Association with lentiginous syndromes suggests a neural crest disorder with genetic influence. A single lentigo simplex on mucocutaneous sites is associated with racial or genetic factors.

Epidemiology

Seborrheic keratosis: Usually in persons older than 30 years of age. Males and females are equally affected. These lesions are common in white persons.

Dermatosis papulosa nigra: Found in 35% of African Americans (in 10%, lesions are numerous). Usually develop during adolescence. Also common in Asians, Hispanics, and other persons of color. They are considered to be variants of seborrheic keratosis. Predominance in females.

Lentigo: Incidence is unknown. More common in skin types I to III.

Special considerations

Seborrheic keratosis: Six types are recognized: irritated, adenoid or reticulated, plane, clonal, melanoacanthoma, inverted follicular keratosis, and benign squamous keratosis. Two clinical variants have been described: stucco keratosis and dermatosis papulosa nigra.

Treatment

Pharmacological treatment

Seborrheic keratosis: Pruritic lesions are often associated with xerotic skin; emollients can be helpful.

Lentigo: Retinoic acid and bleaching agents containing hydroquinone are not effective. To prevent new solar lentigines, protective clothing and sunblocks should be used.

Surgery

Seborrheic keratosis: Light electrocautery, cryosurgery with liquid nitrogen spray, curettage, or shave excision. If these lesions are flat, Q-switched ruby laser can be used. Treatment without histopathologic confirmation should be done undertaken only if skin cancer is not a consideration.

Dermatosis papulosa nigra: Can be removed by several methods, such as light electro-cautery (usually 0.4 to 0.8 W), curettage, cryosurgery with cotton-tip applicator dipped in liquid nitrogen, and excision with Gradle scissors. All three modalities must be approached with caution to avoid hyperpigmentation or hypopigmentation.

Lentigines: Light application of liquid nitrogen (4–10 seconds) or trichloroacetic acid (35%–90%) can lighten these lesions. However, these techniques can cause unwanted hypopigmentation. Laser treatment yields best results. Several lasers are effective, including the pulsed-dye 510-nm, frequency-doubled Nd: YAG (yttrium-argon-garnet) (1064, 532-nm); quasi-continuous wave copper vapor/bromide (511-nm); krypton (520–530 nm); KTP (potassium-titanyl-phosphate) (532-nm), Q-switched ruby (694-nm); and Q-switched alexandrite (755-nm). The carbon dioxide (10,600-nm) and erbium:YAG (2,940-nm) lasers are nonselective, but both can be used to remove epidermal pigment.

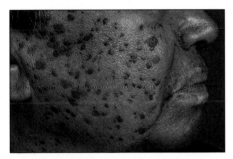

Seborrheic keratoses: gray-brown plaques, cobblestone surface, "stuck-on" appearance.

Treatment aims

These lesions are treated primarily for cosmetic reasons. However, eradication of seborrheic keratosis may be necessary if the lesions are chronically irritated (because of their presence in intertriginous areas or by jewelry and clothing) or are frequently pruritic.

Prognosis

Seborrheic keratosis: Lesions do not spontaneously disappear, and new lesions will continue to appear as patient ages.

Dermatosis papulosa nigra: These lesions can continue to grow in number.

Lentigo simplex: Course is unknown. It has been reported that solar lentigines can evolve into seborrheic keratosis. Atypical types of lentigo simplex may be associated with melanomas on the acral and mucosal regions.

Follow-up and management

Seborrheic keratosis: Internal malignancy (lung, gastrointestinal cancer) should be considered if multiple lesions suddenly erupt (sign of Leser-Trèlat).

Lentigo simplex: Educate patients about changes that suggest melanoma. Patients with solar lentigines should have skin examinations at least annually because of higher risk for skin cancer from photodamage.

General references

Raulin C, Schonermark MP, et al.: Q-switched ruby laser treatment of tattoos and benign pigmented skin lesions: a critical review. Ann Plast Surg 1998, 41:555–565.

Pariser RJ: Benign neoplasms of the skin. Med Clin North Am 1998, 82:1285–1307.

Li YT, Yang KC: Comparison of the frequency-doubled Q-switched Nd:YAG laser and 35% trichloroacetic acid for the treatment of face lentigines. Dermatol Surg 1999, 25:202–204.

Goldberg DJ: Laser treatment of pigmented lesions. Dermatol Clin 1997, 15:397–407.

Grimes PE, Arora S, et al.: Dermatosis papulosa nigra. Cutis 1983, 32:385–386.

Diagnosis

Signs

Epidermoid (epidermal, sebaceous, infundibular) cysts (EC): Firm, round, intradermal or subcutaneous nodules, 1.0 - 5.0 cm, filled with malodorous, cream-colored, keratinaceous material; often connected to surface through keratin-filled pores. Common in areas with numerous sebaceous glands (face, neck, chest, upper back, axillae, scrotum).

Trichilemmal (isthmus catagen) cysts (TC): Clinically similar but lack central punctum. About 90% on scalp.

Acrochordons (A): Three types: **multiple**—1–2-mm-long papules on neck, axillae; **single or multiple**—smooth, 2-mm by 5-mm papules, different locations; **solitary**—baglike, soft exophytic nodules; usually 0.05–1 cm but can be >10 cm; light skin-shades to brown. Papules constricted at base; may have long stalk. Usually asymptomatic. Friction, trauma, torsion may cause irritation, possibly resulting in tenderness, with crusting, hemorrhage. Usually on neck, eyelids, intertriginous areas.

Dermatofibromas (D): Usually asymptomatic, occasionally tender or pruritic; firm, button-like, dome-shaped or depressed papules or nodules; dimple when compressed. Usually on legs; may be on upper extremities, trunk. Typically 5–10 mm; may be 2–3 cm. Color: Flesh-toned, yellow, pink, tan, brown. Center may show postinflammatory hypopigmentation or hyperpigmentation.

Neurofibromas (N): Soft or firm; compressible; light flesh-colored to brown; pedunculated, sessile, or subcutaneous nodules. Usually < 1.0 cm, but may be several centimeters. "Buttonhole" sign (lesion invagination with finger pressure). Solitary or multiple, as in neurofibromatosis (von Recklinghausen's disease).

Investigations

EC biopsy: Sac of stratified squamous epithelium filled with keratinaceous material, a prominent stratum granulosum. **TC biopsy**: Lining of pale, swollen epithelial cells, distinct palisade arrangement resembling follicular outer root sheath in telogen; no stratum granulosum. Keratinous contents may be calcified. **A biopsy**: Thinned epidermis, loose connective tissue stroma. **D biopsy**: Hyperplastic epidermis, whorling fascicles of spindle cells with elongated nuclei and pale-blue cytoplasm in dermis. **N biopsy**: Extraneural, nonencapsulated neoplasm of faintly eosinophilic spindle cells (with elongated nuclei) in a loosely spaced matrix.

Complications

EC, TC: Wall rupture or bacterial infection leads to pain, tenderness. Rare malignant transformation to squamous-cell carcinoma and basal-cell carcinoma. **A**: Irritation (by perspiration), trauma (jewelry, tight clothing). Rare torsion, infarction. Association with clonic polyps. **D**: Almost always asymptomatic. **N**: Lesions may be painful, tender, disfiguring. Neurofibromatosis, an autosomal dominant syndrome, can occur as spontaneous mutation. Cardinal features of the classic type (NF1)—multiple neurofibromas, café au lait macules (>6; 1.5 cm in adults, 0.5 cm in prepubertal children), axillary and inguinal freckling (Crowe's sign), iris hamartomas (Lisch nodules), optic gliomas, distinctive osseous lesions (*eg*, sphenoid dysplasia); first-degree relative with NF1. NF2 (Central neurofibromatosis) features vestibular schwannomas of eighth cranial nerve, first-degree relative with NF2, neurofibroma, meningioma, acoustic neuroma, glioma, schwannoma, and juvenile posterior subcapsular lenticular opacity.

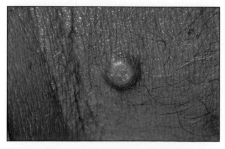

Dermatofibroma may remain static, enlarge gradually; rarely, regress or grow rapidly.

Differential diagnosis

EC, TC: Lipomas, subcutaneous adnexal tumors. **Epidermal inclusion cysts**: Firm, smooth keratin-filled nodules, commonly on palms, soles; usually in a scar. **Mucoid cyst**: Firm, rubbery, translucent nodule formed by extrusion of mucin from underlying joint space, usually on fingers, toes. **Milia**: 0.5- to 2-mm, superficial, white, hard keratinous cysts; arising from pluripotential cells in epidermis, stimulated by follicular epidermal irritation, trauma. Common in periorbital areas, cheeks, forehead, eyelids; rarely, on hands. **Steatocystoma multiplex**: 2- to 20-mm, soft, superficial nodules filled with oily yellow fluid, usually on upper arm, trunk. **A**: Pedunculated seborrheic keratosis, intradermal nevus, neurofibroma, molluscum contagiosum, fibroepithelioma of Pinkus and collagen nevus. **D**: Scar, malignant melanoma, blue nevus, epidermoid cyst, metastatic cancer, Kaposi's sarcoma, dermatofibrosarcoma protuberans, intradermal Spitz nevus, and atypical fibroxanthoma.

N: Neurilemmoma, lipoma, glomus tumor, epidermoid cyst, synovial ganglion.

Etiology

EC: Arise from infundibular portion of hair follicles, "occlusion and inflammation of pilosebaceous follicles" after severe acne vulgaris. **TC**: Arise from isthmus portion of hair follicles; causes—implantation of epidermal cells within dermis after injury; trapping of epidermal cells along embryonal fusion planes. **D**: Possibly related to trauma, *eg*, insect bite. **N**: Genetic defect (for NF1 located on chromosome 17q11.2). In NF2, genetic defect localized to chromosome 22q11-13.1; defect in schwannomin or merlin.

Epidemiology

EC, TC: Rare in children; common in adults. Both sexes affected equally. Multiple cysts, associated with Gardner's syndrome and nevoid basal-cell carcinoma syndrome. **A**: More common in obese patients and in women. **D**: Common in adults; ccur mainly in adults, female preference, 2:1. **N**: Male patients affected slightly more often. Usually appear during third decade. Incidence: NF1, 1:3000; NF2, 1:50,000.

Marina Kuperman Beade and Vicki J. Levine

Treatment

Pharmacological treatment

EC, TC: Distinguishing between rupture and infection may be difficult. Intralesional corticosteroid therapy for inflamed cysts.

Oral antibiotic therapy if infection cannot be excluded. Start oral antibiotic therapy against *Staphylococcus aureus* (the most common pathogen) after cyst incision, drainage, and culturing. Modify antibiotics according to results of sensitivities.

Warm soaks expedite fluctuance. Warm soaks and topical antibiotic ointment are helpful after incision and drainage of infected cyst.

Intralesional corticosteroid therapy may reverse atrophy of small, recently developed facial infected cysts.

Surgery

EC, TC: Surgical excision if no infection or inflammation. Use modified Danna procedure-Excise overlying plug of skin and cyst wall with a skin biopsy punch, then use curette or clamp to remove contents and the cyst wall to minimize scar (if cyst wall is not firmly attached to adjacent connective tissue). If previous infection or inflammation makes dissecting entire lining impossible; excise cyst and surrounding tissue.

M removal options: Use 30-gauge needle; apply trichloroacetic acid with toothpick or calcium alginate applicator; prick surface with sharp scalpel and squeeze with smooth forceps or press down with comedone extractor; light electrodesiccation; applications of tretinoin cream.

A: Excise with curved Gradle scissors; cryosurgery with cotton-tip applicator dipped in liquid nitrogen; light electrodesiccation.

D Surgical excision indications: Repeated trauma, unacceptable cosmetic appearance, uncertain clinical diagnosis. However, the surgical scar is usually more unattractive than the lesions. Cryosurgery with liquid nitrogen can decrease lesion size. Intralesional steroid injections may initiate regression.

N: Surgical excision with scalpel or CO_2 laser. If multiple lesions, subtotal disc resection may provide acceptable cosmetic results.

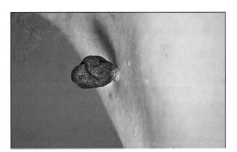

Solitary acrochordon on the axilla of a middle age obese woman.

Treatment aims

Patients seek treatment for cosmesis or because of symptoms. Removing lesions can prevent inflammation or infection of cysts.

Prognosis

EC, TC: No recurrence after surgical excision unless epidermal lining was not completely removed.

A: Lesions tend to increase in size and number, especially during pregnancy or weight gain.

D: Lesions may appear over months and persist without increase in size. They can also increase in size or spontaneously regress.

N: Mortality in neurofibromatosis is higher, due to development of neurofibrosarcoma, and increased incidence of pheochromo-cytoma, rhabdomyosarcoma, leukemia, central nervous system tumors. Annually examine for sarcoma. Consider multidisciplinary approach (internists, neurologists, psychiatrists, orthopedic and plastic surgeons) to treat complications.

General references

Roenigk RK, Ratz JL: CO_2 laser treatment of cutaneous neurofibromas. *J Dermatol Surg Oncol* 1987, **13**:187–190.

Diagnosis

Signs

Congenital (CG)
• Sharply demarcated macules or raised plaques; uniform or mottled pigment, light brown to black; smooth, mammillated, or verrucous; hypertrichosis is often present; on trunk more often than proximal extremities.

Acquired
Nevus spilus (NS): Macular or slightly papular dark brown lesions (speckles) superimposed on uniformly light brown macular background; on trunk more often than proximal extremities.

Simple lentigines (L): Sharply demarcated, evenly pigmented macules; brown to black; 1-6 mm in diameter; varying shapes; over entire integument.

Common (C): *Junctional* (sharply demarcated, uniformly pigmented macules or slightly elevated papules; regular borders; 2-10 mm; preserved skin markings), *intradermal* (skin colored or slightly pigmented, dome-shaped or polypoid papules; smooth or papillomatous surface; <1 cm), or *compound* (more varied than junctional or intradermal; sharply demarcated papules; variable elevation; smooth or papillomatous surfaces; generally uniform light brown to black; usually <6 mm. A few excess hairs may protrude from compound and intradermal nevi. Over entire integument. In dark-skinned people, most easily discerned on palms, soles; in whites, usually no more than 30 lesions.

Dysplastic nevi, atypical moles (DN): Share clinical features (*ie*, asymmetry, border irregularity, color variegation, diameter < 6 mm) with melanoma; severity of clinical features generally worse in melanoma; on trunk, upper extremities, lower extremities, face.

Halo nevi (HN): Typically, 3-6 mm central flat or slightly raised, uniformly brown or pink, melanocytic nevus; symmetrical white depigmentation zone surrounds central lesion; usually on upper back.

Spitz Nevi (SN): Well-circumscribed, dome-shaped papules, 2-2 cm diameter (average 8 mm); uniform color, pink to dark brown. (*pigmented variant*: about 3 mm average diameter; homogeneous dark brown, black color; *agminated variant*: multiple papular lesions, segmental grouping; *congenital agminated lesions* may overlay café-au-lait-like macule.); approximately 40% of cases occur on head, neck; rest on trunk, extremities (*pigmented variant*: 70% on extremities; 20% on trunk; 10% on head, neck.

Blue nevi (BN): *common*: firm, blue-gray or black papule or nodule not more than1 cm; typically solitary, may be grouped; usually on dorsa of hands, feet; also, scalp, sacrum; *cellular*: blue-gray nodule or plaque usually <3 cm diameter, on sacrum, buttocks, also scalp, face, hands, feet; *combined*: typically, common intradermal or compound nevus; small area of a blue nevus within it.

Mongolian spot (MS): Typically, single, light-gray to bluish macule or patch; indistinct borders; lumbosacral, buttocks.

Nevus of Ota; Nevus of Ito (NO; NI): Confluence of small macules forming larger, mottled patch; indistinct borders; brown to gray, blue, or black; NO usually unilateral, on face, following distributions of first and second branches of trigeminal nerve; NI on supraclavicular, deltoid, scapular areas of trunk.

Investigations
• Dermoscopy: visualize skin structures to level of dermoepidermal junction and papillary dermis; differentiate between benign and malignant melanocytic neoplasms.

Complications
CG: Risk of melanoma in large congenital nevi (> 20 cm by adulthood): 5% to 20%; in CG nevi 1.5-19.9 cm: low. **NS**: Melanoma, rare. **L**: Generalized: cardiac abnormalities, developmental defects, Peutz-Jeghers syndrome, xeroderma pigmentosum. **DN**: Melanoma, familial atypical mole multiple melanoma syndrome. **HN**: DN, melanoma rarely. **SN**: Malignant or metastatic SN, very rare. **BN**: Malignant BN may rarely arise in common BN: benign metastatic BN reported in lymph nodes. **NO, NI**: Cutaneous and ocular melanomas, rarely.

Differential diagnosis

CG: Dysplastic nevus, melanoma, epidermal nevus, Becker's nevus, seborrheic keratosis (SK), pigmented squamous cell carcinoma, pigmented Paget's. **NS**: Congenital melanocytic nevus, Becker's nevus, café-au-lait (CAL) spot. **L**: Solar lentigo, C, ephelis, melanoma, pigmented SN, CAL macule, hemangioma, cutaneous hemorrhage. **C, DN**: Dysplastic nevus, melanoma, pigmented SN, SK, pigmented actinic keratosis, basal cell carcinoma (BCC), dermatofibroma, lichen planus–like keratosis, neurofibroma, fibroepithelial polyp, benign adnexal tumors. **HN**: Dermatofibromas, flat warts, molluscum, SK, BCC, lichen planus, psoriasis, sarcoidosis, neuroectodermally derived skin tumors. **SN**: Pyogenic granuloma, hemangioma, verruca, molluscum, juvenile xanthogranuloma, intradermal nevus, dermatofibroma, mastocytoma, melanoma. **BN**: Melanoma, dysplastic nevus, SN, angiokeratoma, venous lake, pigmented BCC, glomus tumor, apocrine hidrocystoma. **MS**: NO, NI, BN, contusion, fixed drug reaction, vascular malformation, argyria, ochronosis. **NO, NI**: BN, contusion, fixed drug reaction, vascular malformation, argyria, ochronosis, melasma, NS, lentigo maligna.

Etiology

Genetic factors may contribute to occurrence or interact with environmental agents to produce clinical lesion.

Epidemiology

NS: Usually acquired in childhood. **C**: More usual in ages 20 to 29. Fair-skinned more often affected; proportion of melanocytic nevi on acral surfaces higher in darker-skinned. **DN**: New lesions may appear into sixth decade. Risk factor for melanoma. **HN**: Typically, 3–42 years (mean, 15). **SN**: Uncommon in patients <40 to 50 years. **BN**: Typically arises in childhood, adolescence. **MS**: Incidence ranges from 100% in Malaysians to <2% in whites; tends to disappear in early childhood. **NO, NI**: More common in darker-skinned people; peaks of incidence at infancy, puberty.

David Polsky and Alfred W. Kopf

Treatment

Diet and lifestyle

• Patients must avoid midday (10am to 4am) sun when possible; protective clothing, high-SPF sunscreen with UVB/UVA protection, especially in DN. Cosmetic cover-ups may help, socially.

Nonpharmacological treatment

• Excise lesions suspicious of melanoma (eg, arising in DN, SN) to narrow margin (2–3 mm). Partial biopsy of large CG nevus suspicious for melanoma acceptable, if problematic; include especially dark or raised areas in specimen.

• MS successfully treated (minimal scarring), with pigment-specific lasers, eg, Q-switched ruby, alexandrite, neodymium/yttrium-aluminum-garnet.

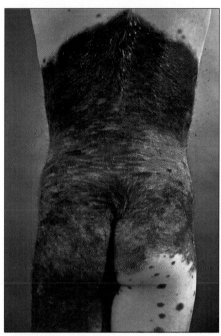

Congenital giant hairy melanocytic nevus extending from upper mid-back to left buttock and right thigh; surrounding satellite nevi.

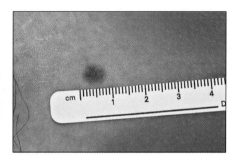

Reddish brown dysplastic (atypical) nevus; darker center, slightly irregular borders.

Treatment aims

Removal of lesions suspicious for malignancy. Patient assurance. Destruction or camouflage of benign lesions

Prognosis:

CG: Morphology changes possible: fading of colors, changing surface texture, development of hairs, halos. Rarely, may regress completely. Development of atypical areas raises suspicion of melanoma. **C**: Believed to evolve from junctional to compound to intradermal. **DN**: Likely to change, disappear. Increasing clinical atypia may indicate biopsy need. Melanoma may arise de novo or within existing nevi. **HN**: Course is highly variable. Central nevus may persist unchanged, change to pink or red, regress completely (about 50% of cases) in months to years. Depigmented zone may repigment. **NO, NI**: Enlarges in childhood, persists through adulthood. Color fluctuates, especially with hormonal changes.

Follow-up and management:

General: Indications for biopsy: changing morphology, symptomatology; features suspicious for malignancy; repeated irritation; cosmetic concerns. **Specific: CG** Large CG with atypia: baseline photographs; physician evaluation every 3 to 12 months. MRI scans of central nervous system for patients with axial lesions. Rule out neurocutaneous melanosis. Other CG may be observed during annual physician evaluation. **C, DN**: Skin self-examamination; routine physician evaluation; total-body photographs for patients with DN syndrome or increased number of common moles and other melanoma risk factors. **HN**: Personal, family history of melanoma, DN, vitiligo; periodic complete skin examinations; close follow up of lesions; biopsy if atypical morphologic features; suspect melanoma especially in patients over 40. **SN**:Remove for step-section histopathologic evaluation, margin evaluation

Support Organizations:

Congenital Nevi: Nevus Outreach, Inc., 1616 Alpha Street, Lansing, MI 48910, 517-487-2306; Fax: 515-684-0953. URL: http://www.nevus.org.; email: info@nevus.org.

Diagnosis

Signs

Primary lesion: Pigmented macules, papules, plaques, nodules (rarely, amelanotic); smooth surface usual; larger lesions may be crusted, eroded, ulcerated. "ABCDs:" (*A*symmetry, *B*order irregularity, *C*olor variability, *D*iameter > 4 mm). Common sites include upper back (men), lower extremities (women); may involve any site.

Metastases: Satellites; in-transit; nodal; systemic.

Symptoms

•Usually asymptomatic; pruritus, tenderness, formication, crusting, bleeding may develop, especially with larger lesions.

Investigations

•Total skin examination. Dermoscopy to differentiate malignant melanoma (MM) from other pigmented lesions. Digitized image analysis. Excisional biopsy remains standard criterion. Histologic diagnosis and appropriate microstaging rely on adequate tissue specimen to measure thickness, level of invasion.

Complications

•Metastases (commonly lungs, brain, liver, bone, intestines). Vitiligo-like hypopigmentation, diffuse hypomelanosis rare.

Clinical staging

American Joint Committee on Cancer staging, based on Breslow thickness; Clark level of invasion; involvement of regional lymph nodes; presence of metastasis. **0**: Melanoma in situ; Clark Level I (Tis [T *in situ*] N0M0). **IA**: Localized melanoma (LM) < 0.75 mm or level II (T1N0M0). **IB**: LM 0.76–1.50 mm or level III (T2N0M0). **IIA**: LM 1.51–4.00 mm or level IV (T3N0M0). **IIB**: LM > 4.00mm or level V (T4N0M0). **IIIA**: Regional lymph node(s) metastasis (RM) < 3 cm in greatest dimension (any T,N1,M0). **IIIB**: RM > 3 cm in greatest dimension and/or in-transit metastasis (any T,N2,M0). **IV**: Distant metastasis (any T, any N,M1).

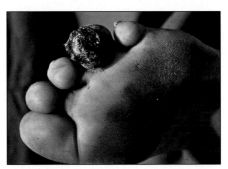

Black nodular acral malignant melanoma on the second toe.

Differential diagnosis

Acquired and congenital melanocytic nevi (especially dysplastic nevi), blue nevi, pigmented basal cell carcinoma; seborrheic keratosis; lichen-planus–like keratosis; solar lentigo; hemangioma; pyogenic granuloma.

Etiology

Solar radiation, especially bursts of sunlight exposure causing sunburn, and cumulative chronic solar radiation causing lentigo maligna melanoma. Melanoma can originate in melanocytic nevi. Giant (> 20 cm) congenital nevi have statistically significant melanoma risk. Dysplastic nevi patients, without personal or family history of melanoma or atypical mole syndrome have a 7-fold to 70-fold increased risk of developing melanoma, and a lifetime risk of 18%.

Epidemiology

Incidence: In the United States, in 1999, 44,200 (25,800 males; 18,400 females) with 7,300 deaths (4,600 males; 2,700 females). Lifetime risk: 1 in 75 in the year 2000. Risk factors: Personal or family history of melanoma or nonmelanoma skin cancer; presence of numerous moles or freckles; blonde or red hair; light eyes; fair complexion (skin phenotypes I, II, III); excessive sun exposure (especially intermittent, intense exposure); sunburns in childhood; presence of precursor lesions.

Elizabeth K. Hale and Alfred W. Kopf

Treatment

Lifestyle

•Sun avoidance or protection; frequent (6 or 12 months) physician skin examinations if increased risk; monthly patient self-examinations.

Nonpharmacological treatment

Surgical excision: Primary treatment; Breslow thickness determines margin of excision: in situ = 0.5 to 1 cm; 0.01 to 0.99 mm = 1 cm; 1 to 4 mm = 2 cm; 4.01 mm or greater = 2 to 3 cm. **Mohs' micrographic surgery**: May be useful for melanomas with indistinct margins. **Lymphoscintigraphy, sentinel node biopsy**: To assess possible lymph node involvement for melanomas 1 mm or thicker, depending on location, etc.; therapeutic lymph node dissection for positive MM to isolated lymph nodes. Discordancy rates between clinical prediction of MM and lymphatic drainage patterns greatest for primary melanomas (PMs) of head, neck, trunk; preoperative lymphoscintigraphy to identify sentinel lymph nodes before dissection is attempted.

Metastatic Work-up: Depending on clinical factors, chest radiograph (CXR); liver function tests (LFTs), especially lactic acid dehydrogenase (LDH); CT/MRI scans; positron emission tomography; blood testing for melanoma-associated antigens (*eg*, TA-90), which may predict subclinical metastatic disease. Most physicians of melanoma patients order no tests for MM in situ; CXR, with or without initial LDH/LFTs, for stages I, II, III, and during follow-up for stages IB, II, III; baseline CT/MRI of chest, abdomen/pelvis, brain for stage III.

Adjuvant therapy: Chemotherapy; most active single agent is dacarbazine (DTIC); combination of DTIC + carmustine (BCNU) + cisplatin + tamoxifen ("Dartmouth regimen") may be more effective than single therapy. Immunotherapy; interferons, vaccines, interleukins, T-cell infusions. Radiation therapy for brain metastatses. Isolation-perfusion procedures for satellitosis. Consider cytoreductive surgery, with postoperative adjuvant immunotherapy, for stage IV MM.

Special therapeutic considerations

•Investigational: melanoma vaccines to slow melanoma progression in patients clinically disease-free by surgical resection but at high risk for recurrence.

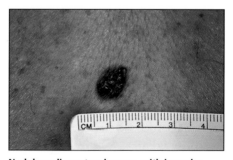

Nodule malignant melanoma, with irregular border and a faint surrounding halo.

Elizabeth K. Hale and Alfred W. Kopf

Treatment aims

Before metastasis, to excise PM. After metastasis to distant sites, attempts to eradicate tumor; palliation; compassionate care.

Prognosis

Poorer-prognosis: increased thickness, level of invasion of primary lesion; older patient age; male gender; axial location; histologically positive nodes; increased mitotic rate; ulceration or regression; diminished host lymphoid response; vertical growth phase. Metastases suggest markedly reduced survival. After distant metastasis, prognosis guarded. Recurrence risk correlates most directly with PM thickness.

Probability of 10-year survival rate (excluding palms, soles subungual lesions)

Thickness < 0.76 mm: Age < 60: women, 0.99 (0.97–1.0); men, 0.99 (0.97–0.99); age > 60: women, 0.98 (0.95–0.99); men, 0.97 (0.93–0.99). **Thickness 0.76 – 1.69 mm**: Age < 60: women, 0.94 (0.91–0.96); men, 0.93 (0.89–0.95); age > 60: women, 0.89 (0.82–0.94); men, 0.87 (0.79–0.93).

Thickness 1.70 – 3.60 mm: Age < 60: women, 0.82 (0.74–0.88); men, 0.79 (0.69–0.86); age > 60: women, 0.69 (0.57–0.79); men, 0.65 (0.52–0.76).

Thickness > 3.60 mm: Age < 60: women, 0.68 (0.55–0.79); men, 0.64 (0.49–0.76); age > 60: women, 0.52 (0.36–0.67); men, 0.47 (0.31–0.63).

Follow-up

Frequency depends on Breslow thickness; thorough history and total cutaneous examinations for original melanoma and new PM(s); diagnostic tests as needed.

Support organizations

American Cancer Society (http://www.cancer.org). Skin Cancer Foundation (www.skincancer.org). American Academy of Dermatology (www.aad.org). E-Room (www.dermnetwork.org).

General references

Friedman RJ, Riegel DS, Kopf AW: Early detection of malignant melanoma. The role of physician examination and self-examination of the skin. *CA Cancer J Clin* 1985, **35**:130–151.

Cutaneous T-cell lymphoma

Diagnosis

Signs

Usually starts as erythematous patches on areas not exposed to sun. Progresses to plaques, tumors. Initial presentation may be plaque or tumor-stage disease or erythroderma.

Investigations

Skin biopsy: May need to biopsy multiple lesions or over a period of time to histologically confirm diagnosis. Plaque-stage lesions characteristically show psoriasiform epidermal hyperplasia, hyperkeratosis, focal parakeratosis, lichenoid infiltrate of mononuclear cells within papillary dermis. Epidermotropism with lymphocytes, singly or in collections within epidermis; surrounded by clear halo (Pautrier microabscesses); hyperchromatic, irregular nuclei. Biopsies for immunophenotying, genotyping helpful; polymerase chain reaction superior to Southern blot for T-cell receptor gene rearrangement. **Initial blood studies**: CBC, complete metabolic panel, LDH and HTLV 1 and 2. **Chest x-ray**; in advanced-stage, biologically active disease: CT of chest, abdomen, pelvis. **Advanced disease**: Analysis of peripheral blood for immunotyping, genotying; lymph-node biopsy of palpable nodes.

Tumor, node, metastasis (TNM) staging

Skin: **T0**: Suggestive of CTCL. **T1** Patches, papules, plaques involving less than 10% body surface area (BSA). **T2**: Patches, papules, plaques involving 10% or more BSA. **T3**: Tumors. **T4**: Erythroderma. **Lymph nodes**: **N0**: No palpable adenopathy; lymph node pathology negative. **N1**: Palpable adenopathy; lymph node pathology negative. **N2**: No palpable adenopathy; lymph node pathology positive. **N3**: Palpable adenopathy; lymph node pathology positive. **Visceral organs**: **M0**: No visceral organ involvement. **M1**: Visceral involvement.

Summary staging classification

Stage IA: T1, N0, M0; **IB**: T2, N0, M0; **IIA**: T1 or T2, N1, M0; **IIB**: T3, N0 or N1, M0; **III**: T4, N0 or N1, M0; **IVA**: T1 through T4, N2 or N3, M0; **IVB**: T1 through T4, N0 through N3, M1.

Differential Diagnosis

Patch-stage or plaque-stage disease: Eczema, atopic or contact dermatitis, xerosis, adult T-cell leukemia/lymphoma. **Tumor-stage disease**: Lymphomatoid papulosis, metastatic disease, leukemia or other lymphomas.

Etiology

Unknown.

Epidemiology

Most often diagnosed during 5th, 6th decade. Affects men almost twice as often as women. Incidence increased from 0.19 to 0.42 cases per 100,000 from 1973 until 1984. Blacks have twice the incidence of whites.

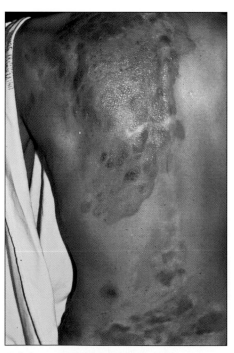

Erythematous, finely scaly patches and thin plaques with central lightening and excoriations around the borders.

Well-demarcated, irregular, dusky red to violaceous infiltrated plaques. Tumors arise within and at the border of the lesions.

Jeremy Rothfleisch and David Ramsay

Treatment

Diet and lifestyle

• Good nutrition with high protein diet and vitamin supplementation for widespread disease and erythroderma.

Pharmacological treatment

Topical

Earlier-stage (IA, IB, IIA) disease: Mid-strength topical steroids. Nitrogen mustard (mechlorethamine) 10 mg vial diluted with 50 mL of water and applied daily. Ointment-based mechlorethamine. Carmustine (BTSU): Daily applications of 10 mg/mL diluted in 95% alcohol followed by maintenance of 2–4 mg/mL solution. Bexarotene gel, 0.1% daily, 2 weeks; then b.i.d., 2 weeks; then 0.5% gel, daily, 2 weeks; then b.i.d., 2 weeks and 1.0% gel, daily, 2 weeks; then b.i.d., 2 weeks.

Systemic

Advanced-stage disease: Interferon α-2a, dose may range from 3 million units three times a week to 18 million units daily. Bexarotene capsules at an initial dose level of 300 mg/m2/day, with food. Denileukin diftitox (ontak) 8 µg/kg to 18 µg/kg, i.v. infusion, 15–60 minutes, 5 days.

Nonpharmacological treatment

Earlier-stage (IA, IB, IIA) disease: Ultraviolet B phototherapy (for patch stage only) Psoralen and long-wave ultraviolet radiation (PUVA) or narrow band UVB (investigational). Localized or total body skin electron beam. Systemic retinoids (acitretin 25–50 mg daily). PUVA coupled with alpha-interferon or systemic retinoids.
Advanced disease: Photopheresis with 8-methoxypsoralen Chemotherapy: Methotrexate can be administered in high i.v. dosages. The purine analogues (*eg*, 2-chlorodeoxyadenosine, fludarabine, pentostatin) promising in refractory CTCL. EPOCH (etoposide, prednisone, vincristine, doxorubicin, and cyclophosphamide) reserved for patients with resistant, extensive, or advanced CTCL. Total skin electron-beam irradiation.

Special therapeutic considerations

• UVB, PUVA, and mechlorethamine have been associated with increased skin cancers. Long-term PUVA may cause an increased risk of melanomas and significantly ages the skin. Individuals using mechlorethamine should avoid excessive sun exposure as together they may increase the incidence of skin cancers.

• Patients in the procreative period should not use BCNU or mechlorethamine.

• Systemic agents have well-established side effect profiles.

• Alternating 3-month cycles of natural lymphoblastoid, natural leukocyte, and recombinant alpha interferon to prevent resistance has been proposed.

• Chlorambucil, 10–12 mg for 3 days, with fluocortolone, 75 mg on day 1, 50 mg on day 2, and 25 mg on day 3. The cycle is repeated every 2 weeks and extended to every 4 weeks after the third cycle and then to every 6 weeks after the sixth cycle and continued until clinical improvement occurs (for unresponsive erythrodermic cases).

Treatment aims

Remission. Reduction in stage. Stabilization. Palliative care

Prognosis

Early stage (T1) mycosis fungoides: Generally indolent, usually a normal survival rate and excellent quality of life. T2 survival rate: About 67% at five years (88% with patch and 61% with plaque stage). More advanced stages: poorer prognosis; survivals often measured in a few years

Follow-up and management

Intensity depends upon stage, method of therapy, biological activity of disease. Patients must be followed for a lifetime. If diagnosis suspected but not confirmed, inform patient of possible diagnosis of mycosis fungoides, and follow for a prolonged time period, even if clearing occurs.

Support organizations

Mycosis Fungoides Foundation; P.O. Box 374, Birmingham, MI 48012-0374
Phone 248-644-9014; FAX 248-644-9014
Moving Forward Foundation; P.O. Box 20388, Houston, Texas 77225-0388
Phone 713-669-0908; FAX 713-592-8656

General references

Hermann JJ, Roenigk HH Jr, Hurria A, *et al.*: Treatment of mycosis fungoides with photochemotherapy (PUVA): long-term followup. *J Am Acad Dermatol* 1995, 33:234–242.

Kuzel TM, Roenigk HH Jr, Samuelson E, *et al.*: Effectiveness of interferon Alfa-2a combined with phototherapy for mycosis fungoides and the Sezary syndrome. *J Clin Oncol* 1995, 13:257–263.

Ramsay DL, Meller JA, Zackheim HG: Topical treatment of early cutaneous T-cell lymphoma. *Hematol Onco Clin North Am* 1995, 9:1031–1055.

Kim YH, Chow S, Varghese A, *et al.*: Clinical characteristics and long-term outcome of patients with generalized patch and/or plaque (T2) mycosis fungoides. *Arch Dermatol* 1999, 135:26–32.

Jeremy Rothfleisch and David Ramsay

Diagnosis

Signs

Diagnosis of dermatomyositis (skin lesions have sensitivity of 94% and specificity of 90% against systemic lupus erythematosus and systemic sclerosis) requires **at least one of the following**:

• Periorbital violaceous edematous erythema (heliotrope rash).

• Erythematous to violaceous papules or plaques overlying extensor surface of joints (Gottron's papules).

• Erythematous patches overlying extensor surfaces of joints (Gottron's sign).

• Linear erythematous patches on extensor surfaces of extremities (linear extensor erythema).

Plus four of the following:

• Proximal symmetrical muscle weakness (upper or lower extremity and trunk).

• Muscle pain on grasping or spontaneous pain.

• Elevated serum creatine kinase or aldolase levels.

• Electromyographic abnormalities (short-duration, polyphasic motor unit potentials with spontaneous fibrillation potentials).

• Positive anti-Jo-1 (histadyl transfer-RNA synthetase) antibody.

• Nondestructive arthritis or arthralgia.

• Systemic inflammatory signs (temperature > 37° C at axilla), elevated serum C-reactive protein level or accelerated erythrocyte sedimentation rate of more than 20 mm/h by the Westergren method).

• Pathologic findings compatible with inflammatory myositis.

Other signs: Malar rash with nasolabial involvement and circumoral pallor, erythema on chest and upper back (Shawl sign), periungual erythema, and telangiectasias with "drop-out" cuticular overgrowth, poikiloderma (late), scaling erythematous scalp, "mechanic's hands" (fissuring and scaling), photosensitivity, calcinosis cutis.

Symptoms

• Weakness (difficulty rising from chair, drooped head, dysphagia), arthralgias, myalgias.

Investigations

• Muscle enzymes (creatine phosphokinase, aldolase, lactate dehydrogenase, alanine and aspartate aminotransferase).

• Antinuclear antibodies: Anti-Jo-1, -PL-12, -SRP, -Mi-2 (R/O MCTD: SSA (Ro), -SSB (La), -Sm, -nRNP).

• Skin biopsy: Epidermal atrophy, liquefaction degeneration of the dermoepidermal junction, mononuclear infiltrate in the dermis, edema of the upper dermis, mucin deposition in the dermis, fibrinoid deposits at the dermoepidermal junction and around the capillaries of the upper dermis.

• Direct immunofluorescence.

• Electromyography.

• Muscle biopsy (quadriceps, deltoid).

• Pulmonary function tests.

• Basic cancer screening in patients >50 years of age, with appropriate follow-up (history, physical examination, routine laboratory evaluation, and age-appropriate cancer screening).

Complications

• Disuse muscle atrophy and joint contractures; calcinosis cutis with secondary infection; interstitial lung disease (10%–30% of cases); greater risk for other autoimmune diseases (arthritis, Raynaud's phenomenon, systemic lupus erythematosus, and Sjögren's syndrome).

• Possible higher rates of cancer in persons with adult dermatomyositis.

Differential diagnosis

Myositis: Polymyositis, scleroderma, mixed connective tissue disease, rheumatoid arthritis, and lupus erythematosus.

Myopathy: Neurologic disorders, muscular dystrophies, infections, toxins, endocrinopathies, inclusion-body myositis.

Dermatitis: Lupus erythematosus, polymorphic light eruption, photo-contact dermatitis, atopic dermatitis, seborrheic dermatitis, rosacea.

Etiology

Genetic factors suggested by histocompatibility antigen prevalence. Immunologic factors suggested by autoantibodies to muscle antigens. Infectious triggers suggested by associations with influenza, rubella, hepatitis B, coxsackievirus and picornavirus infections, and toxoplasmosis.

Epidemiology

Children: 1–3.2 cases/1 million; bimodal, with peaks at 5–9 and 10–14 years of age.

Adults: 1–60 cases/1 million; mean age at diagnosis, 40 (without malignancy) and 55 (with malignancy). Female:male ratio, 1.5–2:1 (without malignancy) and 1:1 (with malignancy). Skin signs in 30%–40% of adults and 95% of children.

Special considerations

Amyopathic dermatomyositis: Rash present > 2 years without weakness; normal muscle enzymes, muscle biopsy findings, MRI scans.

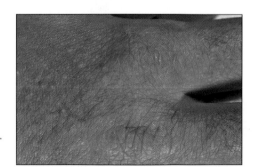

Gottron's papules: Erythematous to violaceous papules on extensor surface of joint.

Macrene Alexiades-Armenakas and Andrew Franks, Jr.

Treatment

Diet and lifestyle
Broad-spectrum sunscreens and sun avoidance. Good nutrition. Periodic cancer evaluation.

Pharmacological treatment

Topical
•Class I or II corticosteroids to involved skin (acute flare).

Systemic
Induction phase:

•Prednisone: Oral—2.0 mg/kg per day until creatine phosphokinase level normalizes, then taper over 1 year after adjuvant therapy initiated.

•Prednisolone: Use in juvenile form; pulsed i.v., 30 mg/kg per dose for 3 days, then as-needed for 4–5 weeks, followed by oral prednisone.

First-line adjuvant:

•Methotrexate: Oral—start at 7.5–10 mg every week increasing by 2.5-mg increments to 25 mg every week (single dose); i.v.—start at 10 mg every week, increasing by 2.5 mg to 0.5–0.8 mg/kg.

•Cyclosporine: Oral—start at 2.5–4.0 mg/kg per day to avoid toxicity; may use dosages as high as 10 mg/kg per day.

Second-line adjuvant:

•Antimalarials: Hydroxychloroquine, 200 mg, twice daily (adult), and 2–5 mg/kg per day (juvenile), orally, with or without quinacrine; chloroquine, 250–500 mg, orally, daily.

Florid or recalcitrant:

•Intravenous gammaglobulin, 2 g/kg, divided dose, every month for 3 months (adult), and 1–2 g/kg, every 2 weeks for 9 months (juvenile).

Tapering:

• Prednisone is tapered, as described above. Once muscle strength, creatine phosphokinase levels, and skin normalize, and the patient is off prednisone, the clinician may slowly taper the steroid-sparing agent in weekly increments, monitoring the noted parameters.

Nonpharmacological treatment

Plasmapheresis.

Physical therapy: Passive stretching, splinting, and strength building.

Surgery: Surgical excision of calcinosis cutis.

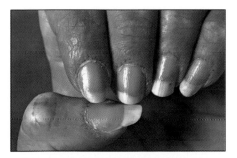

Periungal erythema with telangiectasiae.

Macrene Alexiades-Armenakas and Andrew Franks, Jr.

Treatment aims
To prevent muscle atrophy and joint contractures. Protect against sun exposure, alleviate pruritus, and reverse inflammatory skin changes.

Other treatments
Calcinosis cutis is treated with diltiazem, 240–400 mg/d; probenecid, 250 mg/d; warfarin, 1 mg orally daily; colchicine, 0.6 mg orally two to three times daily; aluminum hydroxide suspension, 15–20 mL four times daily.

Prognosis
Poor prognostic indicators in adults: recalcitrant disease, delay in diagnosis and therapy, old age, malignancy, fever, pulmonary fibrosis, and dysphagia; in juveniles: initial treatment with low-dose prednisone, delay in therapy, recalcitrant disease and pharyngeal involvement. Survival rates: 83% (1 year), 74% (2 years), 67% (3 years), and 55% (9 years). Most common causes of death are malignancy and cardiopulmonary and iatrogenic complications.

Follow-up and management
During the induction phase, creatine phosphokinase levels decrease first, followed by improvement in muscle strength by the third month of therapy. In 25% of patients, no progress is noted by this time and alternative therapies should be initiated.

Special therapeutic considerations
Long-term systemic corticosteroid therapy may result in steroid myopathy, which manifests as progressive weakness despite normalization of creatine phosphokinase values.

Support groups
Dermatomyositis and Polymyositis Support Group; contact Irene Oakley: e-mail, ye72@dial.pipex.com; telephone, 01703-449708; fax, 01703-396402.

Dermatoses of pregnancy

Diagnosis

Signs

Pemphigoid (herpes) gestationis (PG): Pruritic erythematous papules, vesicles, and bullae, initially periumbilically, and then spreading to volar surfaces, and torso; the eruption spares the face and mucous membranes. Erosions and desquamation are often present.

Pruritic urticarial papules and plaques of pregnancy (PUPPP): Eruption begins as pruritic, 1- to 2-mm, erythematous papules that coalesce into erythematous plaques that can be polymorphic; initially on the abdomen (often on striae), then spreading to buttocks and extremities but sparing the face.

Cholestasis of pregnancy (prurigo gravidarum) (CP): Usually begins with intense palmoplantar pruritus, which then spreads throughout the body. Widespread excoriations are present. Jaundice with dark urine and clay-colored stools is evident in 20% of cases. Patients may have fatigue, anorexia, nausea, emesis, and right upper quadrant pain.

Impetigo herpetiformis (IH): Is pustular psoriasis during pregnancy.

Prurigo of pregnancy (prurigo gestationis) and **pruritic folliculitis of pregnancy:** Pruritic diseases of pregnancy with unclear causes and disseminated, erythematous, excoriated, papular eruption in pruritic folliculitis; skin biopsy shows evidence of follicular involvement; may be a variant of acne.

Investigations

PG: Skin biopsy shows a subepidermal blister with basal-cell necrosis over the dermal papillae; a superficial and deep mixed-cell infiltrate of lymphocytes, histiocytes, and eosinophils, with occasional neutrophils; and both dermal and epidermal edema. Direct immunofluorescence shows linear deposition of C3 along the basement membrane zone, with IgG deposition in 30% to 40% of cases. Salt split skin test demonstrates the presence of antibody on the blister roof. Indirect immunofluorescence may detect IgG on the basement membrane zone.

PUPPP: Skin biopsy shows a nonspecific superficial and mid-perivascular lymphohistiocytic infiltrate with occasional eosinophils; variable degrees of dermal edema and spongiosis. Direct immunofluorescence is usually negative.

CP: Elevated serum bile acid levels. Alanine aminotransferase and bilirubin levels can be normal or increased.

IH: Skin biopsy, calcium levels.

Complications

PG: Variable reports of increased fetal mortality, prematurity, and small-for-gestational-age infants.

PUPPP: No serious complications, but pruritus is stressful.

CP: Increased incidence of premature delivery, low-birthweight infants, fetal mortality, postpartum hemorrhage, maternal gall bladder disease, and cholelithiasis.

IH: Hypocalcemia with seizures and tetany; fetal loss.

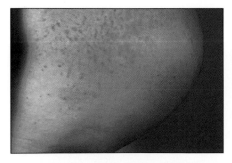

Pruritic urticarial papules, plaques (PUPPP) on abdomen; third trimester.

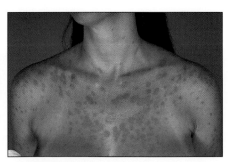

Herpes gestationis papular vesicular eruption: often abdominal; may affect chest, face, extremities.

Rebecca Baxt and Miriam Pomeranz

Treatment

Diet and lifestyle

CP: Rest and low-fat diet. Avoid hot baths.

Pharmacological treatment

Topical
• Corticosteroids class I (for PG), class I or II (for PUPPP; may help CP).

• Antipruritic emollients.

• Colloidal oatmeal baths.

Systemic
• Methylprednisolone or prednisone, 0.05–1.0 mg/kg per day (for PG until delivery, for IH, and for severe PUPPP in short, tapering courses). Dexamethasone, 12 mg/d, for 7 days, may help CP.

• Antihistamines. Dipenhydramine , never hydroxyzine.

• Cyclosporine (postpartum for PG).

• Azathioprine (postpartum for PG).

• Cholestyramine (for CP).

• Ursodeoxycholic acid (UDCA), a bile acid, 15 mg/kg per day, may decrease fetal complications (for CP).

Nonpharmacological treatment

• Conventional or narrow-band ultraviolet B phototherapy (for CP; may help PUPPP).

• Severe CP may be an indication for early (36–38 weeks) delivery.

Special therapeutic considerations

• Vitamin K should be given with cholestyramine to prevent vitamin K deficiency.

• Topical corticosteroids probably present a low risk to the fetus, but because of lack of studies they are classified as category C agents.

• Calcium supplementation and correction of fluid and electrolyte imbalances (for IH).

Treatment aims

PG: To relieve pruritus and cease blister formation.

PUPPP: To relieve pruritus.

CP: To relieve pruritus; decrease bile salts; reduce fetal morbidity and mortality.

Prognosis

PG: About 75% of cases flare at time of delivery. The eruption resolves weeks to months postpartum, although it can flare with menses or hormonal medication and usually recurs with subsequent pregnancies.

PUPPP: Resolves 7–10 days after delivery (mean duration, 6 weeks); usually does not recur. There is no increased risk to fetus or infant.

CP: Pruritus remits within days after delivery, but 60%–70% of cases recur with subsequent pregnancies; can flare with hormonal medications.

Follow-up and management

PG: Monitor infant for signs of adrenal insufficiency if high-dose steroids were used. Fetus is affected 10% of the time, but the disease is mild and self-limited. Disease in mother is self-limited.

PUPPP: Disease is self-limited.

CP: Patients may need intramuscular vitamin K supplementation if prothrombin time is elevated. Monitor for development of gallbladder disease. Rule out viral hepatitis, autoimmune hepatitis, and primary biliary cirrhosis with liver ultrasonography, serologic testing, and autoantibody tests.

General references

Vaughan Jones SA, Hern S, Nelson-Piercy C, *et al.*: A prospective study of 200 women with dermatoses of pregnancy correlating clinical findings with hormonal and immunopathological profiles. *Br J Dermatol* 1999, **141**:71–81.

Shornick JK: Dermatoses of pregnancy. *Semin Cutan Med Surg* 1998 **17**:172–181.

Aronson IK, Bond S, Fiedler VC, *et al.*: Pruritic urticarial papules and plaques of pregnancy: clinical and immunopathologic observations in 57 patients. *J Am Acad Dermatol* 1998, **39**:933–939.

McDonald JA: Cholestasis of pregnancy. *J Gastroenterol Hepatol* 1999, **14**:515–518.

Diagnosis

Signs

Dermatofibrosarcoma protuberans (DFSP): Multinodular cutaneous mass that is slow growing and appears to evolve from an indurated plaque stage. The overlying skin frequently shows a reddish-blue discoloration. About half arise on the trunk, 35% on the extremities, and 15% on the head and neck.

Merkel-cell carcinoma (MCC): Rapidly growing, solitary, red-violaceous-deep purple, dome-shaped nodule or indurated plaque (most < 2 cm) with shiny surface, often with overlying telangiectasia. Most common location is the skin of the head and neck, followed by the extremities and the trunk.

Extramammary Paget's disease (PD): Slow-growing, well-circumscribed reddish-brown plaque, usually in the anogenital region. The plaque may be eroded, moist, or velvety and be pruritic or (rarely) tender.

Investigations

Evaluation

DFSP: Total-body skin examination and palpation of regional lymph nodes. Baseline chest radiograph, if locally recurrent tumor; computed tomography scan if clinical suspicion of metastases.

MCC: Total-body skin examination and palpation of lymph nodes, liver, spleen, liver function tests and baseline chest radiograph; computed tomography scan, if clinical suspicion of metastases.

PD: Palpation of regional lymph nodes, rectal examination. Breast and pelvic examination with Papanicolaou smear for women. Chest radiography, gastrointestinal contrast studies, colonoscopy, and intravenous pyelography.

Skin Biopsy

DFSP: Dermal neoplasm composed of densely packed, monomorphous, plump spindle cells with elongated nuclei showing minimal pleomorphism, and scanty pale cytoplasm. The cells are characteristically arranged in a storiform pattern typified by numerous whorls of cells filling the dermis, often infiltrating the panniculus. On immunocytochemistry, tumor cells are usually diffusely positive for CD34 transmembrane glycoprotein.

MCC: Dermal neoplasm that consists of small undifferentiated monomorphic tumor cells (with scanty cytoplasm and plump, round, or irregular nuclei) closely spaced in sheet and trabecular patterns. Relatively high incidence of mitoses, often with 3–15 mitoses per high-power field. Difficult to distinguish histologically from other poorly differentiated small-cell tumors; therefore, confirmation by immunocytochemistry (juxtanuclear labeling with antibodies to cytokeratins 8, 18, 19, and 20, and cytoplasmic positivity for neuron-specific enolase) and electron microscopy are mandatory.

PD: Infiltration of epidermis by variable numbers of large cells with abundant pale-staining or sometimes eosinophilic cytoplasm containing large vesicular nuclei. Mitotic figures may occasionally be identified. The cells are usually scattered throughout all layers of the epidermis and are present singly or in clusters. Immunocytochemistry: Paget's cells are variably positive for expression of calmodulin 5.2, epithelial membrane antigen, carcinoembryonic antigen, and gross cystic disease proteins; S-100 protein–negative.

Complications

• Metastases.

Differential diagnosis

DFSP: Keloid, dermatofibroma, malignant fibrous histiocytoma, sclerosing basal-cell carcinoma, localized scleroderma.

MCC: Squamous-cell carcinoma, basal-cell carcinoma, pyogenic granuloma, keratoacanthoma, amelanotic malignant melanoma, adnexal tumors, lymphoma, cutaneous metastases of oat-cell carcinoma, leukemia cutis.

PD: Bowen's disease, dermatophytosis, psoriasis, eczema, seborrhea.

Etiology

DFSP: May arise after skin trauma or in scars. **MCC** is associated with other actinically related skin cancers.
PD: In 10% of cases, is a direct extension to the epidermis from underlying adenocarcinoma of the gastrointestinal or urogenital tract.

Epidemiology

DFSP: Accounts for fewer than 0.1% of all malignancies, and about 1% of soft-tissue sarcomas. Presents in the third and fourth decades, slight male predominance.
MCC: More than 600 reported cases, typically in white patients older than 65.
PD: Rare. More frequent in women than in men. Usually starts in the fifth decade or later.

Clinical staging

DFSP: Classic—classic morphologic features; fibrosarcomatous—high-grade fibrosarcomatous change in at least 5% of the lesion.

MCC: Stage 1 (localized disease) —confined to site of primary lesion at time of initial presentation; stage 2 (regional disease) —spread to the primary draining lymph nodes of the primary tumor; stage 3 (systemic disease) —metastases, usually to distant lymph nodes.

Paul Friedman and Roy Geronemus

Treatment

Nonpharmacological treatment

DFSP: Wide local excision with a 3-cm or greater margin down to and including fascia, or Mohs microscopic surgery (permits detection of microscopic tumor elements while maximally conserving normal tissue). No evidence supports prophylactic lymph node dissection. Few data support the value of radiation therapy.

MCC: Wide local excision with 2.5- to 3-cm margins. Mohs microscopic surgery compares favorably to wide excision. Sentinel lymph node lymphoscintigraphy may be useful. Excision of primary tumor followed by therapeutic lymph node dissection, if nodes are involved. Postoperative radiation therapy to the surgical bed and draining lymph nodes has improved local control. Chemotherapy may be administered in patients with regional disease and is the mainstay of stage III disease. Adjuvant chemotherapy regimen most commonly used is cyclophosphamide, doxorubicin, and vincristine. Cisplatin-containing regimens have also been recommended.

PD: If PD is not an extension of an internal adenocarcinoma, wide surgical excision with careful margin control to ensure complete excision, accomplished by intraoperative vertical frozen or vertical paraffin sections of selected margins. PD almost always extends beyond the clinically visibly involved margins, and Mohs micrographic surgery has provided accurate frozen-section margin control with maximal tissue sparing. Lymph node dissections are not indicated unless there is dermal invasion by PD or related lymphadenopathy.

Special therapeutic considerations

DFSP may enlarge more rapidly during pregnancy.

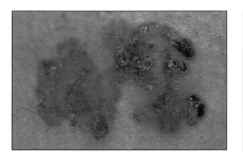

Well-demarcated, dull-red, scaly, serpiginous patch with focal hyperkeratosis, tiny vesicles, crusted erosions; on histopathology, extramammary Paget's disease.

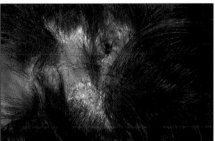

Recurrent nodule lesion of dermatofibrosarcoma protuberans on the scalp.

Treatment aims

Prompt surgical treatment, with tumor-free margins.

Prognosis

DFSP: Natural history: local recurrences 30% within 3 years. Metastases in fewer than 4% of cases, usually in recurrent tumors or the FS-DFSP variant. **MCC**: Local recurrence tends to occur within 1 year of excision in about one-third of patients. Regional lymph node metastases occur in 65% of patients; most of these are palpable at initial presentation. Distant metastases occur in more than one-third of cases, most frequently to liver, bone, brain, lung, and skin. Overall 5-year survival rate ranges from 30% to 64%. **PD**: Local recurrence rates as high as 31%–61% have been reported. It may eventually become invasive and culminate in fatal metastatic adenocarcinoma. Locally aggressive, lymph-node or distant metastases may occur.

Follow-up and management

DFSP: Every 3–6 months during the first 3 years after surgery and then annually (recurrences can develop after several years). Fibrosarcomatous tumors need more aggressive follow-up. **MCC**: Monthly for the first 6 months, every third month for the next 2 years, then biannually. **PD**: Long-term follow-up needed because recurrences may occur up to 11 years after resection.

General references

Coldiron BM, Goldsmith BA, Robinson JK: Surgical treatment of extramammary Paget's disease. *Cancer* 1991, **67**:933–938.

Ratner D, *et al.*: Mohs micrographic surgery for the treatment of dermatofibrosarcoma protuberans. *J Am Acad Dermatol* 1997, **37**:600–613.

Gloster HM Jr: Dermatofibrosarcoma protuberans. *J Am Acad Dermatol* 1996, **35**:355–374.

O'Connor WJ, Brodland DG: Merkel cell carcinoma. *Dermatol Surg* 1996, **22**:262–267.

Diagnosis

Signs

Necrobiosis lipoidica diabeticorum (NLD): Typically, irregularly bordered, pink plaque; gradually enlarges, becoming yellow-brown, atrophic, often with visible telangiectasias. Lesions may have decreased or absent sensation to pinprick and light touch. In 85%, distribution is pretibial or medial malleolar (often bilateral); less often, arms, trunk, face. Usually asymptomatic. **Diabetic dermopathy (DD)**: Asymptomatic, multiple, circumscribed, atrophic pigmented patches over anterior, lower portions of legs. **Diabetic bullae (DB)**: Usually asymptomatic, spontaneous tense blisters on dorsa, lateral aspects of hands, feet, lower legs, arms. Often bilateral. **Limited joint mobility (LJM)** and **waxy skin condition (Rosenbloom's syndrome; RS)**: Tight, thickened, waxy skin over dorsa of hands; limited mobility in small joints. May affect feet. Not painful, but eventual functional limitation of joint movement. **Sclerodema diabeticorum (SD)**: Diffusely indurated, nonpitting skin over posterior, lateral neck, upper back; less often, trunk, arms, legs. Sharply or poorly delineated from surrounding normal skin. Sensation to light touch may be diminished. May be associated with limitation of function.

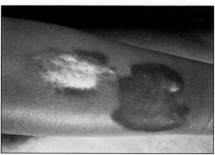

Well-demarcated, atrophic, waxy, yellow-tan patches with hyperpigmented borders in a man with necrobiosis lipoidica diabeticorum.

Investigations

NLD: Generally clinical diagnosis. Biopsy: degenerated collagen in deep dermis, palisading histiocytes, granulomatous vasculitis. Approach leg biopsy cautiously. **DD**: Clinical diagnosis. **DB**: Diagnosis usually clinical. Biopsy: intradermal, subepidermal separation. Direct immunofluorescence test usually negative. **RS**: "Prayer sign" to elicit inability to extend fingers fully and approximate palmar aspects of fingers; inability to flatten hand on level surface. **SD**: Biopsy: thickened collagen bundles, glycosaminoglycan deposition.

Complications

NLD: Up to one third of lesions ulcerate, often from trauma. **DB**: Rarely secondary infection. Associated with microangiopathy. **RS**: ankle LJM may be important in abnormal mechanics of foot, predisposing to injury, ulceration. RS harbinger of retinopathy, other microvascular disorders. **DD**: Associated with retinopathy, nephropathy. **SD**: No associated complications.

Special considerations

Bacterial infections: If diabetes is poorly controlled, immune dysfunction, increased risk for bacterial, systemic fungal infections. Malignant external otitis, caused by *Pseudomonas* in older diabetes patients. Foot fungal infections may function as portals for secondary bacterial infection. Candidal vulvovaginitis, balanitis, paronychia, intertrigo, and oral candidiasis are seen with increased frequency. **Other signs**: Rubeosis facei, pebbling of knuckles, yellow skin. Precise relationship of generalized granuloma annulare (GA) to diabetes is unknown. Acquired perforating disease is associated with DM and renal disease; related to transepidermal extrusion of altered collagen and elastic fibers. Seen in approximately 10% of diabetics on hemodialysis. DM is most common cause of acquired hypertriglyceridemia, which may cause eruptive xanthomas. Acanthosis nigricans: marker of insulin resistance and increased risk for DM. Vitiligo associated with both IDDM and NIDDM at higher-than-expected rates.

Differential Diagnosis

NLD: Granuloma annulare, primarily. **DB**: Bullous diseases, porphyria cutanea tarda, bullous drug or vesicular insect bite reaction. **RS**: Scleroderma, but Raynaud's phenomenon, calcinosis, ulceration, sclerodactyly, systemic involvement absent. **SD**: Scleroderma adultorum of Buschke, which occurs in children following an acute, often streptococcal, infection.

Etiology

Cutaneous manifestations of diabetes mellitus (DM), both insulin-dependent, type 1 (IDDM) and noninsulin-dependent, type 2 (NIDDM) are numerous; may reflect deregulation of glucose, metabolism disorders of collagen and lipid metabolism, immune dysfunction, complications of insulin use and oral hypoglycemic agents, and long-term degenerative changes. Many findings lack easily explainable etiology. **NLD**: Unknown. Proposed: immune-complex–mediated vasculitis, platelet aggregation, microangiopathy. **DD, DB**: Unknown. **SD**: Abnormal deposition of proteoglycans. **RS**: Nonenzymatic glycosylation (NEG) of connective tissue, leading to advanced glycosylation end products (ACE).

Epidemiology

NLD: Females:male predilection (4:1 ratio); often young adults. Insulin-dependent affected at a younger age. Relatively rare; approximately 0.7% of diabetes patients. Approximately two thirds of NLD patients have diabetes; other third will develop abnormal glucose tolerance within 5 years or have at least one first-degree relative with diabetes. Only 1 NLD case in 10 will have no association with diabetes. **DD**: Male:female predilection (2:1 ratio). Most common cutaneous DM manifestation. Affects approximately one third of patients with both IDDM and NIDDM. **DB**: Rare. Only in diabetics, particularly insulin-dependent patients. **RS**: Affects patients with both type 1 and, less commonly, type 2 DM. **SD**: Obese, middle-aged men, usually insulin-requiring with evidence of microangiopathy.

Katherine L. White and J.E. Jelinek

Treatment

Diet and lifestyle

All: Meticulous skin care (twice daily washing with soap, water; careful drying of feet) and properly fitted footwear, especially if neuropathy, which greatly increases risk of injury leading to ulceration and sequelae, including amputation. Daily patient foot inspection; dermatologist foot inspection, every visit. **NLD**: Conservative treatment for nonulcerated lesions. Protection from injury. **DD**: No treatment necessary. **DB**: Prevention of secondary infection. **RS**: Tight glycemic control. **SD**: No effective treatment. High-potency topical corticosteroids proposed.

Pharmacological treatment

Topical

NLD: Topical corticosteroids (with or without occlusion) or intralesional corticosteroids (3–5 mg/mL triancinolone acetonide) in symptomatic cases; avoid atrophy, ulceration. **SD**: High potency topical corticosteroids.

Systemic

NLD: Aspirin, alone or with dipyridamole, (200 mg, b.i.d.), may inhibit platelet aggregation. Pentoxifylline, 400 mg, p.o., t.i.d., decreases blood viscosity, enhances erythrocyte cell flexibility, perhaps improving microcirculation. Improvement may take 6 months. Nicotinamide: 1.5 mg, b.i.d. Clofazimine, 200 mg, p.o., daily. Prednisone, 1 mg/kg/d for a week, followed by 40 mg daily for 4–6 weeks (not beneficial in ulcerated lesions). Cyclosporine, 3–5 mg/kg/d. Low-dose methotrexate, electron beam therapy: Results largely disappointing; analyze risk:benefit ratio. **SD**: No effective treatment. High potency topical corticosteroids may help; monitor closely for epidermal atrophy.

Nonpharmacological treatment

• Split-thickness skin grafts may be necessary for ulcers that fail to respond to treatment. Psoralen plus ultraviolet-A light photochemotherapy (PUVA). Ulcerated lesions may require treatment with systemic or topical antibiotics and active management with dressings and protective padding.

Special therapeutic considerations

• As many as 20% of NLD lesions resolve spontaneously. Multispecialty, multidisciplinary approach to diabetes care ideal.

Treatment aims

Glycemic control important treatment goal; may improve or reverse some cutaneous complications (*eg*, xanthomas, bullae, thickened skin).

Follow-up and management

Ongoing patient education, support essential.

Prognosis

NLD, DD, SD: Chronic.
DB lesions usually heal without scarring in several weeks; may recur.
RS may be marker for microangiopathic complications of DM, including retinopathy, nephropathy.

General references

Jelinek, JE: The skin in diabetes. *Diabet Med* 1993, 10:201–213.

Diabetes Control and Complications Trial Research Group: The effect of intensive treatment of diabetes on the development and progression of long-term complications in insulin-dependent diabetes mellitus. *N Engl J Med* 1993, 329:977–986.

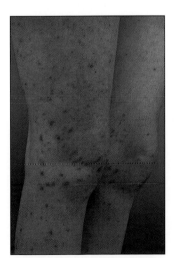

Atrophic, well-circumscribed, hyperpigmented macules characterisitc of diabetic dermopathy.

Diaper dermatitis

Diagnosis

Signs

• This irritant dermatitis is characterized by erythematous patches on convex surfaces of diaper area with sparing of the skin creases. Patches or papules may exhibit punctate erosions, but there are no scales or pustules. With superinfection of *Candida albicans* (*Candida* diaper dermatitis), vivid red erythematous patches and plaques with scaly borders are present and satellite papulopustules crop up at the edges of the eruption. The skin is macerated, and the skin creases are not spared.

Symptoms

• Inflammation of the skin of the lower aspect of the abdomen, genitalia, buttocks, and upper thighs with pain and discomfort during changes.

Investigations

• Skin scrapings for potassium hydroxide examination to rule out *Candida* or dermatophyte infection

• Cultures to rule out yeast or bacterial infection

• Skin biopsy recommended in cases recalcitrant to treatment to exclude other skin diseases

• Zinc serum levels in persistent cases to rule out acrodermatitis enteropathica

Complications

• Secondary bacterial or fungal superinfection, most often with *C. albicans*.

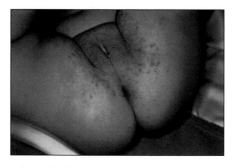

Infant with diaper dermatitis and satellite papullopustules, characteristic of *Candida* superinfection.

Differential diagnosis

Allergic contact dermatitis, atopic dermatitis, psoriasis, congenital syphilis, seborrheic dermatitis, cutaneous candidiasis, dermatophyte infection, Langerhans cell histiocytosis, acrodermatitis enteropathica, perianal streptococcal disease, bullous impetigo, staphylococcal scalded skin syndrome, child abuse.

Etiology

The cause of irritant diaper dermatitis is probably multifactorial. Principle causative factors include: excessive hydration of the skin; chafing and frictional injury to the skin; compromised skin barrier properties and maceration; secondary infection by *C. albicans*; permeation of irritants (ammonia, fecal enzymes, cleansing products, fragrances, and other chemicals) through the compromised skin.

Epidemiology

Most babies develop this dermatitis during their time in diapers.

At any given time, it is estimated that one-third of infants will have diaper dermatitis.

Highest prevalence seen in children aged 6–12 months.

Although most often seen in babies, diaper dermatitis may occur in any person in diapers, such as incontinent children or adults.

Sara L. Tarsis and Seth J. Orlow

Treatment

Diet and lifestyle

- Remove wet diapers and expose skin to air; keep skin cool and dry.
- Change diapers frequently, at least every 3–4 hours.
- Cleanse with mineral oil on a cotton ball, or water and mild soap, after each diaper change.
- Dry the skin thoroughly after cleansing.
- In some children, a change of diet (*e.g.*, addition of high-fiber foods) may lead to firmer stools, which may decrease irritation.
- A change in gastrointestinal flora by dietary supplementation with yogurt that contains live cultures may be beneficial.
- Change in type of diaper being used, such as from cloth to disposable or from one disposable brand to another, may be helpful. Diapers with absorbent gel lining are associated with a lower incidence of diaper dermatitis.
- Avoid occlusive diaper covers, such as rubber or plastic pants.

Pharmacological treatment

Topical

- Application of barrier ointments or pastes containing zinc oxide or petrolatum is essential for treatment and prevention of irritant diaper dermatitis. These include Triple paste (11.5% zinc oxide and aluminum acetate), Desitin (40% zinc oxide , vitamin A, vitamin D, lanolin, talc), Dr. Smith's Diaper Ointment (10% zinc oxide, thymol, petrolatum, mineral oil), and zinc oxide paste (25% zinc oxide, corn starch).
- Rarely, low-potency topical corticosteroids, such as a class VI or VII corticosteroid cream or ointment, may be necessary to treat moderate inflammation. A few applications of 1% hydrocortisone acetate cream is usually sufficient.
- Topical antifungal for treatment of *Candida* or dermatophyte infection. Usually a triazole antifungal (ketoconazole, econazole, oxiconazole, miconazole, clotrimazole) cream is prescribed. However, nystatin, ciclopirox, and terbinafine are also effective against *Candida* infections. Nystatin, 100,000 U/mg, can be mixed in a vehicle containing zinc oxide.
- Mupiricin cream (for bacterial superinfection).

Systemic

- Systemic antibiotics are rarely necessary to treat secondary bacterial infection.

Treatment aims

To decrease inflammation, prevent secondary infection, and educate parents or caregivers to control the condition and limit inciting events.

Prognosis

Usually self-limiting; most cases resolve within 3 days.

Can usually be controlled and prevented with appropriate measures and treatment.

Recalcitrant cases require consideration of alternative diagnoses

General references

Boiko S: Treatment of diaper dermatitis. *Dermatol Clin* 1999, **17**:235–240.

Berg RW: Etiology and pathophysiology of diaper dermatitis. *Adv Derm* 1988, **3**:75–79.

Sires UI, Mallory SB: Diaper dermatitis: how to treat and prevent. *Postgrad Med* 1995, **98**:79–86.

Diagnosis

Signs

Skin Lesions: Macular or papular, urticarial, vesicular and bullous, purpuric macules or papules, bright "drug" red (morbilliform/exanthematous eruptions), dusky red or violaceous (fixed drug eruption; 16% of cases).

Morphology: Morbilliform/exanthematous reactions (39%); urticaria or angioedema (27%); erythema multiforme (5%); fixed drug eruptions (16%).

Other presentations: Photosensitivity eruptions; toxic epidermal necrolysis; acute exanthemous pustulosis; erythema nodosum; drug-induced pemphigus and pemphigoid; dilantin hypersensitivity reaction; coumarin necrosis of the skin; acneform; vasculitis; lichenoid.

Distribution: Varies with morphology.

Symptoms

General: Pruritus, mild to severe, or absent. Pain at sites of erosions,bullae

Severe cutaneous drug eruptions: Fever, chills, lymphadenopathy, arthralgias, shortness of breath, wheezing.

Investigations

• Careful history is essential.

• Skin biopsy may reveal findings characteristic of one of the common morphologic patterns; however, this is rarely useful in identifying a causative agent.

Diagnostic algorithm

• The following elements are the key to determining the probability that a suspected drug is playing a role in a cutaneous eruption:

• Timing of events. Most adverse cutaneous drug reactions occur within 1–2 weeks of initiating treatment with the offending agent. Exceptions: hypersensitivity syndrome (up to 2 months after initiation), fixed drug eruptions.

• Previous experience with the drug. Refer to established relative reaction rates and morphologic patterns.

• Alternative etiologic candidates. Past medical history/investigation may reveal a preexisting disease.

• Dechallenge. Removal of suspected agent that results in resolution of the cutaneous eruption.

• Rechallenge. Perhaps the most definitive evidence on whether or not a drug is causing an adverse cutaneous reaction. However, one must exhibit caution in rechallenging with a suspected agent, to insure the safety of the patient.

Laboratory findings

• No laboratory tests are currently available to establish a diagnosis of a cutaneous drug reaction. Eosinophilia may be a helpful finding in a subset of patients, but is not a common finding. In serious cutaneous drug eruptions, eosinophil levels exceed 1000/*mu*L. Lymphocytosis with atypical lymphocytes: Abnormal liver function tests.

Complications

• Liver, renal and hematologic abnormalities

Differential diagnosis

Erythroderma (psoriasis, cutaneous T-cell lymphoma, pityriasis rubra pilaris, atopic dermatitis), viral exanthems, urticaria, staphylococcal scalded skin syndrome, scarlet fever, allergic contact dermatitis, erythema multiforme related to herpes simplex virus infection, bullous diseases.

Etiology

Hypersensitivity mechanisms (I–IV) are commonest. Photosensitivity (combination of a drug with ultraviolet radiation). Individually idiosyncratic reaction to either a topical or systemic drug. Irritant dermatitis from a topical agent. Accumulation of a systemic drug.

Epidemiology

Can occur at any age. More common in females.

Lesley Clark-Loeser and Ken Washenik

Treatment

Pharmacological treatment

Topical

- Soaks and warm baths with oiled colloidal oatmeal.
- Bland emollients
- Corticosteroid ointments or creams used twice or three times daily.

Systemic

- Start prednisone at 40–60mg/day for adults and 1–2mg/kg/day for children. Treat with prednisone using 10-day taper regimen. However, the efficacy of systemic corticosteroids for severe reactions such as Stevens-Johnson syndrome and toxic epidermal necrolysis has not been scientifically proven. Infection must be ruled out before treating patient with steroids.
- Antihistamines are sometimes helpful for pruritus (hydroxyzine 25–50 mg three or four times daily)

Special considerations

- If cutaneous eruption does not resolve as expected, consider another diagnosis or offending agent. In patients with underlying renal or hepatic insufficiency, drug clearance may be impaired, thereby delaying improvement.

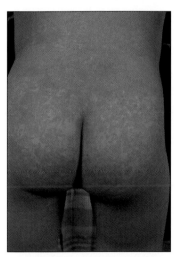

Phenobarbital was the cause of this generalized erythematous eruption.

General references

Litt JZ, Pawlak WA Jr.: *Drug Eruption Reference Manual.* Park Ridge, NJ, Parthenon; 1999.

Stern RS, Wintroub BU: Cutaneous reactions to drugs. In: Fitzpatrick's Dermatology in General Medicine, *edn. 5.* Edited by Freedberg IM, New York: McGraw Hill; 1999:1633–1642.

Diagnosis

Signs

Atopic dermatitis, acute: Poorly defined erythematous, edematous patches, papules, and plaques. Scale, vesiculation, erosions and crusting may be present. **Atopic dermatitis, chronic**: Lichenified, scaly papules and plaques on flexural surfaces (eyelids, neck, wrists, dorsal hands and feet); may be generalized. Dark-skinned patients may have perifollicular accentuation ("follicular eczema"). Infantile disease initially affects scalp, face (with perioral sparing), extensor aspects of extremities; by age 2, flexural surfaces affected; by age 5, facial involvement decreased. Associated findings: ichthyosis vulgaris, palmar hyperlinearity, and, in 10% of patients, keratosis pilaris. **Nummular dermatitis**: "Coin-shaped" or annular, erythematous, scaly papules, patches or plaques, most often on trunk, extensor extremities, particularly lower. Vesiculation, crusting, excoriations possible. **Acute dyshidrotic dermatitis (pompholyx)**: Small (<1.0 mm), deep-seated, "tapioca-like" vesicles; less often, bullae on volar and lateral aspects of fingers, hands, toes, feet (bilateral hand involvement in 80% of cases). **Chronic dyshidrotic dermatitis**: Hyperkeratotic plaques with coalescent vesicles. Crusting, tender fissures, excoriations possible. **Asteatotic dermatitis (eczema craquelé)**: Diffuse, erythematous, mildly scaling patches with fissures, usually on legs, forearms, dorsa of hands. Often superimposed on background xerosis.
Autoeczematization dermatitis (id reaction): Deep-seated, <1.0 mm) "tapioca-like" vesicles (may progress to lichenified); scaly papules, plaques, on forearms, legs, trunk, face, hands, neck, feet (descending order of frequency); may be generalized. Contact dermatitis: See chapter on Allergic contact dermatitis and irritant contact dermatitis.

Symptoms

• Pruritus, fissuring with pain, dryness, scaling.

Investigations

Skin biopsy. Histopathology may not be pathognomonic. Long-standing eczematous dermatitis: biopsy to rule out cutaneous T-cell lymphoma. Recalcitrant eczematous dermatitis: bacterial culture of skin and nares to rule out *Staphylococcus aureus* infection, carriage. **Other**: viral culture; radioallergosorbent test; serum IgE level; fungal smears, culture; provocative pressure test for white or red dermographism.

Complications

All: Lichen simplex chronicus; postinflammatory hypopigmentation or hyperpigmentation; impetiginization. **Atopic dermatitis**: Exfoliative erythroderma; eczema herpeticum (Kaposi's varicelliform eruption) due to herpes simplex virus (life-threatening); keratoconus; bilateral anterior, posterior subcapsular cataracts (up to 20% of severe atopic dermatitis cases); periorbital hyperpigmentation ("allergic shiners"); Dennie-Morgan fold (single or double; lower eyelid); lateral eyebrow thinning (Hertoghe's sign); widespread verrucae, molluscum contagiosum, dermatophytosis. Atopic dermatitis with immunodeficiency disorders, metabolic disorders, genodermatoses. **Dyshidrotic dermatitis**: Dystrophic nail changes (*eg*, irregular transverse ridging, pitting, thickening, discoloration).

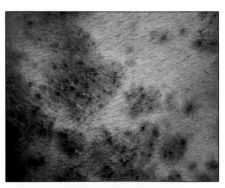

Pruritic, excoriated, coined-shaped, dull-red, plaques, fine scales in collarettes, typical of nummular eczema.

Differential diagnosis

Suspect contact dermatitis in any eczematous dermatitis case. Consider cutaneous T-cell lymphoma and papulosquamous disorders, such as psoriasis, drug eruptions, pityriasis rosea, and tinea. Dyshidrotic dermatitis can resemble palmoplantar pustulosis, pustular bacterid, acrodermatitis continua, bullous tinea pedis, and scabies.

Etiology

Atopic dermatitis: Multifactorial T lymphocyte-mediated response; may involve humoral immunity. Other etiologic factors: genetic predisposition and environmental triggers. Contact allergens, foods, inhalants, frequent bathing and soap use, cold temperature with low humidity, excessive perspiration, emotional stress, hormonal stress (*eg*, pregnancy, menses, thyroid disease), infection (*eg*, S. aureus, group A streptococci, dermatophytosis, candidiasis, herpes simplex virus), Wool clothing, blankets may exacerbate atopic dermatitis. **Nummular dermatitis**: No relation to atopic diathesis; associated with xerosis. **Dyshidrotic dermatitis**: Atopy and emotional stress are factors. **Asteatotic dermatitis**: Poor skin care and suboptimal ambient surroundings (high temperature, low humidity) causing xerosis and irritation. **Autoeczematization dermatitis**: Immunologic response to distant inflammatory dermatosis, usually inflammatory dermatophytosis or stasis dermatitis; less commonly, candidiasis, tuberculosis, bacterial infection.

Epidemiology

Atopic dermatitis: History of atopic diathesis (atopic dermatitis, allergic rhinitis, asthma) in 75%–80%; genetic component suggested. Occurs in 9%–18% of children, usually by age 12 (onset by age 1 year in 50%–60%, by age 5 in 20%–30%, by ages 6 – 20 in <10%). Prevalence increasing. **Nummular dermatitis**: Incidence peaks: young adults, elderly. **Dyshidrotic dermatitis**: Usually affects those aged 12–40. Men, women affected equally. **Asteatotic dermatitis**: Common in persons >60 years.

Treatment

Diet and lifestyle

•Dietary changes are effective in some infants, young children; effects in adults are inconclusive. Foods may exacerbate atopic dermatitis in 10% of children. Dietary management: food challenges, empiric and elimination diets (especially milk, peanuts, eggs, fish, soy, wheat). Nickel-free diet improves dyshidrosis, rarely.

Pharmacological treatment

Topical

Emollients may help; avoid sensitizing agents. **Topical corticosteroids** are mainstay of therapy; also ointments, creams, lotions, impregnated tapes, intralesional injections. **Occlusion** of high-potency corticosteroids with plastic wrap efficacious in recalcitrant eczematous dermatitis; limit to 2-week courses. Asteatotic dermatitis usually responds to medium- or low-potency topical corticosteroids. **Open wet compresses** with saline or aluminum acetate (Domeboro 1:40) for vesiculation, weeping. **Antibiotics (mupirocin)** for impetiginized lesions and to end staphylococcal carriage. **Topical antipruritics** with 0.05% menthol and 0.05% camphor (Sarna), 1% phenol (Schamberg's), or anesthetics (Prax, EMLA, ELA-Max) and crude coal tar (Doak or Neutrogena T-Derm lotions, Balnetar oil). Tacrolimus 0.3% ointment applied twice daily.

Systemic

Systemic antistaphylococcal antibiotics for impetiginized lesions. **Antihistamines** to reduce itching, inflammation. Soporific antihistamines, *eg*, hydroxyzine HCl (Atarax), chlorpheniramine (Chlor-Trimeton), promethazine (Phenergan), for greater pruritus relief; exercise caution for patients operating vehicles or potentially dangerous equipment; and the elderly. Nonsedating antihistamines, such as fexofenadine (Allegra), loratadine (Claritin), and cetirizine (Zyrtec), may increase patient compliance. **Oral corticosteroids** (prednisone, 1 mg/kg/d tapered over 10–14 days) for severe, recalcitrant eczematous dermatitis. Cyclosporine (Neoral), 3–5 mg/kg/d, divided into two doses, for severe, intractable eczematous dermatitis.

Nonpharmacological treatment

Bullae may be drained, but leave bulla roof intact. **Phototherapy** with conventional or narrow-band ultraviolet B or ultraviolet A (UVA) radiation, or photochemotherapy with psoralen plus UVA radiation (PUVA) for severe eczematous dermatitis. Topical PUVA may be useful for lesions on hands, feet. Grenz-ray radiation therapy for palmoplantar disease. **Teach patients** not to scratch, rub; take fewer, shorter showers to maintain skin hydration; minimize hand washing; use soap only in skin folds, nonsoap cleansers elsewhere; use room humidifiers to increase ambient humidity. **Patch test** for allergic contact dermatitis.

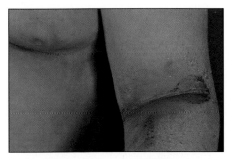

Erythematous, edematous, eroded plaque on child's anticubital fossa, atopic dermatitis.

Treatment aims

Ameliorate inflammation and pruritus; identify and eliminate triggers.

Special therapeutic considerations

Infants, young children, use low-potency topical corticosteroids to avoid hypothalamic-pituitary-adrenal axis suppression. When possible, use noncorticosteroid therapies, such as emollients and tacrolimus. Topical antihistamines may be sensitizing. For autoeczematization dermatitis. Treat inflammatory fungal infection or stasis dermatitis.

Prognosis

Atopic dermatitis: Characteristically presents in infancy. Spontaneous remission usual in childhood; may recur in adolescence. Adult-onset atopic dermatitis is more chronic. Predictors of poor prognosis: early onset; widespread disease in childhood; associated allergic rhinitis; asthma; family history of atopic dermatitis; female sex. Winter flares, summer improvement typical. **Nummular dermatitis, asteatotic dermatitis:** Chronic; often occurs in fall, winter. **Dyshidrotic dermatitis:** Recurrent outbreaks usually for several weeks; may become chronic. More prevalent during hot, humid weather. **Autoeczematization dermatitis:** Resolves with treatment of precipitating condition.

Support organizations

National Eczema Association for Science and Education, 1220 SW Morrison, Suite 433, Portland, OR 97205; tel: 503-228-4430 or 800-818-7546; fax: 503-224-3363; Internet: http://www.eczema-assn.org.

General references

Sidbury R, Hanifin JM: Old, new, and emerging therapies for atopic dermatitis. *Dermatol Clin* 2000, **18**:1–11.

Diagnosis

Signs

Linear verrucous epidermal nevus (LVEN): Skin-colored or brown hyperkeratotic or papillomatous, usually linear plaque(s). May be localized or diffuse: systematized epidermal nevus (lesions generalized throughout body); nevus unius lateris (extensive but limited to half the body); ichthyosis hystrix (lesions extensive, bilateral). Intertriginous areas, nevi may become macerated, malodorous. **Inflammatory linear epidermal nevus (ILVEN)**: Discrete, eythematous, small scaly papules; coalesce into often verrucous linear plaque(s) along Blaschko's lines, usually on left side of body. Lichenification, excoriations, hyperpigmentation possible. Lower extremities most commonly affected; lesions may occur anywhere, specially on buttocks, genitalia, groin. **Nevus sebaceous (NS)**: Well-demarcated, often linear, orange-yellow patch with alopecia during childhood, becomes raised, nodular in adolescence. Usually, single lesion at birth, most common on scalp; less common on face, neck; rarely widespread. **Nevus comedonicus (NC)**: Closely aggregated erythematous papules, central keratotic plugs, usually on face, neck, chest, arm. **Eccrine nevus (EN)**: Skin-colored papules, plaques (may be linear) or discrete, depressed brownish patches, usually on lower extremity. Rare; may be associated with central pore and mucous exudate or localized hyperhidrosis. Eccrine angiomatous hamartoma variant: tan to violaceous solitary plaques, nodules. **Apocrine nevus (AN)**: Solitary or multiple nodule(s) or firm papules on scalp or chest; or soft mass in axillae. **Becker's nevus (BN)**: Large (up to 20 cm), well-demarcated, tan to brown patches with hair, usually on shoulder, chest, scapula; less common on extremities, face. **White sponge nevus (WSN)**: Diffuse white corrugated plaques, usually in oral mucosa.

Symptoms

ILVEN: Usually mildly to moderately (rarely, severely) pruritic. **Other epidermal lesions:** Usually asymptomatic; may be considered disfiguring by patients.

Investigations

• Diagnosis is confirmed with a skin specimen obtained by punch biopsy.

LVEN: Acanthotic epidermis with papillomatosis, hyperkeratosis. Some (especially associated with epidermal nevus syndrome) demonstrate epidermolytic hyperkeratosis (degeneration of granular layer, resulting in vacuolization of granular and upper spinous layers and clumping of keratohyaline granules). **ILVEN**: Moderate psoriasis-like epidermal hyperplasia with slight papillomatosis. Foci of parakeratosis above papillomatous areas, associated with loss of granular layer, which alternate with foci of orthokeratosis, preserved granular layer. **NS**: Papillated epidermal hyperplasia with increased number of normal and abnormal sebaceous lobules and ectopic apocrine glands in dermis. In children, glands are small and poorly developed. **NC**: Large invaginations of the epidermis (occasionally with hair shafts and sebaceous glands) filled with keratin plugs. **EN**: Increased size and numbers of eccrine coils and occasionally eccrine ducts. **AN**: Clustering of mature apocrine glands in dermis and subcutaneous tissue. **BN**: Regular epidermal hyperplasia with basal layer hyperpigmentation with or without increased number of melanocytes, and haphazardly arranged smooth muscle bundles in dermis.

Complications

Epidermal nevus syndrome: Extensive epidermal nevi, generally present at birth; central nervous system involvement (mental retardation, seizures, cranial nerve palsies, hemiparesis, hydrocephalus) skeletal (kyphosis, scoliosis, bone cysts, spina bifida), ocular (muscle dysfunction, nystagmus, colobomas of iris, blindness), cardiovascular (cerebrovascular accidents, vascular malformations), cutaneous (hemangiomas, dermatomegaly, café-au-lait spots, and other pigmentary abnormalities). Mental retardation, seizures, cranial nerve palsies common findings at presentation. Associated malignancies: Wilms' tumor, nephroblastoma, astrocytoma, ameloblastoma, adenocarcinomas. **NS syndrome**: Same abnormalities, associated with linear midline nevus sebaceous. Syringocystadenoma papillilleferum, basal cell carcinoma (BCC) (in about 10%) arise within NS. BCC squamous cell carcinoma (SCC) rare in verrucous epidermal nevi.

Differential diagnosis

LVEN and **ILVEN**: Linear porokeratosis, linear psoriasis, lichen striatus, linear lichen planus, incontinentia pigmenti (verrucous stage), linear Darier's disease, lichen simplex chronicus.
NS: EN, xanthomas.
NC: Acne vulgaris.
BN: Congenital melanocytic nevus
WSN: Oral focal epithelial hyperplasia (discrete white papules), leukoedema (localized, not diffuse), pachyonychia congenita, dyskeratosis congenita.

Etiology

Epidermal nevi: Hemartomas derived from embryonic ectoderm . Possibly, mosaicism of certain lethal genes related to ectodermal development create the various phenotypes of epidermal nevi.

Epidemiology

Epidermal nevi: Occur in about 1:1000 live births, usually sporadically, rarely hereditary. Most are present at birth or within the first year of life and only rarely later in life.
ILVEN typically develops before 5 years of age and rarely in third or fourth decades. It is more common in females (4:1 predilection).

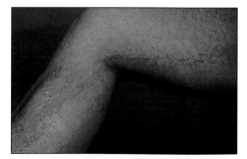

Well-demarcated, pink, linear streak with a finely hyperkeratotic, papillated surface, following Blashko's line from the medial leg to the thigh.

Marisa Baldassano and Hideko Kamino

Treatment

Pharmacological treatment

Topical

Corticosteroids: (class I or II, under occlusion or intralesionally injected) (LVEN, ILVEN); decreased pruritus, atrophy of lesion.

Trichloroacetic acid or phenol peels: (LVEN, ILVEN); destruction of surface

Calcipotriol .0005% ointment: (ILVEN) to relieve of pruritus and erythema.

5-fluorouracil, 5% cream: under occlusive dressing daily with or without tretinoin 1% cream (LVEN, ILVEN); offers improvement but recurrence after treatment cessation.

Systemic

Acitretin, 75 mg daily with reduction of dosage to 50 mg when lesions disappear (LVEN, ILVEN). Recurrence with discontinuation of treatment.

Surgery

Surgical excision (LVEN, ILVEN, NS, NC, EN, AN, BN), dermabrasion (LVEN, ILVEN), and laser (CO2) ablation (LVEN, ILVEN) can be successful but leave potentially disfiguring scars. Surgical excision is recommended for NS (usually around 9–11 years of age) due to risk of BCC.

Q-switched ruby laser is the treatment of choice for Becker's nevus.

585 nm flashlamp–pumped pulsed dye laser at an energy density of 6.5 J/cm2 treatment resulted in disappearance of pruritus and partial resolution of ILVEN.

Cryotherapy: Three to five sprays at 15 to 20 day intervals (ILVEN).

Special therapeutic considerations

• No treatment is indicated for WSN.

• Evaluate new nodules or significant change in EN for development of malignancy, specially in nevus sebaceous.

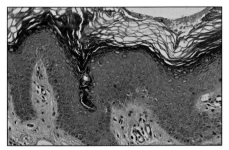

Histopathologic changes include hyperkeratosis, acanthosis, and papillomatosis.

Treatment aims

Removal of EN for cosmetic purposes and of NS to prevent malignant transformation; and to relieve pruritus in ILVEN. Pharmacological therapies attempt to alter the rate of epidermal proliferation and differentiation or to relieve pruritus, but only provide temporary or partial responses.

Prognosis

Most epidermal nevi expand and grow during childhood and stabilize in adulthood. Lesions can be difficult to remove completely, but the prognosis is excellent except for patients with EN syndrome or untreated malignancies.

Follow-up and management

Evaluate patient for signs of EN syndrome. Educate patients about risk for malignancy and evaluate any changes in nevi that develop.

Support groups

Epidermal Nevus Support Group, 19 Benton St., Middleboro, MA 02346; telephone: 508-946-1147; website: http://www.nevus.org; email: www.nevus.org.

National Organization for Rare Disorders, 100 Rt.37, PO Box 8923, New Fairfield, CT 06812; telephone: 203-746-6518; website: www.nord-rdb.com.

General references

Alster TS: Inflammatory linear verrucous epidermal nevus: successful treatment with the 585 nm flashlamp-pumped pulsed dye laser. *J Am Acad Dermatol* 1994, 31:513–514;1994

Happle R. How many epidermal nevus syndromes exist? A clinicogenetic classification. *J Am Acad Dermatol* 1991, 25:550–556.

Zvulunov A, Grunwald MH, Halvy S: Topical calcipotriol for treatment of inflammatory linear verrucous nevus. *Arch Dermatol* 1997, 133:567–568.

Nelson BR, Kolansky G, Gillard M *et al.*: Management of linear verrucous epidermal nevus with topical 5-fluorouracil and tretinoin. *J Am Acad Dematol* 1994, 30:287–288.

Diagnosis

Signs

Epidermolysis bullosa acquisita (EBA): Tense inflammatory or noninflammatory blisters, heal with scarring, milia; usually on acral areas prone to trauma. Often on oral mucosa; also, esophageal, vaginal, urethral, rectal mucosa. Many erosions possible. Scalp lesions result in alopecia; nail dystrophy possible.

Inherited variants

Epidermolysis bullosa simplex (EBS): Most common variant; usually on hands, feet; delayed onset to late childhood, adolescence; hyperhidrosis common. **EBS (Downing-Meara)**: Acral (but may be generalized); herpetiform lesions; may heal with milia, atrophy but no scarring. Nail dystrophy, dental abnormalities possible. Improves with age, but palmoplantar hyperkeratosis prominent. **EBS (Koebner's)**: Generalized; acral, flexor areas prominent. Plantar hyperkeratosis, hyperhidrosis. Improves during adolescence, especially in girls. **EB (Ogna's)**: Generalized, with bruising, onychogryphosis. **EBS (Bart's)**: Congenital partial thickness absence of skin on extremities; heals with fine scarring. **EBS (Mendes da Costa)**: Blistering during first 2 years of life, nonscarring alopecia, reticulated pigmentation and atrophy on face, hands. **EBS (superficialis)**: Just below stratum corneum. **EBS (letalis)**: Generalized; heals with atrophy, milia. Often, death before 20 months. *Other EBS*: **Kallin**: Mottled hyperpigmentation. **Junctional epidermolysis bullosa (JEB) variants**: Gravis, atrophic benign, localized, cicatricial, inversa, progressiva. **Dystrophic epidermolysis bullosa (DEB) variants**: Cockayne-Touraine, minimus, pretibial, albopapuloidea (Pasini's), Hallopeau-Siemens, inversa, EBS transient bullous dermolysis of the newborn.

JEB and **DEB**: Present with tense blisters (often aggravated by trauma), crusted erosions, milia, scar formation, exuberant granulation tissue (Herlitz's). Postinflammatory pigment changes, scarring alopecia, dystrophy or loss of nails possible in variants. Depending on variant, lesions may be localized to acral or inverse regions or may be more generalized.

Symptoms

- Variable pain or pruritus.

Investigations

EBA: Histology: subepidermal blister, may resemble bullous pemphigoid. Direct immunofluorescence: linear bands of IgG, C3, possibly other immunoreactants at dermal-epidermal junction. Indirect immunofluorescence: antibodies binding to dermal side of salted split skin.

Variants: Histology: subepidermal blister. Transmission electron microscopy: level of skin cleavage:

EBS: Blistering at level of basal cells; mutations: keratin 5, 14. **Hemidesmosomal EB**: Blistering at level of basal cells, lamina lucida junction; mutations: *generalized atrophic benign EB*, BPAG2 (Col 17); *EB-pyloric atresia*, alpha6*beta*4; *EB-muscular dystrophy*, plectin. **JEB**: Blistering at level of lamina lucida; mutation, laminin. **DEB**: Blistering at level of sublamina densa; mutation, collagen 7.

Complications

EBA: Skin fragile; many erosions possible in areas of minor mechanical trauma. Scarring can result in alopecia, blindness, esophageal stenosis. **Variants**: Scarring complications may be similar to EBA, but some variants lethal, some have high rates of morbidity. Large areas of denudation can result in fluid imbalance, septicemia; oropharyngeal involvement can lead to airway compromise.

Differential diagnosis

EBA: Bullous systemic lupus erythematosus (SLE), bullous pemphigoid, herpes gestationis, cicatritial pemphigoid, linear IgA bullous dermatosis, bullous drug eruption, porphyria cutanea tarda and dermatitis herpetiformis.

Variants: Disseminated herpes simplex virus, neonatal varicella, disseminated candidiasis, epidermolytic hyperkeratosis, bullous impetigo, staphylococcal scalded skin syndrome, toxic epidermal necrolysis.

Etiology

EBA: Autoantibodies against noncollagenous domain of type VII collagen. Anchoring fibrils also decreased or absent.

Variants: Gene defect (see above).

Epidemiology

EBA: Occurs in fourth to sixth decade. Reported with inflammatory bowel disease, SLE; possible association with human leukocyte antigen-DR2; slightly higher incidence in black and female patients.

Variants: Depending on variant, presents at birth or within 1 year of birth.

Jeanie Chung-Leddon and M. Joyce Rico

Treatment

Diet and lifestyle

•Good nutrition vital; avoidance of trauma to skin imperative.

Pharmacological treatment

Topical

EBA: For mild oral mucosal lesions, potent topical corticosteroid ointments or gels (0.05 % clobetasol propionate ointment).

Systemic

•Systemic therapies not markedly effective in ameliorating fundamental bullous tendency in EB patients; tetracycline, phenytoin not generally used today. Antimalarial preparations, retinoids: usefulness not definitively established. Systemic glucocorticoids have not proven useful.

EBA:Prednisone (0.5 to 2 mg/kg/d): Severe mucosal or inflammatory cutaneous lesions may respond, recur on tapering or discontinuation. Noninflammatory lesions: addition of cyclosporine (above 6 mg/kg). Other immunosuppressants, plasma exchanges not consistently effective, but may be steroid-sparing. Mycophenolate mofetil and autologous keratinocyte grafting reported. Colchicine 0.6–1.5 mg/d effective in some cases. Dapsone disappointing. High-dose i.v. immune globulin (40 mg/kg for 5 days) may be effective and reduce required dose of corticostroids; must be continued indefinitely.

Variants: Corticosteroids for compromised airway. Skin lesions rarely responsive to any systemic treatment.

Nonpharmacological treatment

DEB: Finger splinting, appropriate hand protection against trauma, surgical release of fused digits followed by splinting.

JEB, **DEB**: Ophthalmologic evaluation, follow up.

General: Stool softeners. Management of chronic wounds. Protection from trauma to skin. Protective footwear. Heat avoidance. Biologic dressings, grafting with skin explants for chronic ulcers. Extracorporeal photochemotherapy (refractory EBA).

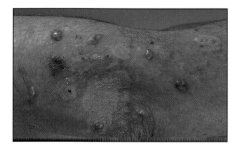

Serosanguinous tense bullae, which heal with scarring in the upper extremity of a patient with epidermolysis bullosa acquisita.

Treatment aims

EBA: To minimize blister and scar formation, particularly in ocular, oral mucosa.

Variants: To prevent new blister formation, enhance healing of erosions, provide relief of pain, prevent infection, and provide supportive care (nutritional support) to reduce morbidity, mortality.

JEB:Keratinocyte autografts in chronic hypertrophic granulation tissue.

Prognosis

Chronic disease; periods of partial remissions, exacerbations. Spontaneous resolution rare; in some, disease intensity may decrease with time.

Follow-up and management

Base follow-up, treatment adjustment on disease activity.

JEB: Observe lesions closely for squamous cell carcinomas, which can behave aggressively.

Support organizations

Dystrophic Epidermolysis Bullosa Reasearch Association of America, Inc., 40 Rector Street, Suite 140, New York, NY 10006. Telephone: (212) 513-4090; fax: (212) 513-4099.

General references

Fine J, Bauer EA, Briggaman RA, *et al*.: Revised clinical and laboratory criteria for subtypes of inherited epidermolysis bullosa. *J Am Acad Dermatol* 1991, **24**:119–135.

Rico MJ: Autoimmune blistering diseases in children. *Semin Dermatol* 1995, **14**:54–59.

Hall RP, Rico MJ, Murray JC: Autoimmune skin disease. In *Clinical Immunology*. Edited by Rich RR, Fleisher TA, Schwartz BD, *et al*. St. louis: Mosby; 1996:1316–1342.

Diagnosis

Signs

• Malaise, fever, myalgias; often precede skin, mucous membrane lesions by 1–3 days. "Prodromal" sore throat, cough, conjunctivitis: first manifestations in mucosal areas. **Erythema multiforme (EM)**: Self-limited. Symmetrically distributed, round, erythematous macules; evolve into edematous (even urticarial) papules. May enlarge, become confluent into plaques, which can have central bullae. Some become target or iris lesions; dusky (necrotic) centers, pale edematous ring, peripheral red margin. Infestations of lesions tend to erupt centripetally on extensor extremities, palms, then trunk, face. Bullous EM: is less than 10% epidermal detachment with typical or atypical target lesions. **Stevens-Johnson syndrome (SJ)**: Flat, atypical target lesions; scattered, erythematous, irregular macules; blisters possible. Epidermal detachment: about 10% of skin. Severe painful, erythematous erosions, often yellow pseudomembranes, crusting; usually oropharyngeal (especially labial); less often, anogenital. **Overlap SJ–toxic epidermal necrolysis (TEN)**: Epidermal detachment 10% to 30%; atypical target flat lesions, erythematous macules (usually with central bullae). **TEN**: Painful, burning, blotchy erythema.

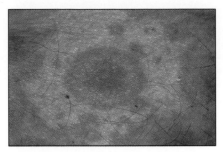

One of several early lesions of erythema multiforme showing discrete oval or circular, pink urticarial plaques, darker centers, thin, slightly raised, more edematous outer borders. With time the center may become purpuric, necrotic or vesiculate.

Spreads from face, trunk, to extremities; throughout body in 2–5 days, occasionally 24 hours. Should be more than 30% epidermal detachment (bullae) when atypical flat targets present. Nikolsky sign markedly positive. Chest, upper back, shoulders, are heavily involved.

Symptoms

• Pain and burning (especially on mucosal surfaces and areas with epidermal detachment), dysphagia, conjunctival burning, photophobia and visual impairment, leukopenia, high fever, excessive salivation, and painful micturation.

Investigations

EM: Superficial perivascular infiltrate of mononuclear cells, occasionally eosinophils (drug-induced cases, especially); edema of papillary dermis, vacuolar degeneration of epidermal junction, spongiosis, epidermal intracellular edema, subepidermal vesiculation, necrotic keratinocytes with eosinophilic cytoplasm (Civatte's bodies), which may be surrounded by mononuclear cells (satellite necrosis). **SJ, TEN**: Groups of necrotic keratinocytes (may involve entire epidermis except stratum corneum), satellite necrosis; exocytosis of mononuclear cells, neutrophils. Frozen sections for immediate diagnosis and to exclude TEN (Lyell's disease) from staphylococcal scalded skin syndrome (Ritter's disease); epidermal detachment subepidermal in former, subcorneal in latter.

Complications

Chronic: Morbidity high when mucosal surfaces affected. Ophthalmologic sequelae, in 30% to 50% with severe SJ or TEN, and can include keratitis siccae, conjunctival scarring, symblepharon, synechiae, blindness. Other chronic complications include deformed or missing nails, variegated skin pigmentation. **Acute**: Massive edema, electrolyte abnormalities, pneumonia, hepatitis, nephritis, anemia, septicemia (most common cause of death). Esophageal sloughing may cause gastrointestinal bleeding, strictures. Tracheobronchial erosions can lead to acute respiratory disease syndrome. **Mortality**: TEN, 25% to 30%; SJ, 5%.

Robert Auerbach and Miguel Sanchez

Treatment

Pharmacological treatment

Topical
•Biologic wound coverings, biosynthetic skin substitutes. Silver nitrate solution (0.5%)–impregnated dressings. Avoid silver sulfadiazine because of potential absorption.

Systemic
Systemic corticosteroids appear to increase mortality in TEN; possibly effective in EM, SJ, only if administered early and in high doses (prednisolone, 80–120 mg daily). If no improvement evident in 24–48 hours, discontinue. **Intravenous immune gammaglobulin**: 0.2–0.75 g/kg/d, 4 consecutive days; interrupts disease progression in 24–48 hours. **TEN**: Cyclosporine with granulocyte colony stimulating factor; cyclophosphamide reported beneficial. Antibiotic prophylaxis, only if increasing numbers of bacteria cultured from skin, single pathogenic bacterial strain cultured, hypothermia develops, or clinical condition deteriorates. **EM**: Thalidomide, levamisole, cyclosporine reported to help some cases.

Nonpharmacological treatment

•Plasmapheresis. Antacid prophylaxis, sedatives for anxiety; analgesics for pain; anticoagulants to prevent thromboembolism during recovery. Oral cleansing with antiseptic agents. Ophthalmic lubricants and antibiotic/antiseptic eye drops; ophthalmologist consultation and daily follow-up during acute eye disease. Prophylaxis with antiviral medications effective against herpes simplex for recurrent EM.

Special therapeutic considerations

SJ, **TEN**: Immediate hospitalization upon suspicion; TEN optimally treated in burn unit, intensive care unit. General: isolation to minimize infection; strict adherence to aseptic technique by health care personnel; aggressive control of fluid, electrolyte imbalance; volume replacement; nutritional support; prevention of wound superinfection; environmental temperature control; optimal wound care.

Treatment aims
To reduce morbidity, mortality and long-term complications.

Patient support
Stevens Johnson Syndrome Foundation, 9285 N. Utica Street, Westminster, CO 80030; 303-430-9559.

General references
Roujeau J-C, Chosidow O, Saiag P, et al.: Toxic epidermal necrolysis (Lyell syndrome). *J Am Acad Dermatol* 1990, **23**:1039–1058.

Rzany B, Correia O, Kelly JP, et al.: Risk of Stevens-Johnson syndrome and toxic epidermal necrolysis during first weeks of anti-epileptic therapy. *Lancet* 1999, **353**:2190–2194.

Kokuba H, Imafuku S, Huang S, et al.: Erythema multiforme lesions are associated with expression of a herpes simplex virus (HSV) gene and qualitative alterations in the HSV-specific T-cell response. *Br J Dermatol* 1998, **138**:952–964.

Toxic epidermal necrolysis with diffusely erythematous skin and sheet-like epidermal separation from underlying skin.

Robert Auerbach and Miguel Sanchez

Diagnosis

Signs

All panniculidities: Inflammation in subcutaneous tissue.

Erythema nodosum (EN): Multiple, erythematous, warm, tender, bilateral infiltrated plaques, nodules; acquire bluish-violaceous coloration; never ulcerate. Usually on anterior aspects of lower legs, but any area with subcutaneous fat; remain 2–4 weeks. Fever, malaise possible.

Erythema induratum (Bazin's disease; BD): Lesions similar; usually posterior aspect of lower extremities, particularly calves.

Idiopathic lobular panniculitis (Weber-Christian disease; WC): Erythematous, edematous, tender subcutaneous, usually 1–2 cm, usually on lower extremities; heal in weeks, leaving atrophic, hyperpigmented scars. Oily, yellow-brown exudate may drain from lesions. Fever (often high), malaise, arthralgias, myalgia, fatigue, nausea, abdominal pain, hepatomegaly, bone pain. Lungs, intestine, pericardium, kidneys, adrenal glands may be affected. Variants: Rothman-Makai syndrome (cutaneous lesions; no systemic manifestations): suppurative granulomatous eosinophilic panniculitis.

Histiocytic cytophagic panniculitis (HCP): Large violaceous, occasionally purpuric, subcutaneous nodules, infiltrated plaques; usually on upper, lower extremities, occasionally trunk, face. Spontaneous ulceration common. Fever, hepatosplenomegaly, weight loss, diffuse adenopathy usually prominent. Bone marrow involvement may lead to pancytopenia, lethal hemorrhages.

Investigations

All panniculitis (P): Histologic examination key to diagnosis. Inflammatory infiltrate may be septal or lobular, with or without vasculitis. Detailed history, including antecedent infection, medications, systemic diseases. Complete blood count (anemia, neutrophilic leukocytosis frequent), erythrocyte sedimentation rate, chest radiographs. Amylase, lipase levels (for pancreatic P) and alpha-1 antitrypsin level (to detect deficiency), direct immunofluorescence (for lupus P). Most important: Deep-tissue (at least 6 mm) skin biopsy with adequate amounts of fat. **EN**: Antistreptolysin titers, pharyngeal culture, purified protein derivative testing for tuberculosis, stool examination.

HCP: Bean-bag cells on biopsy.

Complications

EN: Localized pain, lower-extremity swelling. **WC**: Focal necrosis of liver, spleen, myocardium; adrenals, death. **HCP**: Pancytopenia, lethal hemorrhages.

Differential diagnosis

Histologic patterns may overlap.

Septal P, with no vasculitis: EN.

Septal P, with vasculitis: Superficial migratory thrombophlebitis; polyarteritis nodosa (PAN), cutaneous PAN.

Lobular P, with no vasculitis: WC, HCP, alpha-1-antitrypsin deficiency, physical P, P associated with systemic disease (including pancreatic disease [eg, pancreatitis and pancreatic carcinoma] and lupus erythematosus), sarcoidosis, calciphylaxis associated with renal failure and secondary hyperparathyroidism, lymphoma and leukemia.

Lobular P with vasculitis: Nodular vasculitis (may be associated with *Mycobacterium tuberculosis* infection) (BD).

Etiology

EN: Drugs; infections; inflammatory diseases; pregnancy; malignancy, particularly lymphoproliferative diseases; postradiation therapy. Approximately 50% of cases are idiopathic.

Epidemiology

EN: Any age, but peak incidence 20–30 years. Female-to-male ratio is 4:1. Age, gender distribution differ worldwide.

WC: Mostly in women 30–60 years of age.

Katherine L. White and J.E. Jelinek

Treatment

Diet and lifestyle

• Bedrest, cool compresses, leg elevation may provide relief.

Pharmacological treatment

Systemic

EN: Nonsteroidal antiinflammatory drugs (NSAIDs), including aspirin or indomethacin, 50 mg, orally, three times daily; despite high toxicity, may produce best results. Newer COX-2 inhibitors may be beneficial; studies lacking. Systemic corticosteroids for severe, disabling cases, if infectious etiologies excluded. Potassium iodide, 300–600 mg, daily, may be effective. Colchicine, 0.6 mg, three times daily, in refractory cases.

PAN, cutaneous PAN: Cutaneous lesions may spontaneously regress. Oral corticosteroids, antisuppressive agents, NSAIDs, colchicine.

WC: Systemic corticosteroids, NSAIDs in acute phases. Azothioprine, cyclosporine, cyclophosphamide, mycophenolate mofetil, thalidomide reported beneficial in some. Rothman-Makai syndrome: tetracycline.

α-1 antitrypsin deficiency-associated panniculitis: Dapsone, 25–200 mg, daily, alone or with prednisone; alpha-1 antitrypsin infusion can be added.

Lupus P: Intralesional corticosteroids controversial; lesions typically heal with atrophy. Antimalarial drugs routinely administered.

Nodular vasculitis: If associated with tuberculosis, full anti-tubercular therapy required. Otherwise, systemic steroids are mainstay. Potassium iodide is treatment of choice. Success reported with tetracycline, NSAIDs.

HCP: Prednisone with cyclophosphamide, chlorambucil, vincristine, adriamycin, busulfan; variable results. Addition of cyclosporine to courses of cyclophosphamide, doxorubicin, vincristine, and prednisolone (CHOP) reported beneficial. Anecdotal: high-dose chemotherapy with cyclophosphamide, doxorubicin, and vincristine on day 1, prednisolone on days 1–5, and etoposide on days 1, 3, and 5 (CHOP-E) followed by autologous peripheral blood stem cell transplantation (one case); corticosteroid pulse therapy plus oral cyclosporine.

Treatment aims

To provide symptomatic relief during acute episodes. To identify and address underlying etiology.

Prognosis

EN: Lesions usually resolve spontaneously, without scarring or atrophy, in three to six weeks.

WC: If systemic disease is prominent, prognosis is guarded. If predominantly cutaneous, permanent remission after years of recurrent exacerbations, remissions.

HCP: Death by hemorrhage common but spontaneous; therapeutically-induced remissions occur.

α-1 antitrypsin deficiency: Prognosis good with treatment, if no pulmonary or hepatic disease.

Follow-up and management

Successful management depends on identifying, treating underlying diseases, conditions.

General references

White WL, Wieselthier JS, Hitchcock MG: Panniculitis: recent developments and observations. *Semin Cutan Med Surg* 1996, **15**:278–299.

White WL, Hitchcock MG: Diagnosis: Erythema nodosum or not? *Semin Cutan Med Surg* 1999, **18**:47–55.

White JW Jr, Winkelman RK: Weber-Christian panniculitis: A review of 30 cases with this diagnosis. *J Am Acad Dermatol* 1998, **39**:56–62.

Craig AJ, Cualing H, Thomas G, *et al>*: Cytophagic histiocytic panniculitis—a syndrome associated with benign and malignant panniculitis: case comparison and review of the literature. *J Am Acad Dermatol* 1998, **39**:721–736.

Watanabe T, Tsuchida T: Lupus erythematosus profundus: A cutaneous marker for a distinct clinical subset? *Br J Dermatol* 1996, **134**:123.

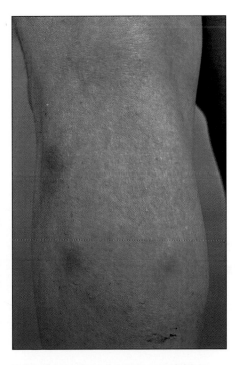

Tender nodular plaques with violaceous bluish color on the anterior shin due to erythema nodosum.

Bluish pink, tender, subcutaneous nodules on the calf area in a woman with nodular vasculitis. In contrast to lesions of erythema nodosum, these nodules, have a tendency to ulcerate.

Katherine L. White and J.E. Jelinek

Diagnosis

Definition

•Dark-skinned patients may develop various pigmentary conditions, including melasma, postinflammatory hyperpigmentation or hypopigmentation, hyperpigmentation of palmar creases, pigmentary demarcation lines (Voigt and Futcher's lines), lichen planus pigmentosus, familial periorbital melanosis, Mongolian spot, ochronosis, pigmented gums.

Asians: Predisposed to nevus of Ota (trigeminal), nevus of Ito (unilateral on distribution of posterior supraclavicular, lateral cutaneous brachial nerves), acquired bilateral nevus of Ota–like melanosis (bilateral on face), late-onset dermal melanosis (bilateral on upper back), prurigo pigmentosa.

Hispanics: More often develop actinic prurigo, erythema dyscrhomicum perstans.

Blacks: Commonly develop leukoedema, punctate palmar keratosis, alopecia due to traction or chemicals, inherited patterned lentiginosis.

Signs

Pseudofollliculitis barbae (PFB): Scattered inflammatory papules, pustules on beard area; moustache region usually spared.

Acne keloidalis nuchae (AKN): Follicular pustules become small (occasionally large) keloids in nuchal region; abscesses, sinus tract involvement, alopecia, polytrichia possible.

Postinflammatory pigmentation (PIP): Brown to bluish gray patches at previous sites of inflammation.

Postinflammatory hypopigmentation (PIH): Patches with varying degrees of diminished pigmentation, but not complete depigmentation. Pityriasis alba variant common in school-age children (incidence as high as 1 in 20); appears as hypopigmented patches with fine scales, involving face alone in half the cases; also common on neck, shoulders.

Erythema dyschromicum perstans (EDP): Early lesions are hypopigmented or hyperpigmented patches with erythematous raised borders, most common on back, neck, chest, forearms, possibly face. Lesions flatten, develop the slate gray hue of "ashy dermatosis."

Investigations

PFB: Bacterial, fungal cultures; histology shows foreign-body granulomatous reaction, dermal abscess, epidermal microabscesses in area of follicle.

AKN: Bacterial, fungal cultures; histology shows dense perifollicular, follicular inflammatory infiltrate and, as lesions progress to follicular rupture, transepidermal elimination of necrotic tissue, hair fragments, dermal fibrosis.

PIP: On Wood's-light examination, epidermal pigmentation darkens lesion; no significant dermal pigmentation change. Histology shows concentration of melanin in basal-cell layer (epidermal type) or melanin in dermis, within melanophages (dermal type).

PIH: Biopsy to exclude inflammatory diseases, cutaneous T-cell lymphoma.

EDP: Biopsy from border of early lesion shows basal cell-layer pigmental incontinence, lichenoid, superficial perivascular chronic inflammatory infiltrate, melanin deposition in dermis.

Complications

•Disfigurement may decrease patients' self-esteem.

PFB: Postinflammatory pigmentation, secondary bacterial infection, shallow criss-cross scarring, hypertrophic or keloidal scarring.

AKN: Bacterial infection, keloid formation.

Nevus of Ota: Intraocular melanomas are more common.

Differential diagnosis

PFB: Bacterial folliculitis, acne, tinea barbae.

AKN: Bacterial folliculitis, pomade acne, tinea capitis, papular sarcoidosis.

PIP: Tinea versicolor, café-au-lait spots, ashy dermatosis, melasma, other pigmentation disorders.

PIH: Vitiligo, tinea versicolor, hypopigmented CTCL, nevus anemicus, guttate hypomelanosis.

Epidemiology

PFB, AKN: Predominantly in black men; possible in any curly-haired man.

PIP, PIH: Common in darkly pigmented skin.

Etiology

PFB: Intrafollicular or extrafollicular penetration of shaved tip of hair into dermis generates foreign-body reaction.

AKN: Follicular inflammation results in follicular rupture, subsequent foreign-body reaction; may be precipitated by close haircut.

PIP: Inflammation causes pigmentation, possibly through stimulation by chemical mediators of inflammation of melanogenesis and melanin granule transfer.

PIH: Unknown.

Sumayah Jamal

Treatment

Pharmacological treatment

Topical

PFB: Depilatory every 2 to 4 days, instead of shaving; glycolic acid lotion twice daily. Shave with Benzashave, 5% to 10% shaving cream (more effective than benzoyl peroxide preparations, probably because of vehicle), or Glytone Serious Shave Cream (contains glycolic acid, potassium hydroxide hair softener).

AKN: Intralesional triamcinolone acetonide, 10 to 40 ml, depending on size of keloids; hypopigmentation may develop.

PFB, **AKN**: Erythromycin 2% solution or clindamycin 1% solution, followed by corticosteroid gel or cream (class I for AKN; class VI or VII for PFB). Tretinoin, 0.25% to 0.1% cream, or 0.125% to 0.25% gel, daily or every other day.

PIP: Prevent lesions by avoiding aggressive treatment of acne, eczema, arthropod bites, drug eruption or any skin-disease–causing pigmentation. Use UVA and UVB sunscreens; protective clothing.

Systemic

AKN: Oral antibiotics (tetracyclines, macrolides, cephalosporins); isotretinoin, 0.5–1.0 mg/kg daily for severe cases.

Nonpharmacological treatment

Physical modalities

PFB: Cease shaving; as beard grows out, patient can release hairs trapped under skin, using toothpick or sterile needle and magnifying mirror. Subsequent shaving options include electric shaver, shaving gently, never pulling skin taut; electric clippers, leaving short stubble; single, foil-guarded blade (PFB razor) or adjustable razor at low setting to prevent close shave. Wait at least 5 minutes after application of shaving cream, for hairs to soften; shaving during or after shower; hot compress to soften hairs before shaving; never shave upward; pass over each area only once.

AKN: Avoid shaving, very short hair cuts of nuchal region, applications of hair oils. Allow hair to grow long.

Surgery

PFB: Hair-removal laser.

AKN: Elliptical excision of affected area down to subfollicular level with healing by secondary intention or by primary intention with use of extensive undermining, tissue expansion (for very severe cases) or laser hair removal.

Special therapeutic considerations

EDP: Anecdotal, unsubstantiated reports suggest improvement with dapsone or griseofulvin, Clofazimine, 200 mg daily for 1 year was found beneficial in one small series and single case reports.

Nevus of Ota, **Nevus of Ito**: Excellent responses achieved with Q-switch ruby, Q-switched neodymium–yttrium-aluminum-garnet lasers.

| **Treatment aims** |
| To prevent development of lesions and to eradicate such lesions once formed. |

Sumayah Jamal

Diagnosis

Signs

• Diffuse erythema, scaling and shiny, thickened skin involving at least 90% of the total skin surface. Edema of legs and feet is common. Commonly begins in the genital area, trunk, or head and progresses to total body. The disease may be acute or chronic. Secondary signs include onycholysis, shedding of nails, dermatopathic lymphadenopathy (less than 50%), alopecia (approximately 25%), spared mucous membranes, areas of pigmentation and hypopigmentation, palmoplantar involvement, hepatomegaly (7% to 37%), splenomegaly (3% to 23%), fever or hypothermia.

Symptoms

• Pruritus, burning, chills, shivering, malaise, and anorexia

Investigations

• Exfoliative erythroderma is a clinical diagnosis.

• In 20% of patients, the cause cannot be determined from either the history or histopathologic findings. Repeated biopsies may be needed.to determine cause.

• Blood cultures should be performed in acute erythoderma or during fever spikes.

• Serum prealbumin and albumin are low.

Complications

• Secondary infections/septicemia, dehydration, high output cardiac failure, severe hyperthermia and hypothermia, tetany, pneumonia

Etiology

Cutaneous T-cell lymphoma (CTCL), psoriasis, atopic dermatitis, contact dermatitis, pityriasis rubra pilaris (PRP, characterized by sharply defined islands of sparing), drug hypersensitivity, seborrheic dermatitis, leukemia. In 50%, there is a history of preexisting dermatosis.

Other special tests for the identification of specific diseases include lymph-node biopsy, immunophenotyping, special histopathology stains, flow cytometry, immunofluoresence, and T-cell receptor gene–rearrangement studies.

Epidemiology

Generally affects those older than 50 years; mean age: sixth decade. Uncommon in children.

Male predilection.

A patient with exfoliative erythroderma showing diffuse, confluent erythema and desquamation.

Lesley Clark-Loeser and Jerome Shupack

Treatment

Diet and lifestyle

• When drug reaction is suspected, withdrawal of the offending agent often results in rapid clearing.

• Avoid dehydration due to increased extrarenal water loss from exfoliating skin, monitor fluid intake and output and restore hydration.

• High-protein diet to prevent negative nitrogen balance.

• Minimize recurrent environment irritants (*ie, soaps, detergents, fabric softeners, fragrances, and high humidity*)

Pharmacological treatment

Topical

• Emollients (for dryness)

• Corticosteroid ointments (high-potency corticosteriods may result in systemic side effects if applied to more than 30% if body surface area).

• Coal-tar ointments (use cautiously because they may exacerbate dermatitis and irritation).

Systemic

• Antihistamines (for pruritus).

• Corticosteroids (for idiopathic/primary exfoliative erythroderma). Initially 100–300 mg cortisone equivalents/day, then 50 mg/day (use caution in debilitated or elderly patients).

• Retinoids (Acitretin is specially useful for psoriasis, PRP, and CTCL. Bexarotene for CTCL is being investigated).

• Systemic immunosuppressants when appropriate to treat an underlying pathologic process (*ie*, methotrexate for PRP or psoriasis, and cyclosporin for psoriasis).

Nonpharmacological treatment

• Psoralens and UVA photochemotherapy (for CTCL, seborrheic dermatitis, and psoriasis)

• UVB narrow or broad band phototherapy (for CTCL, seborrheic dermatitis, and psoriasis).

• Extracorporeal photophoresis (for erythrodermic CTCL).

Treatment aims

Diagnosis of underlying cause and appopriate treatment of the condition.

Prognosis

Varies with underlying cause:

Idiopathic: Variable.

Acquired PRP: 4 years (with retinoids, possibly only 1year).

Psoriasis: Recurrent.

CTCL: Progressive, ultimately leading to death.

General references

Abel EA, Lindae ML, Hoppe RT, Wood GS: Benign and malignant forms of cutaneous erythroderma: Cutaneous immunophenotypic characteristics. *J Am Acad Dermatol* 1988, **19**:1089–1095.

Freedberg IM: Exfoliative dermatitis. In: *Dermatology in General Medicine*, edn. 5. Edited by Freedberg IM, *et al*. New York: McGraw-Hill; 1999:534–537.

Pal S, Haroon TS: Erythroderma: a clinico-etiologic study of 90 cases. *Int J Dermatol* 1998, **37**:104–107.

Diagnosis

Signs

• Transient reddening of face and, frequently, other areas (*eg*, ears, neck, upper chest, epigastric region), especially noticeable in persons with fair complexion.

Symptoms

• Sensation of warmth, occasionally pruritus; rarely, associated pain, paresthesias, or burning (*eg*, with antidromic sensory neural flushing); may be associated with sweating, tachycardia, dry mouth, diarrhea, headache, pruritus (depending on cause).

Investigations

• History: Inciting factors (drugs, foods, emotions), temporal relationships (timing, frequency), other symptoms (sweating, pain, tachycardia, diarrhea, headache).

• Exclusion diet: Foods high in histamine (*eg*, fish), food or drugs that affect urinary 5-hydroxyindoleacetic acid (5-HIAA) tests (*eg*, bananas), foods that cause flushing (*eg*, spicy foods); if flushing resolves, may try reinstating items.

• Plasma histamine and 24-hour urine for histamine, *N*-methylhistamine, and prostaglandin D_2 metabolites for mastocytosis; 24-hour urine for 5-HIAA, preferably while patient is on an exclusion diet, for carcinoid syndrome; 24-hour urine for vanillylmandelic acid (VMA) and metanephrines for pheochromocytoma; plasma vasoactive intestinal peptide (VIP) for Verner-Morrison syndrome (VIPoma).

Complications

• Frequent, intense flushing may lead to loss of vascular tone, erythema, and telangiectases. Complications of systemic diseases, if present.

Differential diagnosis

Rosacea, seborrheic dermatitis, atopic dermatitis, physical erythemas (*eg*, sunlight, wind, heat), contact/photo-contact dermatitis, systemic lupus erythematosus, dermatomyositis, erythropoietic protoporphyria, chronic actinic dermatitis, drugs, cutaneous lymphoma, erythroderma.

Etiology

Transient increase in cutaneous blood flow; limited distribution due to greater capacity and greater visibility of superficial cutaneous vasculature at involved sites. "Wet flushes" (autonomic neural-mediated): accompanied by eccrine sweating (*eg*, induced by exercise, hot food or beverages, menopause, drugs, emotions). "Dry flushes" (direct vasodilator-mediated): antidromic sensory neural-mediated, associated with pain, paresthesias, burning (*eg*, cluster headaches, Parkinson's disease); circulating vasodilator agent, no dysesthesia, exogenous (*eg*, alcohol, drugs, food) or endogenous (*eg*, carcinoid syndrome or mastocytosis) agent.

Epidemiology

Common occurrence; usually idiopathic.

Edwin Joe and Nicholas A. Soter

Treatment

Diet and lifestyle
• Avoid precipitants that cause or that lower the threshold for flushing (*eg*, alcohol, spicy foods).

Pharmacological treatment

Systemic
Antihistamines: H_1-antihistamines—first-generation (*eg*, hydroxyzine) or second-generation, low-sedating (*eg*, loratadine); start at low dose, increase as tolerated; if an agent from one therapeutic group is ineffective, try another therapeutic group; agents from different groups may be combined. A combination of H_1- and H_2-antihistamines may be helpful.

• Contraindications: Monoamine oxidase inhibitors (prolong and augment anticholinergic effects); pregnancy: limited guidelines (mostly category B and C). Exercise caution with alcohol use (central nervous system depressant) and driving of motor vehicles; first-generation antihistamines and prostatic hypertrophy.

• Main drug interactions: Exercise caution with other central nervous system depressants (*eg*, benzodiazepines); cimetidine: many drug interactions, especially warfarin, quinidine, nifedipine, theophylline, phenytoin.

• Main side effects: Central nervous system (*eg*, drowsiness) and anticholinergic (*eg*, dry mouth), gastrointestinal (*eg*, nausea).

Other pharmacological agents
• Nadolol (emotional flushing); hormone replacement or clonidine (climacteric flushing); aspirin (*eg*, before niacin, which provokes flushing); rarely, carbamazepine and gabapentin.

Nonpharmacological treatment
• Biofeedback and hypnosis for emotional flushing.

Treatment aims
To identify underlying cause and prevent recurrences; targeted to specific cause.

Prognosis
Varies according to underlying cause.

Follow-up and management
Individualized, depending on underlying cause.

General references

Griffiths WAD: The red face—an overview and delineation of the MARSH syndrome. *Clin Exp Dermatol* 1999, **24**:42–47.

Murray AH: Differential diagnosis of a red face. *J Cutan Med Surg* 1998, **2(Suppl 4)**:S411-S415.

Wilkin JK: The red face: flushing disorders. *Clin Dermatol* 1993, **11**:211–23.

Diagnosis

Signs

Gout: Soft nodules (tophi) on the helix and antihelix of the ear and index fingers. Erythema, swelling and warmth surrounding the joints. Nephrolithiasis, elevated serum urate level, leukocytosis, elevated sedimentation rate, hemolytic anemia, abnormal calcium levels.

Calcinosis cutis (CC): Subepidermal calcified nodules overlying joints, muscles, tendons, scrotum, vulva and breast; verrucous nodules on the head or extremity in children; nodules and papules in heels in neonates. Pain associated with ulceration

Symptoms

Gout: Excruciating, throbbing pain in the affected joint, most commonly the great toe (podagra), but multiple joints may be involved; renal colic; fever.

Investigations

Gout: Joint fluid examination reveals needle-shaped and strongly negative birefringent crystals. Serum urate level more than 7 mg/dl or normal. Radiographs reveal soft tissue or bony tophi with or without calcification and erosive arthropathy.

CC: Skin biopsy (may need special stains); serum calcium, phosphate ,and parathyroid hormone levels.

Complications

Gout: Nephroliathiasis, hemolytic anemia, erosive arthropathy.

CC: Ulceration of the nodules, infection. Kidneys, lungs, stomach, and the media of arteries may be affected.

Differential diagnosis

Gout: Chondrocalcinosis (pseudogout), osteoarthritis, Reiter's disease, psoriatic arthritis, multicentric reticulohistiocytosis, rheumatoid arthritis.

CC: Calciphylaxis, osteoma cutis, epidermal cysts, gout.

Etiology

Gout: Primary gout results from increased circulating levels of uric acid because of overproduction or underexcretion of uric acid. Secondary gout may be associated with diuretic therapy, renal disease, polycythemia rubra vera, lymphoma, myeloma, in patients with leukemia receiving active chemotherapy, and psoriasis.

CC: Occurs in various clinical settings. Initially, there is calcium phosphate deposition that progresses to hydroxya-patite crystal formation within a collagen matrix. Four subsets: **Metastatic calcinosis (MC)**: High levels of serum calcium or phosphate, with precipitating crystals in tissues. **Dystrophic calcinosis (DC)**: tissue damage followed by intracellular calcium influx. **Idiopathic calcinosis**: Normal serum calcium, no preceding trauma. **Iatrogenic calcification**: Following intravenous extravasation of calcium chloride and phosphate, as well as calcium salt exposure. Heel sticks in neonates.

Epidemiology

Gout: Prevalence of gout increases with age and is higher in blacks than whites. Genetic predisposition; higher incidence in US blacks, Filipinos, South Pacific Islanders.

MC: Renal failure, hypervitaminosis D, milk-alkali syndrome.

DC: Inflammatory lesions, such as acne, stasis ulcers, granulomas, and benign and malignant neoplasms. Calcinosis circum-scripta in scleroderma, crest or systemic lupus erythematosus. Inherited diseases, such as Ehlers-Danlos syndrome and pseudoxanthoma elasticum. Tumoral calcinosis is a familial disorder associated with hyperphosphatemia.

Dina Began

Treatment

Diet and lifestyle

Gout: Avoid alcohol consumption, lead exposure, limit diuretic use.

CC: Low calcium, phosphate diet.

Pharmacological treatment

Systemic

Gout: Nonsteroidal antiinflammatory agents for acute gout at a high initial dose followed by rapid taper over 2–8 days (indomethacin, 50 mg, orally, every 6 hours, for 2 days; followed by 50 mg, orally, every 8 hours, for 3 days; followed by 25 mg, orally, every 8 hours, for 2–3 days. Observe renal function and do not prescribe in the presence of active peptic ulcer disease).

• Colchicine, 0.6 mg, every 1–2 hours, or 1.0–1.2 mg, every 2 hours, until symptoms abate; maximum dosage recommended is 6.0 mg in 24-hour period. Observe for gastrointestinal side effects, myleosuppression. Intravenous preparations may give faster relief with fewer side effects. Treatment is most effective if given in first 12–24 hours of an acute attack.

• Prednisone, 40–60 mg, orally, four times daily, with a rapid taper; for acute gout. Monitor for side effects of steroids.

• Intra-articular injections of glucocorticoids.

• Allopurinol, 300 mg, orally, four times daily, for chronic gout. Adjust dose for decreased creatine clearance.

• Probenecid, 500 mg, orally, four times daily.

CC: Warfarin, 1 mg/kg/d. Early, limited calcinosis may responded, but extensive disease rarely improves.

• Colchicine, 5 mg, orally, twice daily, for ulcers associated with calcinosis.

• Aluminum hydroxide (may reduce calcification in dermatomyositis).

• Diltiazem, 60 mg, orally, three times daily. Ttitrate dose as blood pressure tolerates. Mmay be effective.

Surgery

CC: Surgical excision is indicated for painful masses, recurrent infection, ulcerations, functional impairment, cosmetic concerns.

Special therapeutic considerations

Gout: Adjust treatments appropriately for decreased renal function.

CCB: Reduce dialysate calcium in dialysis patients

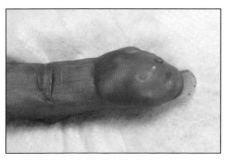

Calcinosis cutis presents as firm lesions that commonly ulcerate and exude a chalk-like material.

Treatment aims

Gout: To alleviate pain and decrease frequency of episodes.

CC: To reduce calcification and heal ulcers.

Prognosis

Gout: Excellent relief of pain with medications over days. Recurrences are common.

CC: Often recalcitrant to treatment.

General references

Touart D, Sau P: Cutaneous deposition diseases. Part II. *J Am Acad Dermatol* 1998, 39:538–541.

Walsh JS, Fairley JA: Cutaneous mineralization and ossification. In: *Fitzpatrick's Dermatology in General Medicine* edn 5. Edited by Freedberg IM, Eisen AZ, Wolff K, *et al.* New York: McGraw-Hill Health Professions Division; 1999:1829–1833.

Graft-versus-host (GVH) disease

Diagnosis

Signs

Hyperacute GVH disease (H): Generalized inflammation.

Acute GVH disease (A): Macular erythema of palms, soles, pinnae, neck, upper back. Severe reactions may progress to bullae, generalized erythroderma, or total epidermal sloughing.

Chronic GVH disease (C): Widespread morbilliform eruption with violaceous lichen planus–like papules, often on palms, soles; papules later become generalized. Sclerodermoid changes of trunk, proximal extremities. Bullae, atrophic or papulosquamous plaques, mucosal atrophy or ulceration possible.

Symptoms

H: Fever, hepatitis, fluid retention, vascular leakage, shock.

A: Pruritus or burning in affected areas, nausea, vomiting, abdominal pain, paralytic ileus, diarrhea (voluminous, often bloody).

C: Pruritus, abdominal pain, diarrhea, xerostomia, jaundice, bronchitis, keratoconjunctivitis, polymyositis, sinusitis.

Investigations

A: Skin biopsy: superficial, diffuse, sparse, lymphocytic dermal infiltrate and necrotic eosinophilic keratinocytes scattered throughout epidermis.

C: Skin biopsy: Epidermal acanthosis, scattered Civatte-like eosinophilic keratinocytes, cell necrosis in basal layer, mononuclear lichenoid dermal infiltrate; sclerotic stage: epidermis atrophic, dermis shows thickened hyalinized collagen bundles.

• Total bilirubin, alkaline phosphatase, and aminotransferase levels.

Complications

• Graft failure. Death.

Differential diagnosis

A: Chemotherapeutic reactions, radiation recall phenomenon, acral erythema, neutrophilic eccrine hidradenitis, eruption of lymphocyte recovery, drug eruptions, toxic epidermal necrolysis, viral exanthems, infectious enteritis.

C: Lichen planus, lichen sclerosis, subacute cutaneous lupus, morphea, eosinophilic fasciitis.

Etiology

Develops in setting of viable immunocompetent cells to host, incompetence of host to reject foreign cells, and antigenic disparity between host and donor tissues (HLA mismatch). Engrafted donor cells proliferate and attack in response to foreign antigens on host tissues.

Epidemiology

Patients who receive allogenic bone marrow transplants, autologous and syngeneic bone marrow transplants, blood product transfusions, solid-organ transplants, neonates with graft-versus-host disease.

Special considerations

Clinical grading of acute graft-versus-host disease
Grade I: Erythematous macular and papular eruption < 25% body surface area.

Grade II: Erythematous macular and papular eruption 25% to 50% body surface area.

Grade III: Generalized erythroderma.

Grade IV: Bullae or generalized epidermal necrolysis.

Treatment

Pharmacological treatment

Topical
Corticosteroids for mild acute graft-versus-host disease.

Systemic
Corticosteroids: Methylprednisolone, tapering dose beginning at 2 mg/kg, for acute disease; or oral prednisone, 1 mg/kg, tapered after 9 weeks, but continued for 9 months, for chronic disease.

Cyclosporine and antithymocyte globulin for corticosteroid-resistant graft-versus-host disease.

Thalidomide for recalcitrant chronic cases.

Acitretin for sclerodermoid chronic disease.

Nonpharmacological treatment

Physical modalities
- Psoralen plus ultraviolet A may be used in both acute and chronic disease.
- Extracorporeal photophoresis.

Supportive methods
- Grade IV disease may necessitate care in a burn unit.

Treatment aims

Suppression of graft-versus-host response.

Prognosis

Systemic disease continues to be a major source of morbidity and death after bone marrow transplantation.

General references

Horn TD: Graft versus host disease. In: *Dermatology in General Medicine*. Edited by Freedberg IM, *et al*. New York: McGraw-Hill; 1999:1426–1433.

Johnson ML, Farmer ER: Graft-versus-host reactions in dermatology. *J Am Acad Dermatol* 1998, 369–384.1

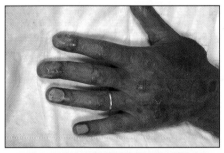

Chronic graft-verus-host disease: violaceous lichenified papules over proximal phlalangeal joints; pink, hyperpigmented, scaly papules over knuckles; healing erosions and shiny, darkly pigmented patches on hand; periungual erythema, loss of several nails with atrophic scarring of the nail bed; remaining nail plates are thin and ridged.

Diagnosis

Signs

Granuloma annulare (GA)

Localized (LG): Skin-colored, erythematous or violaceous, annular plaques, 1–5 cm in diameter, often formed from grouped dome-shaped papules or erythematous patches. No epidermal change distributed on extremities, particularly on dorsal hands or feet.

Generalized (GG): (15% of cases):More than 10 lesions, sometimes innumerable; skin-colored, erythematous, violaceous, yellow, or gray; usually smaller than 5 cm in diameter; discrete or confluent macules or papules, which may form reticulate and circinate patterns and which are distributed most commonly on the trunk but also on the forearms, legs, or elbows

Subcutaneous: Solitary or multiple, painless, skin-colored nodules distributed on palms, soles, legs, buttocks, and scalp. Lesions can exist near joints ("pseudorheumatoid nodules") and may ulcerate.

Perforating: Small papules with central umbilication, plugs, or crusts. Lesions often localized; occur most commonly on hands.

Other lesions

•Rare, arcuate or circinate erythematous plaques resembling erythema multiforme; and large annular plaques on actinically damaged skin. Follicular pustular granuloma annulare presents as an eruption of generalized follicular pustules and, in some cases, also scaly papules and pseudovesiculous lesions over the palms.

Granuloma faciale (GF): Round, erythematous to violet-colored plaques, usually on the cheeks.

Actinic granuloma (AG): Usually multiple pink or violaceous, slow-growing, infiltrated papules or nodules, often in the eyelids, in photodamaged skin. Annular elastolytic granuloma is considered to be an annular or serpiginous variant, with erythematous, brown, either solitary or multiple annular papules or plaques with elevated borders occurring predominantly but not exclusively over sun-exposed areas. Lesions may begin as lichenoid papules that gradually evolve into annular lesions of about 0.5–1 cm in diameter.

Granuloma disciformis chronica et progressiva of Miescher (GD): Gradually enlarging, discoid plaques with slight central sclerosis, usually on the legs.

Symptoms

GA: Benign, self-limited infiltration of the skin; usually asymptomatic.

Investigations

GA: Histopathologic examination shows sharply-demarcated areas of degenerated collagen (necrobiosis) surrounded by infiltrate composed of histiocytes in a pallisading arrangement, lymphocytes and fibroblasts. Mucin is usually present. The epidermis is normal except in the perforating variant.

GF: Histopathologic changes include a dense superficial and mid-dermal perivascular inflammatory infiltrate composed of histiocytes, lymphocytes, plasma cells, neutrophils, and eosinophils.

AG: Biopsy shows a mid-dermal, noncaseating granulomatous reaction centered around elastotic fibers, with giant epithelioid and multinucleated cells engulfing the fibers throughout the lesion. In annular elastolytic granuloma, fibers are engulfed predominantly at the edge of the lesion.

GD: Biopsy reveals small foci of necrobiotic collagen and new collagen formation and an infiltrate composed of macrophages and lymphocytes.

Differential diagnosis

Rheumatoid nodules, tinea corporis, erythema migrans, sarcoidosis, syphilis, annular lichen planus, cutaneous tuberculosis, lymphocytic infiltrate of Jessner, arthropod bite, xanthomas, lipoid proteinosis, erythema multiforme, subacute cutaneous lupus erythematosus, amyloidosis, necrobiosis lipoidica, erythema elevatum diutinum, granuloma multiforme (Mkar disease), alopecia mucinosa, Miescher's actinic granuloma (possibly a variant of GA).

Etiology

Unknown, for all these diseases.

Epidemiology

Granuloma annulare

Most commonly in children and young adults, but occurs in all age groups; 2:1 female predilection.

Systemic associations

Patients with GA generally have normal health otherwise.

GG frequently coexists with diabetes mellitus.

The disease may also coexist with necrobiosis lipoidica or rheumatoid arthritis.

Anecdotal reports suggest a relationship between HIV infection and GG.

Arcuate and annular papules with smooth surfaces, erythematous firm, raised borders, and central clearing characteristic of granuloma annulare.

Bruce E. Strober and Roy L. Stern

Treatment

Pharmacological treament

Localized GA
• Intralesional triamcinolone :Most effective treatment.

• Potent topical corticosteroids with or without occlusion.

Generalized GA
• PUVA: Treatment of choice.

• Acitretin (alone or with PUVA)

• Dapsone 100–200 mg daily

• Isotretinoin 1–1.5 mg/kg/d

• Antimalarials (plaquenil 200–400 mg daily).

• Potassium iodide 0.6 mg three times daily.

• Pentoxifylline, 400 mg three times daily.

• Cyclosporine 3–6 mg/kg/d

• Systemic corticosteroids are highly effective but rarely required.

• Low-dose recombinant human interferon-*gamma*, niacinamide, and chlorpropamide have been anecdotally reported to be beneficial.

Physical modalities

• Cryosurgery with liquid nitrogen or nitrous oxide , with one freeze-thaw cycle of 10–60 seconds. If necessary, treatment is repeated after 20–30 days.

Surgery

• Excision of tumor-size lesions.

Other

GF: Cryotherapy, surgery, and CO_2 laser can be effective but recurrences are common. Dapsone at 100 mg daily and intralesional corticosteoids may be beneficial in some cases. Cryosurgery and pulse dye laser have been proposed as the treatment of choice.

AG may respond to intralesional corticosteoids or isotretinoin at usual doses. Some cases have responded to dapsone.

GD responds to topical corticosteroids under occlusion. Patients do not have diabetes.

Treatment aims

GA is a benign condition, and treatment is dictated by cosmetic concerns.

Prognosis

Granuloma annulare
Spontaneous resolution of individual lesions is the rule, usually within 2 years. Almost half of patients display recurrence, often at original site.
Resolution less likely in older patients with generalized disease.

General references

Smith MD, Downie JB, DiCostanzo D: Granuloma annulare [review]. *Int J Dermatol* 1997, 36:326–333.

Penas PF, Jones-Caballero M, Fraga J, *et al*.: Perforating granuloma annulare [review]. *Int J Dermatol* 1997, 36:340–348.

Diagnosis

Signs

Erythema annulare centrifugum (EAC): Begins as one or more pink, urticarial papules that spread peripherally while clearing centrally and gradually enlarge by peripheral extension to form annular, arcuate, or polycyclic plaques with flat or slightly raised, scaly or smooth margins (4-6 mm in width) that usually advance 2-5 mm daily. Rarely vesicles appear at the edges. Lesions appear predominantly on the trunk, thighs, legs; less often on upper extremities, face, never on palms and soles. *Superficial type* has indistinct border, trailing scale; is more likely to be pruritic. *Deep type* has a firm border, lacks scale, and is rarely pruritic.

Familial EA (FEA): Lesions similar to (EAC), develop as early as a few days after birth, are more transitory, and the disease persists for many years.

Erythema gyratum repens (EGR): Concentric, annular, and serpiginous bands of erythema frequently surmounted by a fine marginal desquamation, which move in waves about 1 cm daily to form a pattern that resembles grain in wood. Erythematous bands may be flat or raised.

Necrolytic migratory erythema (NME): Lesions usually begin in perioral, perinasal, and perineal areas; in genitalia, groin, ankles, shin, and feet; less often in lower abdomen, thighs, buttocks, and fingers with areas of bright erythema, which heal centrally, resulting in annular lesions (with pigmented centers) that extend peripherally to form geographic, circinate, and serpiginous patterns. Vesiculopustular lesions arise from the areas of erythema and rupture, leaving superficial, crusted erosions. Painful glossitis and cheilitis are common.

Symptoms

EAC, FEA, and **EGR** may be pruritic.

NME: Symptoms of gucagonoma include weight loss (71%), diarrhea (29%), malabsorption, cheilitis or stomatitis (29%), anemia, and adult onset diabetes mellitus (38%).

Investigations

• Skin biopsy shows a superficial perivascular lymphohistiocytic infiltrate in the *superficial type*. In *deep type*, infiltrate is superficial and deep dermal with dense cuffing around the vessels. *Superficial type* may have slight papillary edema, epidermal spongiosis, and parakeratosis. *Deep type* has no epidermal changes and the infiltrate is superficial and deep.

• Consider Lyme antibody titer, antinuclear antibody test with anti-Ro/anti-La antibodies, complete blood count with differential, chest radiograph, fungal smear and culture, purified protein derivative.

NME: Skin biopsy shows acute necrosis of spinal layer, which may become detached from the rest of the epidermis (necrolysis), Neutrophilic collections, when present, form pustules. Chronic lesions have psoriasiform hyperplasia and hydropic changes within epidermis. Immunochemical stains specific to peptide are available. Evaluations include serum glucagon levels, CT scan for pancreatic tumor, fasting glucose level, oral glucose tolerance tests, and hepatic enzymes.

Differential diagnosis

Tinea corporis, eczema, erythema chronicum migrans, urticaria, annular urticarial phase of bullous pemphigoid or linear IgA disease, erythema marginatum rheumaticum (an evanescent, nonscaling gyrate erythema, which spreads in hours, present in 10% to 18% of patients with rheumatic fever. Histologically, infiltrate is neutrophilic rather than lymphohistiocytic), granuloma annulare, sarcoidosis, cytotoxic T-cell lymphoma, subacute lupus erythematosus, Hansen's disease, trypanosomiasis, and erythema multiforme.

NME: Acrodermatitis enteropathica, pustular psoriasis, Basex disease should be considered in addition to other gyrate erythemas.

Etiology

Cause obscure, but may result from a type-IV hypersensitivity reaction to triggers, such as fungi (tinea pedis, tinea corporis, Candidiasis, tinea versicolor, ingestion of moldy cheeses), parasites (*Ascaris*), viruses (Epstein Barr, molluscum contagiosum), bacteria (*Streptococcus* species) systemic disease (sarcoidosis, Graves' disease, cholestatic liver disease), connective tissue diseases (Sjögren's sundrome), arthropod bites, malignancy (Hodgkin's disease, squamous cell carcinoma, ovarian carcinoma, leukemia, dysproteinemias), vaccination, and drug hypersensitivity (antimalarials, penicillin, cimetidine, gold, piroxicam, salicylates, amitryptilline).

Erythema gyratum repens: Associated with cancers of breast, lung, bladder, prostate, cervix, stomach, esophagus; thymomas; and multiple myeloma.

NME: Most often associated with an alpha-2-glucagon–producing islet cell tumor of the pancreas. Eruption occurs in 67% of glucagonoma cases; may precede detection of tumor by years. Also reported in cases of hepatic disease, jejunal adenocarcinoma with hepatic dysfunction, pancreatic insufficiency, gluten-sensitive enteropathy, heroin abuse, and malabsorption with villous atrophy. Defect may result from inhibition or underproduction of delta-6-desaturase, which results in phospholipid fatty acid abnormalities; enzyme inhibited by zinc deficiency, excessive ethanol ingestion.

Epidemiology

EAC found in 1:100,000; no race or gender predilection.

Miguel Sanchez

Treatment

Diet and lifestyle
• Infusion of essential fatty acids and amino acids causes temporary resolution of necrolytic migratory erythema.

Pharmacological treatment

Topical
• Corticosteroid creams, ointments, and gels (Class III–VII) may clear the eruptions but have to be continued indefinitely.

Systemic
• Prednisone usually suppresses EAC, but recurrence is common on discontinuation. Antihistamines (for pruritus): Streptozotocin, a peptide antagonist (for necrolytic migratory erythema); lanreotide (long-acting somatostatin analogue) or octeotride (somatostatin analogue) (for necrolytic migratory erythema). Other antibiotics and antifungal agents, administered empirically, sometimes beneficial.

EGR: Removal of the malignant tumor usually resolves erythema gyratum repens completely within 6 weeks.

NME: Surgical excision of glucagonoma results in resolution. Metastasis to liver treated with surgery, hepatic arterial chemoembolization, and systemic chemotherapy.

Treatment aims

Most cases resolve spontaneously.

Prognosis

EAC: Excellent, if not associated with malignancy or systemic disease. Mean duration of eruption 11 months (4 weeks–34 years).

NME: Approximately 60% of glucoganomas are malignant. Metastasis to the liver is common.

Diagnosis

Definition
Paucibacillary HD: Indeterminate (IT), tuberculoid (TT), borderline tuberculoid (BT).
Multibacillary HD: Borderline (BB), borderline lepromatous (BL), lepromatous (LL).

Signs
IT: Hypopigmented or erythematous macule or small patch. **TT**: One to three, usually anesthetic, anhidrotic annular plaques <10 cm, sharp, raised borders, hypopigmented centers. Nerves (great or posterior auricular, ulnar, peroneal, posteriortibial) usually thickened, palpable. **BT**: Sharply marginated anesthetic papules, plaques; annular configuration, but less erythema, elevation, induration. Plaques may exceed 10 cm; satellite papules. Nerves enlarged. **BB**: Large annular plaques, well-demarcated margins or large plaques with punched out areas of normal skin (Swiss-cheese plaques; SCP). **BL**: Annular plaque, poorly marginated outer border, sharply demarcated inner border (in half of cases); SCP; poorly demarcated papules, nodules. Lesions often hypesthetic. **LL**: Hyperpigmented, hypopigmented, flesh-color or erythematous macules, papules, plaques or nodules; predilection for cooler areas of skin. Facial skin may be indurated with flattened nasal bridge; lateral to medial loss of eyebrows, eyelashes.

Symptoms
• Nasal stuffiness, eye irritation in BL, LL.

• Numbness, paresthesias, usually over extremities.

• Further neurologic involvement: muscle weakness, neuropathic pain.

• Reactional states may cause acute tenderness, pain, loss of function along affected nerves.

Investigations
• Biopsy: From active margin of lesion, Fite stain to identify bacilli. Tuberculoid is paucibacillary and lepromatous is multibacillary in skin sections.

• Slit skin smears: Scrape, stained skin lesion tissue fluid to quantify bacteria.

• Lepromin skin test: To classify. Patients closer to TT spectrum show > 3-mm induration; those with BL and LL disease show < 3-mm induration.

• Culture: Grows on mouse foot pad, not in vitro; main use: cases of resistance.

Complications
LL: Conjunctivitis, iritis, keratitis; atrophy of thenar, hypothenar muscles. Traumatic ulcers, tissue mutilation from anesthetic extremities; cosmetic disfigurement, especially face, nasal septal cartilage; glaucoma, cataracts, uveitis, corneal damage from ocular involvement. Hypogonadism from testicular involvement.

TT, BL: Muscle atrophy, nerve palsies (foot drop, claw hand). Reactional states: immune responses; sudden clinical status changes, spontaneous or during therapy.

Type I (reversal reaction): Inflammation (redness, edema, pain) within existing skin lesions. Fever, satellite lesions, neuritis, usually with worsening (upgrading) or treated (downgrading) BT disease, but may occur as part of borderline spectrum.

Type II (erythema nodosum leprosum):– Widely disseminated tender nodules, mainly on extremities, with fever, arthralgias, lymphadenitis, and neuritis in patients with BL or treated LL disease.

Type III (Lucio's reaction): Generalized edema and shallow ulcerations (mainly on legs) from hemorrhagic infarcts in patients with LL from Mexico; bacterial superinfection and septicemia may develop.

Differential diagnosis
Tinea corporis or versicolor, cutaneous sarcoidosis, granuloma annulare, pityriasis rosea, vasculitis, cutaneous lymphoma, cutaneous tuberculosis or atypical mycobacterial infection, morphea, vitiligo, psoriasis, cutaneous lupus erythematosus.

Etiology
Mycobacterium leprae.

Epidemiology
Worldwide prevalence:12 million; incidence: 650 000 annually. US: 4000 patients, almost all in immigrant populations with nasorespiratory transmission. Predisposition: Male:female ratio, 2:1. Median age of onset, < 35 years.

Special considerations
Consider patients with simultaneous fifth- and seventh-cranial-nerve palsies to have leprosy until proven otherwise. Nasorespiratory transmission apparent typical route of infection. Patients with multibacillary disease have many mycobacteria in nose, mouth. Armadillo transmission unproven. Incubation period appears to be up to 5 years for TT, 20 years or longer for LL. Prolonged close contact needed.

Narayan S. Naik and Rena Brand

Treatment

Diet and lifestyle

• Patient education regarding regular self-inspection of body sites for injury.

Pharmacological treatment

Systemic, for infection

• World Health Organization (WHO) recommendations. **Paucibacillary**: Dapsone, 100 mg/d, plus supervised rifampin, 600 mg/month for 6 months. **Multibacillary**: Dapsone, 100 mg/d, plus clofazimine, 50 mg/d, plus supervised rifampin, 600 mg/month, plus supervised clofazimine, 300 mg/month for 5 years.

• Other recommendations. **Paucibacillary**: Dapsone, 100 mg/d for 3–5 years. **Multibacillary**: Dapsone, 100 mg/d, for life plus rifampin, 600 mg/d for 3–5 years.

• Main side effects. **Dapsone**: Anemia universal, can be severe in G6PD-deficient patients. **Clofazamine**: Reddish-brown skin discoloration, gastrointestinal effects. **Rifampin**: Red secretions, hepatotoxicity, decreased effect of other drugs.

• Reactional states. **Type I reactions**: Prednisone, 0.5–1.0 mg/kg per day, tapered over 3–6 months. **Type II reactions**: Thalidomide, 100–200 mg orally every night, tapered slowly with or without prednisone, 0.5–1.0 mg/kg per day, tapered over 6–8 weeks. **Type III reactions**: Mild disease usually self-limiting; severe disease, corticosteroids with supportive topical care.

Nonpharmacological treatment

• Wound care, secondary infection prevention. Protective padding, orthotic shoes. Physical and occupational therapy for muscle weakness, skeletal deformities, neuropathy. Cosmetic and orthopedic surgery for tissue disfigurement. Eye surgery for ophthalmic complications.

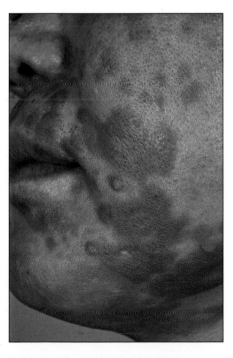

Brownish-red nodules and plaques that on biopsy proved to be lepromatous leprosy.

Treatment aims

To cure paucibacillary disease and treat multibacillary disease. To prevent and treat complications and reactional states. To facilitate patient integration into society.

Prognosis

High cure and low relapse rate reported with WHO treatment regimens in paucibacillary disease. Treatment for multibacillary disease is recommended for life.

Follow-up and management

Monthly during therapy; more frequently, if complications. After therapy: Paucibacillary—every 12 months for at least 2 years; multibacillary —every 12 months for at least 5 years, with clinical, microbiological examinations each visit.

Special therapeutic considerations

During pregnancy, dapsone therapy may continue; type II reactions must be treated with corticosteroids, never thalidomide. Infants of infected mothers should never be breast-fed. Multibacillary disease should be followed ophthalmologically.

Support organizations

Hansen's Disease Center, Carville, LA, assistance and management information about investigational treatment protocols (telephone: 800-642-2477). Internet information on leprosy can be found at http://www.who.int/lep.

General references

Rea TH, Modlin RL: Leprosy. In *Dermatology in General Medicine*, edn 5. Edited by Freedberg IM, *et al*. New York: McGraw-Hill; 1999:2306–2318.

Wathen PL: Hansen's disease. *South Med J* 1996, **89**:647–652.

Jain S, Sehgal VN: Multidrug therapeutic challenges in leprosy. *Int J Dermatol* 1997, **36**:493–496.

Whitty CJM, Lockwood DNJ: Leprosy—new perspectives on an old disease. *J Infect* 1999, **38**:2–5.

Jacobson RR: Leprosy. *Lancet* 1999, **353**:655–660.

Narayan S. Naik and Rena Brand

Diagnosis

Signs

Hemangioma: Pale macules with thread-like telangiectases in newborn. The tumor becomes bright red, slightly elevated, noncompressible plaque or nodule, 1.0–8.0 cm. Hemangiomas deeper in the skin are soft, warm masses with bluish hue. More common areas are the head and neck (50%), and trunk (25%).

Lymphangioma: Localized malformations of cutaneous, subcutaneous, or submucous lymphatic vessels; subcategorized as microcystic (lymphangioma circumscriptum), macrocystic (cavernous lymphangioma or cystic hygroma), or combined.

Superficial lymphatic malformation (lymphangioma circumscriptum): Numerous small, discrete vesicle-like lesions, often with a verrucous surface; grouped into plaques resembling frogspawn. Vesicles may contain blood, weep clear fluid. Asymptomatic, unless irritated. Most commonly on axillary folds, shoulders, flanks, proximal parts of limbs or perineum.

Diffuse (deep cavernous) lymphangioma: Large, diffuse, ill-defined swelling, usually on head and neck region, extremities.

Cystic hygroma: Large, fluid-filled cystic mass, a few millimeters to several centimeters; sometimes tender. Usually diagnosable by transillumination. Most common sites: lateral (mainly left side) neck (at least 75%), axillae, inguinal region.

Investigations

•Cutaneous, mucosal examination for other hemangiomas. Measurement of hemangioma (including superficial and deep components). Liver palpation. Ophthalmologic examination if periorbital area is affected.

•Skin biopsy if diagnosis is in question.

•MRI scan to evaluate structural brain abnormalities in infants with large facial hemangiomas, to differentiate between hemangiomas and venous or arteriovenous malformations, to evaluate depth of lymphangiomas.

•Platelet count, ultrasonography to evaluate potential complications.

•Soft-tissue ultrasonography and color Doppler imaging.

Complications

Hemangioma: Skin ulceration most common. Symptomatic airway hemangiomas common with mandibular lesions. Cardiac failure may occur with large lesions. Other: permanent disfigurement (lip, ear hemangiomas), deformation of nasal cartilage or nasal obstruction (nasal lesions), amblyopia (hemangiomas of periorbital region), and auditory canal obstruction (ear lesions). Large cervicofacial hemangiomas are associated with posterior fossa malformations (including Dandy-Walker malformation). Lower-spine hemangiomas are associated with occult spinal dysraphism.

Lymphangioma: Infection is most serious. Squamous-cell carcinoma may arise within lymphangioma circumscriptum. Cavernous lymphangiomas on face or extremity may be associated with bony involvement. Cystic hygromas have been reported in Maffucci's syndrome. Lesions of the posterior triangle of the neck are associated with hydrops fetalis, Turner's syndrome, other congenital malformations, several varieties of chromosomal aneuploidy, and fetal death.

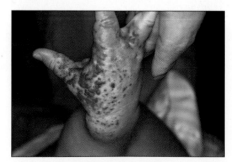

Hemangioma of the hand.

Differential Diagnosis

Hemangioma: Tufted angioma, port-wine stains, venous malformations, lymphatic malformations, arteriovenous malformations, Kaposiform hemangioendothelioma, adrenal carcinoma, pyogenic granuloma, nasal glioma, myofibromatosis, spindle and epithelioid (Spitz) nevus, dermoid cysts.

Lymphangioma circumscriptum: Herpes simplex, herpes zoster, dermatitis herpetiformis.

Deep cavernous lymphangioma and cystic hygroma: Lipomas, neurofibromas, branchial cleft cyst, other soft subcutaneous masses.

Etiology

Hemangioma: Benign proliferation of vascular elements. Growth factors, hormonal and mechanical influences may affect focal abnormal growth of endothelial cells.

Lymphangioma: Most arise from deep contractile lymphatics that are malformed and not in continuity with normal lymph-conducting pathways. Some arise after dissection of regional lymph nodes, radiation therapy, trauma, infection.

Epidemiology

Hemangioma: 1% to 2% of newborns; 10% of 1-year-olds. More common among whites; increased incidence in premature infants; 3:1 predilection for females.

Lymphangioma circumscriptum, cystic hygroma: Usually noted at birth or during childhood.

Cavernous lymphangiomas: Present at birth; may go unnoticed for years until accidental injury, surgery, infection. Equal sex distribution.

Paul Friedman and Robin Ashinoff

Treatment

Pharmacological treatment

Topical

•Triamcinolone acetonide, 10–40 mg/mL (for hemangiomas), sometimes mixed with dexamethasone sodium phosphate, 4 mg/mL.

•Interferon-α 2a; initial dose, 1 million U/m² per day, subcutaneously, for hemangiomas. For nonresponders, this is increased to 3 million U/m² per day, if tolerated. Spastic diplegia is a possible side effect.

•Intralesional administration of sclerosant, such as doxycycline or picibanil (OK-432) for lymphangioma circumscriptum not amenable to surgery. Results are variable.

Systemic

•Prednisone, 2–4 mg/kg per day in single morning dose or divided doses in emergency cases of hemangiomas; indicated mainly in growth phase.

•Systemic corticosteroid therapy plus pulsed-dye laser, (for hemangiomas).

Nonpharmacological treatment

•Cryosurgery.

•Flash-lamp pulsed-dye laser, early treatment of hemangiomas may prevent ensuing proliferation, irreversible cutaneous changes, disfigurement.

•Early surgical excision (especially eyelid and nasal hemangiomas).

•Radical surgery is treatment of choice for lymphangioma circumscriptum.

•CO₂ laser surgery has provided palliative benefit for lesions localized to dermis.

•Surgery, cryotherapy, laser phototherapy for small cystic hygromas, deep cavernous hemangiomas. Larger, subcutaneous lesions may be observed for possible spontaneous regression, unless symptomatic or compressing vital structures.

Special therapeutic considerations

•Antiangiogenic therapy for large, unresponsive hemangiomas.

•Recurrences of lymphangiomas are common, usually within 3 months of excision.

•Bacterial infection should be promptly treated with antibiotics (often require prolonged intravenous administration).

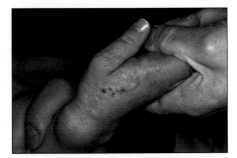

Same hand after several pulsed-dye laser treatments.

Treatment aims

Prevent or reverse any complications. Minimize psychosocial distress for patient and family.

Prevent permanent disfigurement left by residual skin changes after hemangioma involution. Cautious observation is recommended for most hemangiomas, providing no impending danger is associated with the lesion. Small hemangiomas are unlikely to leave permanent disfigurement or cause functional impairment. Large hemangiomas on prognostically poor locations and lesions that involve extracutaneous structures or cause functional impairment should be treated.

Prognosis

Proliferation of hemangiomas is most rapid in patients between 3 and 6 months of age; growth may continue until 12 months of age. After proliferative phase, virtually all hemangiomas of infancy undergo spontaneous involution (50% to 60% by age 5; 90% by age 9). May resolve entirely or leave residual atrophy, depigmentation, infiltration. Lip, nose involvement suggests poor outcomes after involution.

Follow-up and management

Hemangioma: High-risk lesions require multidisciplinary team of pediatrician, dermatologist, plastic surgeon, ophthalmologist, otolaryngologist, interventional radiologist, psychologist, and social worker.

Lymphangioma: Followed initially, monthly, or bimonthly with photographs and measurements, then, when growth is stable, semiannually or annually.

Support organizations

Children Anguished with Lymphatic Malformations (CALM). A nonprofit organization helping children born with lymphatic abnormalities. 11411 Prestige, Frisco, TX 75034. Phone: 877-570-2256; fax: 972-377-4326; Internet: http://web2.airmail.net

General references

Frieden IJ, Eichenfield LF, Esterly NB, **et al.**: Guidelines of care for hemangiomas of infancy. **J Am Acad Dermatol** 1997, **37**:631–637.

Blei F: New clinical observations in hemangiomas. **Semin Cut Med Surg** 1999, **18**:187–194.

Drolet BA, Esterly BA, Frieden IJ: Hemangiomas in children. **N Engl J Med** 1999, **341**:173–181.

Diagnosis

Signs

Primary infection: 2- to 3-mm vesicles/pustules on erythematous base. On moist surfaces, such as mouth or vagina, vesicles quickly rupture, leaving moist erosions or ulcers, which may be only signs. Most commonly affects face, especially lips oral mucosa; in men: penile shaft, groin, perianal area, buttocks; in women: vulva, perineum, perianal area, buttocks. Bilateral tender adenopathy possible. Course, from onset of symptoms to development of crusting, may be up to 21 days.

Recurrence/first episode: Unilateral, 4–8 grouped 1- to 2-mm vesicles on erythematous base. Vesicles may turn into pustules, then crusts, before erosions form. Genital lesions crust in 4–5 days, average; heal in 9–10 days.

Immunocompromised patients: Reactivated latent HSV infection common in HIV-infected and other immunosuppressed patients. Erosions can enlarge, form painful scalloped ulcers, even at atypical sites. Severity of HSV infection reflects degree of immuno-suppression. Lesions can last weeks or months.

Symptoms

Primary infection (*ie*, no prior antibodies to herpes simplex virus 1 [HSV-1] or HSV-2): Low-grade fevers, malaise, myalgias 1–2 days before eruption; pain, tenderness, itch, dysuria. **Recurrence or first episode**: Prodrome—tingling or itching sensation, lips or genital area—1–2 days before eruption. Lesions are less tender than in primary infection.

Investigations

Viral culture: Viral typing helpful for prognosis (genital HSV-2 more likely to recur than HSV-1); 60% to 90% sensitive. **Tzanck smear** (Wright stain, Giemsa stain, methylene blue): Multinucleated giant cells in 60% of lesions with positive cultures. **Skin biopsy:** Intraepidermal vesicle with multinucleated giant cells, ballooning degeneration, acantholytic cells. **Serologic testing: False-positive results are due to cross-reactivity between HSV-1 and HSV-2.**

•Evaluate for other sexually transmitted diseases.

Complications

• Gingivostomatitis may cause difficulty swallowing and eating.

• Primary genital infections are accompanied by aseptic meningitis in 35% of women and 12% of men. Urinary retention common.

• Acquisition of HSV during third trimester associated with increased rates of neonatal herpes. Neonatal herpes affects one in 2000 US live births. Herpes cervicitis has been linked to spontaneous abortion.

• Ocular involvement (keratoconjunctivitis) can be devastating. Patients with suspected corneal involvement require slit-lamp examination.

• Skin dissemination may occur in atopic patients or with compromised skin barriers. Herpetic whitlow of the finger or hands is dental and medical occupational hazard. Herpes gladiatorum occurs among athletes (especially wrestlers).

Differential diagnosis

Syphilis, chancroid, folliculitis, fixed drug eruption, trauma, herpes zoster (most cases diagnosed as recurrent herpes simplex are actually zosteriform herpes simplex), insect bites, candidiasis, impetigo, aphthous ulcer, Behçet's disease.

Etiology

HSV-1 and HSV-2 are double-stranded DNA–enveloped viruses. Virus may cause primary skin infection or silently ascend to dorsal root ganglia, establishing latency; during reactivation, descends to epithelial or mucosal surface.

Epidemiology

(HSV-1 seropositivity rate is 70% by age 30. Most oral-labial HSV-1 infections occur in childhood (ages 1 to 5 years). HSV-2 seropositivity (generally indicative of genital infection) rate is 22%; HSV-1 is increasingly seen. Recurrent genital herpes simplex affects 25 million US adults. Sexually active young adults at greatest genital herpes risk; seropositivity higher among ethnic minorities and men who have sex with men.

Infectivity/incubation period

Primary episodes occur 2–10 days after contact with an infected individual. Most patients do not experience primary episodes, and are silently infected. Recurrent episodes are usually infectious 1 day before outbreak until 4 days after the onset of lesions. Vesicles and moist erosions are more infectious than dry crusts. Asymptomatic shedding (positive culture in absence of visible lesions) appears between clinical episodes, and may account for most transmissions.

Typical herpes simplex lesions: grouped vesicles on erythematous base.

Barry Goldman

Treatment

Diet and lifestyle

• Efficacy of over-the-counter and home remedies, lysine, undecylenic acid cream, zinc, vitamin C or E unsupported. Topical steroids may promote viral replication, shedding, satellite-lesion formation. Stress-outbreak connection doubtful.

Pharmacological treatment

Topical

•In patients with oral herpes: Acyclovir cream, q.i.d., decreases viral shedding by 1 day; penciclovir cream, q.i.d. decreases time to healing by 1 day.

Topical anesthetic agents (*ie*, benzocaine): May be soothing for a few days, but may cause contact dermatitis.

Topical antiviral agents: Have limited efficacy, and are not indicated in genital herpes.

Systemic

First clinical episode: Acyclovir, 400 mg, p.o., t.i.d., 7–10 days; acyclovir, 200 mg, p.o., five times daily, 7–10 days; famciclovir, 250 mg, p.o., t.i.d., 7–10 days; valacyclovir, 1 g, p.o. t.i.d., 7–10 days.

Episodic recurrent infection: Acyclovir, 400 mg, p.o. t.i.d., 5 days; Acyclovir, 200 mg, p.o., five times daily, 5 days; acyclovir, 800 mg, p.o., b.i.d., 5 days; famciclovir, 125 mg, p.o., b.i.d., 5 days; valacyclovir, 500 mg, p.o., b.i.d., 5 days.

Daily suppressive therapy for patients with > 6 episodes per year or difficult psychological adjustment: Acyclovir, 400 mg, p.o., b.i.d.; famciclovir, 250 mg, p.o., b.i.d.; valacyclovir, 250 mg, p.o., b.i.d.; valacyclovir, 500 mg, p.o., b.i.d.

Daily suppressive therapy for patients with > 10 recurrences per year: Valacyclovir, 1000 mg, p.o., daily.

Immunocompromised patients: Acyclovir, 400 mg 3–5 times daily, may be necessary. Consider continuous suppressive therapy if frequent relapses or slowly healing severe lesions. Initial suppressive acyclovir dosage: 400 mg, p.o., b.i.d.; may be increased. Famciclovir, 500 mg, p.o., b.i.d., may lessen recurrences, decrease viral shedding by 80% in HIV-infected patients. Valacyclovir, 500 mg, p.o., b.i.d., may be equivalent to acyclovir, 400 mg, p.o., b.i.d. Valacyclovir: 8 g/d associated with thrombotic microangiopathy during clinical trials for cytomegalovirus; no other patients, receiving up to 3 g/d developed this syndrome.

Severe disease: Acyclovir, 5–10 mg/kg, i.v., q.8h., 5–7 days.

Nonpharmacological treatment

• Warm baths, saline soaks. Bacitracin may help prevent bacterial superinfection.

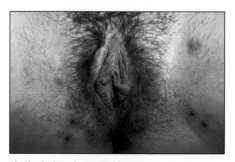

Similar lesions in genital herpes.

Herpes simplex

Treatment aims

Relieve symptoms, decrease healing and viral shedding times. Oral-labial and genital herpes episodes self-limiting, usually heal without treatment.

Special therapeutic considerations

Immunosuppressed patients: Continue therapy until all lesions heal. Most acyclovir-resistant cases are thymidine kinase–deficient; consider foscarnet (40–60 mg/kg, i.v., q.8h.), but watch for nephrotoxicity. Topical cidofovir gel appears promising. **Pregnancy and HSV**: *In neonatal herpes*, usually no clinical history of maternal genital herpes. Risk of transmission to neonate 30% to 50% with last-trimester maternal acquisition, >2% if recurrent or acquired earlier in pregnancy. Maternal antibodies provide neonate protection. Viral culturing in pregnancy does not predict viral shedding at delivery. *In pregnancy*, safety of acyclovir (category C drug) not established; famciclovir and valacyclovir are category B. Acyclovir often given to reduce duration of active primary-episode lesions; no increased risk for major birth defects found, but routine use in pregnancy not recommended.

Asymptomatic shedding and transmission

Antiviral medication may decrease number of culture-positive days by as much as 95%; HSV detectable on 8% of days during suppressive acyclovir therapy.

Prognosis

Facial-oral herpes: Annually, as many as 15% of young adults have at least one episode, usually a cold sore; 20% of patients have 4–5 recurrent episodes. **Genital herpes**: *Recurrence after primary infection*. Men, 50% within 4 months; women, 50% within 8 months. Within first year, HSV-2, 95%; HSV-1, 50%. *Average episodes per year*: HSV-2 infection, 4; HSV-1 infection, 1–2. About 15% with recurrent genital herpes average > 8 episodes.

Follow-up and management

Genital herpes: Provide supportive counseling about natural history of disease, recurrences, asymptomatic transmission, and pregnancy.

Support organizations

American Social Health Association, telephone: 800-230-6039; www.ashastd.org.

Diagnosis

Signs

Verruca vulgaris (common warts; VV): Well-demarcated, hyperkeratotic papules, plaques, nodules; usually on hands, distal fingers, knees.
Verruca plana (flat warts; VP): Small (usually 1–4 mm), flat or slightly elevated papules; usually on face, dorsal hands.
Palmoplantar warts (PP): Thick, endophytic, callused plaques; palms, soles.
Condyloma acuminata (genital warts; CA): Single or multiple, skin-colored or pigmented, papules or plaques; penis, vulva, vagina, cervix, perianal region. External lesions range from pinpoint, flat or hyperkeratotic, papillated papules to cauliflower-like nodules. Cervical warts usually flat, white, plaquelike lesions, best visualized by colposcopy.

Symptoms

• Human papillomavirus (HPV) infection usually asymptomatic, but pain, pruritus, burning, from pressure, irritation may occur. Discharge possible with urethral or vulvovaginal warts.

Investigations

Diagnosis usually clinical; black dots (thrombosed capillaries) after paring distinguishes warts from calluses. Subclinical lesions better visualized through acetowhitening.
Biopsy to diagnose lesions, exclude skin cancer. Filter hybridization, in situ hybridization, polymerase chain reaction (PCR) to determine HPV typing.
Papanicolaou smear if vaginal or cervical warts and for sex partners of infected men; for cervical dysplasia at diagnosis, then annually against high grade dysplasia, cervical cancer.
Anal smear for dysplasia in HIV-infected men with history of anal warts.
All: Evaluate for gonorrhea, chlamydia, syphilis, HIV infection other sexually transmitted diseases (STDs), based on history, physical examination. If perianal warts, evaluate by anoscopy.

Complications

• Bleeding after trauma. Warts may spread; if immunocompromised, may disseminate. Malignant transformation can occur, particularly on cervix of women, anal/perianal area of HIV-infected men. HPV-DNA in 80% to 90% of CIN-3 lesions, invasive cervical cancers. Bowenoid papulosis: cellular atypia, cell crowding, pleomorphic, hyperchromatic nuclei. Lesions difficult to distinguish from squamous cell carcinoma (SCC); cell markers have shown single polyclonal population of keratinocytes. Buschke-Lowenstein tumor: fungating, locally invasive, HPV-induced low-grade carcinoma.

Differential diagnosis

CA: Condyloma lata, SCC, seborrheic keratoses
PPB: Calluses, corns, poromas.
VP: Syringomas, sebaceous hyperplasia, fibromas, trichoepitheliomas,

Etiology

Infection occurs when the HPV enters basal keratinocyte, most likely through breaks in normal epithelium. Viral DNA migrates into nucleus of infected cell to reproduce.
Transmission: Direct contact required. Genital HPV usually sexual contact; rare reports suggest mother-to-infant transmission during childbirth.

Epidemiology

Genital HPV most common STD. Annual CA incidence, 1%; prevalence exceeds 50%, highest between older adolescence, third decade. Estimated 75% of sexually active women infected at some point. Overt disease more common in men, but risk of infection may be higher in women. HPV infection rate in asymptomatic, healthy men estimated 7%, but 69% to 77% in partners of women with detectable infection.

Skin-colored, oval or round, slightly elevated, flat-topped papules on the face; verruca plana.

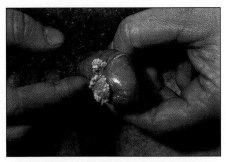

Exophytic, pink condyloma acuminata with papillated surfaces covered with macerated, gray-white scales growing on the penile frenulum.

Casey Gallagher and Louis Vogel

Treatment

Diet and lifestyle

• No proven way to prevent transmission. Condom use encouraged, but active infection may lie outside area covered by condom. Sexual partners of patients with CA at risk of infection. Cigarette smoking associated with diminished response to treatment.

Pharmacological treatment

Topical

Salicylic acid, 17% in polyacrylic solution or 40% plaster (plantar warts), daily; pare before application. **Podophyllin**, 25% to 50% resin or alcohol solution, once or twice a week, directly to condyloma, washed off with soap and water 4–6 hours later. Contraindicated in pregnant women. Cure rate about 40%. **Podophylotoxin**, 0.5% solution or gel, b.i.d., 3 consecutive days each week, maximum of 4 weeks. No more than 0.5-ml solution or 0.5-g gel in 1 day. Thorough hand-wash after each application. **Trichloroacetic acid**, 25% to 100%, directly to warts, alone or with podophyllin. Cure rate about 50%. **Imiquimod cream**, 5%, to condyloma areas, three times weekly, 10–16 weeks May be useful in nongenital warts especially applied more frequently and under occlusion. **Cantharadine**, 0.7%, or 1% (with 30% salicylic acid and 5% podophyllin) solution painted on wart under occlusion; good for hyperkeratotic, nongenital warts. **Tretinoin** liquid, 0.05%; cream, .025% to 1.0% or gel, .025% to 0.5% for flat warts; effective in warts not responsive to more common treatment. **5-Fluorouracil**, 5% cream, daily, as tolerated, 10 weeks, or 1% cream, twice daily, 2–6 weeks; useful to prevent recurrence in immunocompromised patients; risk of vaginal adenosis, clear-cell adenocarcinoma. **Cimetidine** has had more measured long-term results. **Bleomycin**: A 15-U vial reconstituted with 1–5 mL sterile water or normal saline, injected into wart. Pain may be severe after treatment. Disappearance of remaining warts reported after treatment of one. **Formalin**, 10%, with aggressive paring, plantar warts. **Interferon-α-n3**, 250,000 U injected into each wart, twice weekly, up to 8 weeks, maximum dose of 2.5 million U per treatment session; may be more effective (cure rate 50% versus 34%) than interferon-α-2b, 1 million U, intralesionally, three times weekly, 3 weeks. Relapse: 20% to 40%. **Cidofovir gel**, 1%, daily, 5 consecutive days per week, up to 12 weeks

Systemic

Retinoids (Isotretinoin, 1.0–2.0 mg/kg/d or acitretin, 0.5–1.0 mg/kg/d) in immunocompromised patients with disseminated warts who fail other treatment; recurrance after discontinuation. **Cimetidine**, 30 mg/kg/d, 3 months, alone or with levamisole, 150 mg, b.i.d.. Reports: No efficacy or complete or marked responses in up to 75%.

Nonpharmacological treatment

Immunotherapy with topical application of dinitrochlorobenzene (DNCB) or squaric arid (SA); intralesional mumps, *Candida* antigens. **Cryosurgery** with liquid nitrogen; cure rates: 60% for condymoma, 80% for warts in nonacral skin. Excision reasonable to treat one or few lesions resistant to topical therapy. **Electrosurgery**: Cure rate approximately 90% in warts smaller than 1 cm and in condyloma. **CO_2 laser** ablation: Cure rate approximately 90%; treatment of choice for large warts. **Pulsed dye laser**, 585-nm, effective against flat warts; may be reasonable against recalcitrant warts.

Special therapeutic considerations

• Warts in immunosuppressed patients often require more aggressive therapy.

Treatment aims

To eradicate pathologic tissue. Three general modalities against warts: cytodestructive, chemotherapeutic compounds, antiviral medicines; none is curative.

Prognosis

Extremely variable. Incubation period 1 to 6 months, but as long as 2 years. About two thirds develop condylomas within 3 months of sexual contact with a partner with active lesions. Warts often resolve spontaneously. Some recur after years, despite appropriate treatment. Condyloma recurrence rates exceed 50% after 1 year from reinfection by sexual contact; persistence of virus in surrounding skin, hair follicles; incomplete treatment; subclinical lesions; underlying immunosuppression.

Follow-up and management

Regularly observe warts to ensure complete treatment of infected tissue. Advise that lesions may recur; if so, retreatment necessary as soon as possible.

General references

Sedlacek TV: Advances in the diagnosis and treatment of human papillomavirus infections. *Clin Obstet Gynecol* 1999; 42:206–220.

Vogel, LN: Epidemiology of human papilloma viral infections. *Semin Dermatol* 1992, 11:226–228.

Fazel N, Wilczynski S, Lowe L, Su LD: Clinical, histopathologic, and molecular aspects of cutaneous human papillomavirus infections. *Dermatol Clin North Am* 1999, 17:521–536.

Diagnosis

Signs

• Profuse sweating, beyond what is necessary to maintain thermal regulation, affecting areas with eccrine sweat glands.

• May be generalized or localized (axillae, palms and soles, groin). Skin may become macerated in affected areas. Primary hyperhidrosis usually affects the palms, soles, and axillae.

• Emotionally induced hyperhidrosis is usually localized to the palms, soles, and forehead. These patients tend to sweat normally during sleep.

• Unilateral circumscribed hyperhidrosis is a variant with a sharply demarcated hyperhidrotic area (less than 10 x 10 cm²), usually on the face and upper extremities.

Investigations

• Evaluate both systemic and local causes of underlying disorders.

• Starch iodine test: For localized hyperhidrosis. Paint starch iodine on areas of most severe sweating; areas of greatest eccrine activity will show blue color. Also: Drape tissue paper over axillae to localize area of hyperhidrosis.

Complications

• Skin maceration, superimposed fungal or bacterial infection, occupational or functional disability due to excess sweat on hands, social embarrassment due to wet clothing, foul odor, stained and damaged clothes.

Differential diagnosis

Generalized hyperhidrosis
Exposure to heat, humidity and exercise; febrile illness, infection, malignancy; metabolic disease (hyperthyroidism, diabetes mellitus, hypoglycemia, gout, hyperpituitarism, pheochromocytoma, menopause); sympathetic discharge (shock and syncope, intense pain, alcohol and drug withdrawal); neurologic (Riley-Day syndrome [familial dysautonomia], hypothalamic lesions); vascular (Raynaud's phenomenon, erythromelalgia, arteri-ovenous fistula, cold injury); drugs (propanolol, physostigmine, pilocarpine, tricyclic antidepressants or selective serotonin reuptake inhibitor antide-pressants, venlafaxine, mercury).

Localized hyperhidrosis
Heat exposure; primary or essential hyperhidrosis; neurologic lesions (spinal cord injury, post-traumatic syringomyelia, peripheral neuropathy, brain neoplasm, Parkinson's disease); dermatological conditions (nail-patella syndrome, keratosis palmaris et plantaris, Unna-Thost keratoderma).

Etiology

Sweat glands are innervated by sympathetic postganglionic fibers of nerves using acetylcholine as neurotransmitter. Sweat control centers in the hypothalamus contain neurons that respond to changes in temperature and cerebral cortical events. Although the glands are morphologically normal, patients with hyperhidrosis have an abnormal neurological response to hypothalamic stimuli (heat, anxiety). The hypothalamic sweat centers of patients with primary hyperhidrosis are more sensitive to emotional stimuli. Excessive sweating of the hands and feet leads to a cycle in which the lowered skin temperature caused by evaporative cooling increases the reflexive sympathetic outflow, thus aggravating the hyperhidrosis.

Epidemiology

Primary hyperhidrosis affects 0.6% to 1.0% of population. May be inherited. Unlike generalized hyperhidrosis, develops in adolescence, rarely in childhood.

Lance H. Brown

Treatment

Diet and lifestyle
- Avoid excessive heat and humidity.
- Evaluate and treat anxiety.
- Avoid citric acid, coffee, chocolate, peanut butter, and spicy foods

Pharmacological treatment

Topical
- Aluminum chloride, one of the most common first-line therapies, is thought to work by mechanical obstruction of the eccrine sweat gland pores, resulting in atrophy of the eccrine glands and reduced sweating. Over-the-counter preparations are available. For more severe sweating, 20% aluminum chloride hexahydrate dissolved in anhydrous ethyl alcohol is applied to dried skin to prevent formation of hydrochloric acid. This treatment is applied at night, when sweat glands are inactive. Occlusion with plastic wrap or a transparent dressing may be used.
- Glutaraldehyde, tannic acid, or formaldehyde, painted on affected skin, may be useful but can lead to staining of the skin and sensitization (in the case of formaldehyde).
- 0.5% topical glycopyrrolate solution for facial hyperhidrosis

Systemic
- Benzodiazepines (lorazepam, alprazolam) are useful for anxiety-induced hyperhidrosis.
- Systemic anticholinergics: Propantheline, 7.5 mg three times daily or glycopyrrolate, 1–2 mg twice or three times daily. Benztropine has been used for hyperhidrosis induced by selective serotonin reuptake inhibitors.
- Nonsteroidal anti-inflammatory drugs have been used successfully in a few instances (mechanism is unclear).
- Calcium-channel blockers (eg, diltiazem) presumably inhibit calcium influx into sweat gland cells.
- Clonidine has been found to be effective for hyperhidrosis induced by tricyclic antidepressants.
- Propoxyphene (for hyperhidrosis associated with autonomic dysreflexia).

Nonpharmacological treatment

Physical modalities
- Iontophoresis: Causes plugging of pores and is effective for palmoplantar hyperhidrosis (80% response that remains for about 30 days) and less effective for axillary and groin hyperhidrosis. Used daily until response; then every 1–2 weeks for maintenance.
- Botulinum toxin: Inhibits the release of acetylcholine at both the neuromuscular junction and the postganglionic sympathetic fibers to sweat glands. Effect lasts from 4 months to 1 year, but treatment is relatively painful and can lead to weakness of neighboring muscles. Intradermal injections (as many as 50 per palm or sole), 2 units each, are given in a grid-like pattern. For axillary treatment, total amount used may be up to 100 units (50 units per axilla).

Surgery
- Surgical excision with extensive undermining and resection of exposed sweat glands for axillary hyperhidrosis that is unresponsive to other treatments. Surgical repair should include Z-plasty or other closure methods to avoid cicatricial contracture.
- For severe palmar hyperhidrosis, endoscopic transthoracic sympathectomy is preferred to upper-dorsal sympathetic ganglionectomy (T2) because of equal effectiveness (>95%), fewer complications, and higher satisfaction (60%). However, both procedures are associated with high rates (65%–85%) of compensatory hyperhidrosis, which may be more disturbing than the initial problem. Other complications include gustatory sweating, permanent Horner's syndrome, wound infection hemothorax, intercostal neuralgias, and recurrence of hyperhidrosis.
- Lumbar sympathectomy for plantar hyperhidrosis can lead to sexual dysfunction.
- With tumescent liposuction (for axillary hyperhidrosis), tunneling is performed in the superficial subcutaneous layer to avoid brachial plexus injury. The underside of overlying dermis may be scraped with the open end of the cannula to promote additional sweat gland fibrosis and injury.

Treatment aims
To reduce excessive sweating, once systemic or local causes are excluded.

Prognosis
Identification and treatment of underlying causes or elimination of inciting medication may lead to improvement of condition.

Patients with primary or essential hyperhidrosis should be offered a trial of conservative therapy, especially iontophoresis, before aggressive surgical methods are attempted.

Follow-up and management
Primary hyperhidrosis is a chronic condition that requires regular follow-up and treatment.

General references
Stolman LP: Treatment of hyperhidrosis. *Dermatol Clin* 1998, **16**:863–867.

Shelley WB, Talanin NY, et al.: Botulinum toxin therapy for palmar hyperhydrosis. *J Am Acad Dermatol* 1998, **38**:227–229.

Glogau RG: Botulinum A neurotoxin for axillary hyperhidrosis. *Dermatol Surg* 1998, **24**:817–819.

Coleman WP, Sato K, et al.: Hyperhidrosis. In *Cutaneous Medicine and Surgery: An Integrated Program in Dermatology*. Volume 2. Edited by Arndt KA, LeBoit PE, Robinson JK, Wintroub BU. Philadelphia: WB Saunders ; 1996:1311–1317.

Lance H. Brown

Diagnosis

Signs

Hyperthyroidism (H): Warm, moist, soft skin; persistent facial flushing; erythematous palms; soft, fine scalp hair; onycholysis; clubbing; asymmetric and lobular thyroid.

Graves' disease (GD): Associated with **pretibial myxedema (PTM)**, preradial myxedema, acropachy, and proptosis (periorbital swelling with lid lag and lid retraction).

PTM develops in 5% of patients (in half of those after initiation of thyroid treatment) with GD; begins as yellow or white, infiltrated, waxy plaques and nodules on legs, feet; usually becomes confluent. In time, nonpitting edema resembling orange peel is seen throughout lower extremity (most common presentation). Subsequently, skin becomes thicker, more nodular, verrucous (elephantiasic variant). Lesions occasionally localized, may become polypoid. PTM may develop in patients with chronic lymphocytic thyroiditis, who may be euthyroid or hypothyroid.

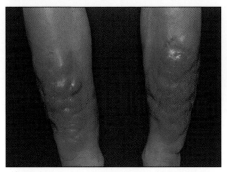

Pretibial myxedema, showing bilateral, pink nodules that coalesce into thick, indurated, plaques with a dry, hyperkeratotic surface.

Generalized myxedema (M): Diffuse dry, pale skin; nonpitting edema in acral parts; dull, listless facies; edematous eyelids; broadened nose; thick lips; brittle, dry, coarse hair; alopecia of lateral third of eyebrow; brittle nails; large tongue; palpable thyroid.

Symptoms

H: Nervousness, emotional lability, insomnia, tremors, weight loss, increased appetite, dyspnea, palpitations; angina pectoris in elderly.

M: Lethargy, cold intolerance, constipation, weight gain, deepening of voice.

Investigations

H: Thyroid-stimulating hormone (TSH) undetectable; free thyroxine (T_4), tri-iodothyronine resin uptake (T_3RU) elevated; antithyroid antibodies (antithyroglobulin, antimicrosomal, anti-TSH receptor antibodies) present in thyroiditis.

PTM: Skin biopsy: markedly thickened dermis, separation of collagen bundles and individual fibers due to huge deposition of mucin.

GM: TSH markedly elevated in primary hypothyroidism; T_3RU, free T_4 decreased; serum cholesterol increased. Skin biopsy: abnormalities, only in severe cases, include swelling, splitting of collagen bundles into individual fibers, possibly small amount of mucin between fibers; mucin also around blood vessels, hair follicles on special stains (colloidal iron, alcian blue, toluidine blue).

Complications

H: Arrythmias; hypothyroidism secondary to treatment for hyperthyroidism.

M: Coma; pericardial effusions; hypothermia; respiratory depression; megacolon.

Etiology

H: May be caused by GD, toxic multinodular goiter; induced by iodine, TSH.

GD: An autoimmune disease thought to be caused by antibodies (long acting thyroid stimulators; LATS), which stimulate the thyroid through their action on TSH receptors.

PTM: Late manifestation of GD. Onset usually followed by diagnosis of hyperthyroidism and ophthalmopathy; less commonly, diagnosis of hyperthyroidism or onset of ophthalmopathy. The cause believed to be stimulation of fibroblasts by thyroid antibodies to produce abnormally high amounts of glycosoaminoglycans (especially hyaluronic acid).

M: Dysfunction at level of hypothalmus, pituitary, or thyroid gland; may be secondary to circulating antibodies.

Epidemiology

H: Develops in third, fourth decade. Female predominance. Human leukocyte antigen (HLA)-B8 and and HLA-DRw3 increased in whites; HLA-Bw36, in Japanese; HLA-Bw46, in Chinese.

M: Age 40–60; female predominance.

Dina Began

Treatment

Pharmacological treatment

H: Symptomatic therapy for palpitations, tremor, anxiety: beta-adrenergic antagonists. Radioactive iodine. Thionamides (methimazole and propylthiouracil inhibit thyroid hormone synthesis).

GM: Synthetic levothyroxine, orally, daily.

PTM: Class I topical corticosteroids under occlusion may be effective in early disease. Less potent corticosteroids may then be administered (38% have long term partial remissions). Intravenous steroid pulse therapy followed by oral therapy with gradual tapering. High-dose intravenous immunoglobulin. Plasmapheresis followed by immunosuppressive therapy.

Surgery

H: Subtotal thyroidectomy.

PTM: Excision of a pseudotumorous manifestation

Special therapeutic considerations

H: May become hypothyroid.

M: Comanagement with internal medicine/endocrinology. Monitor patient closely; monitor replacement therapy by checking TSH level.

Treatment aims

H: To correct the hyperthyroidism.
M: To correct the hypothyroidism.

Prognosis

H and **M**: Good.

PTM: May persist for months or years. Often regresses spontaneously; however, some patients progress to elephantiasis.

General references

Wartofsky L. Diseases of the thyroid. In: *Harrison's Principles of Internal Medicine*, vol. 2, edn. 14. Edited by Fauci AS, Braunwald E, Isselbacher KJ, *et al*. New York: McGraw-Hill Health Professions Division; 1998:2012–2034, 2053–2054.

Fatourechi V, Pajouhi M, Fransway AF: Dermopathy of Graves' disease (pretibial myxedema). Review of150 cases. *Medicine* 1994, 73:1–7.

Ohtsuka Y, Yamamoto K, Goto Y, *et al*.: Localized myxedema, associated with increased serum hyaluronic acid, and response to steroid pulse therapy. [review] *Intern Med* 1995, 34:424–429.

Diagnosis

Signs

Hypertrichosis: Excessive growth of androgen-independent hair, anywhere on body; either sex. Associated with anorexia nervosa, malnutrition, porphyria, hypothyroidism; can be drug-induced.

Hirsutism: Excessive growth of androgen-responsive terminal hair on upper lip, chin, chest, upper arms, thighs, abdomen, back. Usually benign. Rare in men. Associated with androgen overproduction or virilization (acne, deepening of voice, temporal balding, clitoris > 1.0 cm in diameter, increased muscle mass in limb girdles), cortisol excess (plethora, centripetal obesity, striae, dorsocervical/supraclavicular fat pads, easy bruising), or insulin resistance (obesity, acanthosis nigricans).

•In polycystic ovarian syndrome (PCOS), irregular menses very common. In hyperprolactinemia, galactorrhea occurs, even if normal menstrual cycle.

Investigations

•Review for onset (acute *vs.* chronic), obesity, secondary amenorrhea, galactorrhea, symptoms of virilization, medications, personal/family history of diabetes, excessive hair.

Laboratory testing

•Not warranted for mild, gradually progressive hirsutism, acne, or androgenic alopecia responsive to simple topical therapy and not associated with menstrual abnormality.

•Laboratory tests for hirsutism associated with acne that is resistant to simple therapies or is of rapid onset in a nonpubertal female include **testosterone** (measured as free or total, best overall estimate of androgen production; normal values exclude ovarian/adrenal tumor), **dehydroepiandrosterone sulfate** (DHEA-S; especially important in rapidly progressing hirsutism; normal values exclude adrenal tumors), and **follicle-stimulating hormone** (elevated levels indicate declining ovarian function, or premature ovarian failure).

Evaluation

•If both serum testosterone and DHEA-S levels are normal and neither menstrual abnormalities nor galactorrhea is present, no further tests are warranted.

•If DHEA-S level > 800 ng/dL or testosterone level is > 200 ng/dL, with rapid-onset hirsutism or virilization, perform a CT scan of the adrenals and ovaries. If DHEA-S level is high but < 800 ng/dL or testosterone level is high but < 200 ng/dL and patient has galactorrhea or menstrual irregularities, measure serum prolactin level.

•If prolactin level is elevated, perform a brain MRI scan for prolactinoma. If normal (or if high clinical suspicion of Cushing's syndrome), perform an overnight dexamethasone suppression test.

•In PCOS and idiopathic hirsutism, testosterone level is probably normal. Diagnose PCOS by 5-day dexamethasone suppression test (0.5 mg, p.o., q.6h.), with before-and-after measurements of plasma-free testosterone, cortisol, and DHEA-S.

Additional laboratory tests

Serum 17-hydroxyprogesterone: More important in younger girls, women with early-onset hirsutism, associated hyperkalemia, positive family history; elevated level suggests 21-hydroxylase deficiency; draw blood between 7 a.m. and 9 a.m.

Thyroid-stimulating hormone (TSH).

Fasting serum glucose: Elevated insulin level, seen in insulin resistance, stimulates ovarian androgen production.

Luteinizing hormone (LH): Elevated level suggests, but is not specific for PCOS; 25% of patients with PCOS have normal LH levels.

Hypertrichosis: Only TSH determination is recommended.

Complications

•Complications are related to underlying cause.

Etiology

Hirsutism
An androgen excess or increased androgen sensitivity of the skin; most cases are idiopathic or caused by PCOS. Causes of androgen excess: **Pituitary/adrenal**, including pituitary adenomas (tumors that secrete adrenocorticotropic hormone, *eg*, small-cell lung carcinoma, pancreatic islet-cell carcinomas, thymus tumors); congenital adrenal hyperplasia (deficiencies of 21-hydroxylase, 11-hydroxylase, 3β-hydroxysteroid dehydrogenase); androgen-producing adrenal tumors (adrenal adenomas and carcinomas); **ovarian**, including virilizing ovarian neoplasms (granulosa-stromal cell tumors, Sertoli-Leydig cell tumors); insulin resistance; **combined adrenal and ovarian**, including PCOS and idiopathic hirsutism (including increased androgen sensitivity of the skin); **medications/drug use**, including anabolic steroids, danazol, some oral contraceptives, medications that cause hyperprolactinemia (metoclopramide; high-dose phenothiazines; butyrophenones, such as haloperidol, thioxanthenes, methyldopa, reserpine, estrogens, opiates).

Hypertrichosis
Hypothyroidism (causes an increase in free testosterone level); anorexia nervosa, porphyria (porphyria cutanea tarda, variegate porphyria, erythropoietic porphyria), medications, including phenytoin, minoxidil, diazoxide, cyclosporine, hexachlorobenzene, psoralen plus ultraviolet A.

Epidemiology

Benign (non-neoplastic) hirsutism progresses slowly over years, often affects peripubertal females, can begin after period of weight gain or discontinuation of oral contraceptives. Rapidly worsening hirsutism not occurring during puberty should prompt a higher suspicion for androgen-secreting neoplasms.

Women tend to gradually develop more body hair until menopause, after which a slow depilation occurs. In postmenopausal women, combined estrogen-androgen hormone replacement may be the cause.

Bruce E. Strober and Christopher Nanni

Treatment

Diet and lifestyle
•Weight loss essential to decrease secretion of gonadotropin, androgen, insulin, decrease insulin resistance. Systemic treatments contraindicated in pregnancy. Cosmetic measures may be helpful.

Pharmacological treatment

Topical
•Cosmetic therapy should commence concomitantly with medical therapy.

•Chemical depilatories with calcium thioglycolate are effective but can irritate face, and are malodorous, messy; some brands are better tolerated than others. Mild corticosteroid may be necessary after depilatory removal, to avert irritation.

•Eflornithine cream, 15%, b.i.d., reduces facial hair growth in 60% of women.

Systemic
•Ovarian suppression effective against ovarian hyperandrogenism, including PCOS. Preferred: oral contraceptives using lowest effective dose of estrogens (30–50 µg ethinyl estradiol) and synthetic progestins with less androgenicity (eg, norgestimate, desogestrel). Avoid androgenic 19-nortestosterone progestins (eg, norgestrel, norethindrone). Cyproterone acetate antiandrogen, in combination with ethynylestradiol (available in Europe), effectively reduces androgen production. If condition unresponsive, give analogue of gonadotropin-releasing hormones subcutaneously, estrogen/progesterone supplementation.

Adrenal suppression: Glucocorticoids (ie, prednisone, 2.5–5.0 mg, p.o., q.d.; dexamethasone, 0.25 mg, p.o., q.a.m.; hydrocortisone, 10–20 mg, p.o., q.d.) for congenital adrenal hyperplasia; efficacy varies, enhanced by concomitant antiandrogen.

Antiandrogens: **Spironolactone**, 25–100 mg, p.o., b.i.d. Improvement in 70% of women within 6 months. Combine with oral contraceptive to reduce irregular menstrual frequency. Drug of choice for obese or hypertensive patients. Avoid in patients with renal insufficiency or patients prone to hyperkalemia. **Cyproterone acetate**, 25 mg, p.o., q.d., or 25–100 mg, p.o., during first 10 days of cyclical 21-day course of estrogen, or 25–100 mg during first 10 days of oral contraceptive cycle. Benefits patients with PCOS with increased testosterone. Cyclic administration reduces chance of adverse effects. Not approved in United States. **Flutamide**, 250 mg, p.o., b.i.d., given with oral contraceptive: potent, nonsteroidal, selective antiandrogen; efficacy similar to spironolactone and cyproterone. Expensive, associated with serious, potentially fatal hepatocellular necrosis, cholestasis in approximately 0.5% of patients. **Finasteride**, 1 mg, p.o., q.d., a 5α-reductase inhibitor, may be useful in postmenopausal women. Risk of ambiguous genitalia in male fetus exposed during first trimester.

Nonpharmacological treatment

Bleaching.

Shaving: Electric razor preferred.

Plucking: Effective for eyebrows, around nipples; pain, folliculitis, postinflammatory hyperpigmentation may occur.

Waxing: Removes hairs from beneath skin; results last longer (2–6 weeks).

Electrolysis: Can permanently prevent subsequent growth, but painful and can cause scarring, hyperpigmentation.

Laser epilation: With long-pulsed ruby, Nd:YAG, alexandrite, intense pulse light, or diode laser; effectiveness varies in direct proportion to number of anagen hairs in body site (upper lip, 65%; legs, bikini line, 20% to 30%; ears, eyebrows, 10% to 15%). Several treatments required. Light-skinned persons best candidates; treat dark-skinned persons using lower energy levels, cooling system. Minimal effect on hair lacking target chromophore (melanin), unless dyed black. Not inexpensive. Proven long-term results.

Bruce E. Strober and Christopher Nanni

Treatment aims
To prevent further hair loss. Depending on underlying cause, objectives include suppressing androgen production, blocking androgen effect. @SIDEHEAD:Prognosis Pharmacological therapy must continue longer than the growth cycle of the hairs involved. Improvement with medical management may continue for 2–3 years.

Prognosis
Pharmacological therapy must continue longer than the growth cycle of the hairs involved. Improvement, with medical management, may continue for 2–3 years.

General references
Rittmaster RS: Hirsutism. *Lancet* 1997, **349:**191–195.

Sakiyama R: Approach to Patients with Hirsutism. *West J Med 1996,* **165:**386–391.

Watson RE, Bouknight R, Alguire PC: Hirsutism: Evaluation and Management. J Gen Intern Med 1995, **10:**283–292.

Nanni CA, Alster TS: A practical review of laser-assisted hair removal using the Q-switched Nd:YAG, long-pulsed ruby, and long-pulsed alexandrite lasers. *Dermatol Surg* 1998, **24:**1399–1405.

Hughes CL: Hirsutism. In *Disorders of Hair Growth.* Edited by Olsen EA. New York: McGraw-Hill; 1994:337–351.

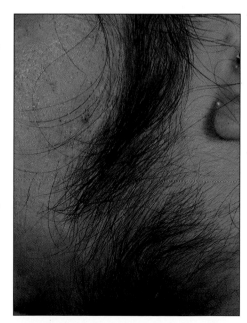

Hirsutism: Excessive, long terminal hairs on woman's face, neck.

Diagnosis

Definition

• Most common ichthyoses:

DOC1, ichthyosis vulgaris (IV).

DOC2 (steroid sulfatase deficiency), X-linked recessive ichthyosis (XLI).

DOC3 (bullous type), epidermolytic hyperkeratosis (EH) or congenital ichthyosiform erythroderma (bullous form).

DOC4 (recessive lamellar icthyosis).

DOC6 (dominant lamellar ichthyosis; LI).

DOC5, nonbullous form of congenital ichthyosiform erythroderma (CIE).

•Xerosis is dry skin.

Signs

Xerosis: Localized or diffuse fine, small white scales.

IV: Fine white or translucent scales; hyperlinear palms, soles. Affects extremities more often than trunk; flexor parts of extremities are relatively spared.

XLI: Thick, brown, variably-sized scale make skin appear dirty; asymptomatic corneal opacities (50% to 100% of males, less often in heterozygotic females). Flexor involvement in 10%. Involvement of neck, preauricular regions aids diagnosis.

EH: Variable morphology, may represent several distinct disorders. Generally, blistering and erythroderma are present at birth, wane in childhood. Linear, palmoplantar, flexural keratoses become more prominent through childhood, persist in adulthood.

CIE Often born as "collodion babies." Generalized fine white scale with flexural prominence, diffuse erythroderma develops. Ectropion and eclabium may be seen.

LI Collodion babies. Shedding reveals large, brown, plate-like scales over entire body. Often, alopecia, ectropion, erythroderma between scales. Scale generalized but more pronounced on forehead, flexors, legs. Thickened palms, soles.

Symptoms

Xerosis and **IV**: Occasionally pruritus.

EH: Foul odor secondary to bacterial colonization.

CIE and **LI**: Heat intolerance/hyperpyrexia due to hypohidrosis.

Investigations

•Diagnosis usually by clinical features. Biopsy may be needed to rule out ichthyosis or determine type. Histologically, all ichthyoses show hyperkeratosis.

IV: Granular layer thin or absent, follicular plugging seen.

XLI: Granular layer normal or thickened.

EH: Many keratinocytes have clear halos around nuclei, granular layer markedly thickened, mitotic figures increased, inflammatory infiltrate in upper dermis.

CIE and **LI**: Histologically similar; CIE—generally, mildly thickened stratum corneum with parakeratosis; LI—markedly thickened stratum corneum but no parakeratosis.

Complications

IV: 50% of patients have atopic dermatitis.

XLI: Cryptorchidism occurs in 12% of patients, resulting in a higher incidence of testicular cancer.

EH: Recurrent skin infections. **LI** and **CIE**: Hyperpyrexia. Incidence of squamous and basal-cell carcinomas increased in CIE.

Differential diagnosis

Ichthyoses can be misdiagnosed as severe xerosis, atopic dermatitis, or mycosis fungoides.

Etiology

Xerosis: Combination of genetic, environmental factors likely. Increased incidence with age likely from age-related skin changes that impair barrier function.**IV** (autosomal dominant): Molecular defect has not been identified. Filaggrin concentration is decreased in tissue. **X-linked ichthyosis**: Retention hyperkeratosis linked to deletion or mutation of the gene for steroid sulfatase (*Xp22.3*). This leads to increased cholesterol sulfate and decreased cholesterol in the stratum corneum. Elevated cholesterol sulfate may slow degradation of desmosomes and impair desquamation. **EH** (autosomal dominant): Classic form has been linked to point mutations in keratins 1 and 10 that provide mechanical stability in the epidermis above the basal layer. Siemens type has been linked to keratin 2e. Epidermolytic palmar/plantar keratoderma of Voerner type has been linked to mutations of keratin 9. **LI** (autosomal recessive): Not hyperproliferative. In many families, the disease locus maps to 14q11 and mutations of the *TGM1* gene have been found. The tgase 1 enzyme cross-links loricin and involucrin, which form the scaffold for the "cell envelope" (the protein layer on the inner surface of stratum corneum keratinocytes that provides a physical barrier in the epidermis). In some families, another disease locus mapping to 2q33-35 (ICR2B locus) has been identified. **CIE** (autosomal recessive): Hyperproliferative process. Bullous form has been linked to mutations of keratins 1 and 10. Nonbullous CIE has been mapped to the same transglutaminase 1 (*TGM 1*) gene as LI in families from Norway and in other subsets.

Epidemiology

Xerosis: Very common, especially in dry climates, cold weather months, elderly persons. **IV**: Incidence, 1:250–2000. **XLI**: Incidence, 1:2000–6000 males. Prenatal diagnosis is available. **EH**: Prevalence, 1:100 000–300 000. 50% of cases may be due to new mutations. Prenatal diagnosis is available. **LI**: Incidence, 1:300 000. Prenatal diagnosis is available. **CIE**: Incidence, 1:300 000.

Chrysalyne Delling Schmults and Irwin M. Freedberg

Treatment

Diet and lifestyle
•Humidifier or humid climate often improves xerosis and ichthyosis. Important to avoid heat, prolonged strenuous exercise in CIE and LI, especially for infants, small children, as decreased perspiration impairs thermoregulation.

Pharmacological treatment

Topical
•Emollient lotions, creams, and ointments (for xerosis and as adjuvants for ichthyoses); with lactic acid or glycolic acid.

•Keratolytics: 10% to 40% urea, 5% to 10% salicylic acid in hydrophilic petrolatum or propylene glycol-base, or 60% propylene glycol. Absorption and effect can be increased with occlusion, but toxicity (even death) from increased systemic absorption can occur in children.

•Topical retinoids (tretinoin, tazarotene): Irritating to skin, disappointing in effectiveness.

•Antifungals: If tinea corporis, capitis, versicolor, or onychomycosis is present.

•Antibacterials (4% chlorhexidine, antibiotic ointments): For bacterial superinfection and malodor.

Systemic
•Retinoids, such as acitretin (25–50 mg/d) or isotretinoin (0.5–1.5 mg/kg), improve ichthyosis; despite need for long-term use, may be indicated for LI, CIE. Adverse effects at higher doses may preclude long-term treatment.

•Antibiotics against *Staphylococcus aureus* for infected bullous lesions of CIE.

Nonpharmacological treatment
LI, **CIE**: Surgical correction of ectropion.

Xerosis: Brief, infrequent, cool-to-lukewarm showers; emollients to minimize transepidermal water loss.

Ichthyosis: Long baths with mineral oil-based or cottonseed oil-based products; emollients to hydrate stratum corneum and prevent moisture evaporation. Mild abrasives (loofa sponges) to thin stratum corneum.

Special therapeutic considerations
• In acquired ichthyosis, exclude underlying malignancies (Hodgkin's disease most commonly), drug reactions (nicotinic acid, nafoxidine, haloperidol, antilipid drugs, protease inhibitors), endocrine (especially thyroid) disease, metabolic disease, sarcoidosis, connective tissue disease (systemic lupus erythematosus, dermatomyositis), AIDS, graft-versus-host disease. Gene therapy for ichthyoses is investigational.

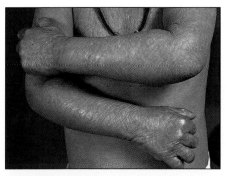

Child with typical large, plate-like scales of lamellar ichthyosis.

Treatment aims
Amelioration and remission. Curative treatments are not available. Topical treatment with emollients or mild keratolytics and good skin care are generally sufficient to improve xerosis. However, a combination of topical and systemic therapy may be necessary to treat ichthyosis.

Prognosis
Xerosis can be well-controlled with treatment. All ichthyoses are chronic, although X-linked ichthyosis may improve during adulthood. Lamellar ichthyosis generally most severe and debilitating ichthyosis.

Follow-up and management
Individualized by patient on the basis of disease severity.

Support organizations
Foundation for Ichthyosis and Related Skin Types, Box 669, Ardmore, PA 19003, Phone: 800-545-3286; fax: 610-789-4366, e-mail: ichthyosis@aol.com, Internet: http://www.libertynet.org/ichthyos/.

General references
Ammirati CT, Mallory SB: The major inherited disorders of cornification. *Dermatol Clin* 1998, **16**:497–508.

Bale SJ, DiGiovanna JJ: Genetic approaches to understanding the keratinopathies. *Adv Dermatol* 1997, **12**:99–113.

Diagnosis

Signs

Phase I
- Acute febrile period, with an average duration of 12 days.

- A polymorphous eruption, seen in 92% of patients, appears 1–3 days after onset of fever, usually starting as erythematous macules on palms and soles that spread to trunk and extremities within 2 days.

- Urticaria-like lesions are most common, followed by morbilliform, scarlatiniform, and erythema multiforme–like patterns (< 5% of cases).

- Confluent erythematous plaques on perineum can persist after other lesions disappear.

- Other findings include reddening of palms and soles (90%); firm, indurated edema of hands and feet (75%); deeply erythematous to violaceous brawny edema of palms and soles, with fusiform swelling of digits, bilateral vascular dilatation of bulbar conjunctivae (begins 2 days after onset of fever and persists 1–3 weeks) (90%); diffuse oropharyngeal erythema, and erythema with protuberance of papillae of tongue (strawberry tongue) (77%).

Phase II
- Subacute phase, during which the risk of sudden death from coronary thrombosis is highest.

- Starts 14–20 days after onset of fever and continues for about 1 week.

- Findings include fever resolution, thrombocytosis, elevated erythrocyte sedimentation rate (ESR), cardiac findings (pericardial tamponade, dysrhythmias, rubs, congestive heart failure, left ventricular dysfunction), and a highly characteristic pattern of desquamation (94%), which begins at the tips of the fingers and toes, and progresses to desquamation of sheets of palmar/plantar epidermis.

Phase III
- Convalescent period; begins approximately 8–10 weeks after onset of illness, from the time when all signs of illness have disappeared until ESR normalizes.

- Beau's lines and telogen effluvium may be present.

Symptoms

- Fever of sudden onset

- Constitutional symptoms, including diarrhea, arthralgias, photophobia, and complications, *eg*, arthritis, hepatic dysfunction, meatitis, tympanitis, and aseptic meningitis.

Investigations

- Diagnostic criteria: Temperature >39.4 °C, lasting > 5 days, without other known cause, plus four of the five following criteria:

1. Bilateral conjunctival injection.

2. At least one mucous membrane abnormality, *ie*, injected or fissured lips, injected pharynx, strawberry tongue.

3. At least one extremity involvement, *ie*, palmoplantar erythema, edema of hands and feet, generalized or periungual desquamation.

4. Polymorphous exanthem.

5. Cervical lymphadenopathy, usually unilateral and ≥1.5 cm in diameter.

Laboratory monitoring: Complete blood count, with differential, liver function tests, urinalysis, cardiovascular monitoring (baseline echocardiography, cardiac angiography).

Complications

- Leukocytosis (leukocyte count >18,000 cells/mm³); polycythemia; mild anemia; elevated hepatic enzyme levels; thrombocytosis; elevated ESR; pyuria; prolonged PR and QT intervals; ST-segment and T-wave changes; coronary aneurysms; sudden death due to myocardial infarction or dysfunction.

Differential diagnosis
Infectious mononucleosis, viral exanthems, scarlet fever, leptospirosis, Rocky Mountain spotted fever, Lyme disease, toxic shock syndrome, erythema multiforme, serum sickness, systemic lupus erythematosus, juvenile rheumatoid arthritis, Reiter syndrome, drug reaction.

Etiology
Unclear; infectious etiology has been implicated.

Epidemiology
Most patients (85%) are younger than 5 years of age; 50% are younger than 2.5 years. Some patients are older than 10 years.

Special considerations
Highest mortality seen in boys younger than 6 months of age.

Sara L. Tarsis and Mary W. Chang

Treatment

Pharmacological treatment

Systemic

• Aspirin: 100 mg/kg per day until fever is controlled or until day 14 of illness; then, 5–10 mg/kg per day, until ESR and platelet count normalize (approximately 6–12 weeks after onset of illness) plus a single dose of intravenous gamma-globulin: 2 g/kg in a 10- to 12-hour infusion.

• Systemic corticosteroids are contraindicated because of higher rate of coronary aneurysms.

Nonpharmacological treatment

Supportive methods

• Cool compresses for fever.

• Topical emollients or low-potency topical corticosteroids for skin eruption, if pruritic.

Surgery

Surgical revascularization for severe artery abstruction.

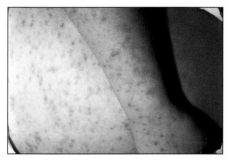

Kawasaki syndrome presents as a generalized, morbilliform (measles-like) eruption.

Treatment aims

Prompt diagnosis to prevent cardiovascular complications. Hospitalize patient during acute febrile stage to monitor for cardiac and vascular complications.

Prognosis

Uneventful recovery in most patients. Coronary artery abnormalities develop in 20%–25% of patients with untreated disease.

Treatment with intravenous gamma-globulin in the acute phase decreases this risk three-to fivefold.

Coronary aneurysms resolve in 5–18 months in approximately 50% of affected patients.

Overall mortality, originally 1%; with institution of prompt therapy, now estimated at 0.04%.

Follow-up and management

Follow-up echocardiogram between 21 and 28 days after onset of fever.

Long-term follow-up of all patients with Kawasaki disease is necessary; delayed complications have been reported.

General references

Laupland KB, Davies HD: Epidemiology, etiology and management of Kawasaki disease: state of the art. *Pediatr Cardiol* 1999, **20**:177–183.

Taubert KA, Shulman ST: Kawasaki disease. *Am Fam Phys* 1999, **59**:3093–3102.

Hurwitz S: Kawasaki disease. In *Clinical Pediatric Dermatology*, edn 2. Edited by Hurwitz S. 1993:543–549.

Diagnosis

Signs

- Primary lesions are scaly, rough-textured, flesh-colored papules that develop a yellow-tan crust. Papules often coalesce into crusted, thickened, and even verrucous plaques.

- A seborrheic distribution is common (on forehead, nasolabial folds, scalp, chest, back, ears, groin). Multiple punctate keratotic papules (acrokeratosis, verruciformis-like) develop on the palms and soles, and white punctate papules with a cobblestoning pattern develop on mucosal surfaces.

- Nail findings include thin brittle nails, V-shaped nicks (paronychia), and longitudinal red and white lines with ridging.

- Variants include vesiculobullous, hypertrophic, erosive, and hemorrhagic forms. The linear or zosteriform type probably results from genetic mosaicism and often follows Blaschko's lines.

Symptoms

- Pruritus can be intense. Foul odor is secondary to bacterial overgrowth.

Investigations

- Biopsy shows suprabasal acantholysis, often with lacunae formation, villous projections of basal cells into the lacunae, and dyskeratosis. Cells with basophilic pyknotic nuclei surrounded by clear or eosinophilic halos (corps ronds) are present in the granular and horny layers. Large parakeratotic cells in the stratum corneum (grains) are also characteristic.

- Bacterial culture, if bacterial superinfection is suspected.

- Tzank stain and viral culture, if herpes virus infection if suspected.

Complications

- Impetigo and other pyodermas.

- Disseminated, painful herpes simplex infection with vesicles and crusted erosions.

- Salivary-gland obstruction, if ductal epithelium is involved.

- The disease is especially disfiguring when the face and scalp are involved. Pigmentation and scarring from chronic scratching may occur.

- Retinitis pigmentosa, presence of bone cysts, encephalopathy, epilepsy, and affective disorders have been reported, rarely, in association with Darier's disease.

Differential diagnosis

Seborrheic dermatitis, benign familial pemphigus, pemphigus foliaceous, epidermal nevi (for linear and localized variants of Darier's disease).

Etiology

Inheritance is autosomal dominant. Disease penetrance is H 95%, but new mutations are common.

The disease is caused by mutation of the *ATP2A2* gene on chromosome 12q. *ATP2A2* codes for the calcium pump SERCA2 (sarco/endoplasmic reticulum Ca^{2+}-ATPase isoform 2), which is believed to be involved in a calcium-mediated signal transduction pathway that regulates cell adhesion in keratinocytes.

Electron microscopy studies of Darier's lesions show disruption of tonofilament attachments to cell membranes and decreased numbers of basal-cell desmosomes.

Epidemiology

Begins in the first or second decade of life.

Incidence varies: 1:36,000 (United Kingdom) to 1:100,000 (Denmark).

Lesions may be precipitated by heat, humidity, ultraviolet B light, friction, systemic bacterial infection, herpes virus infection, oral lithium therapy, exposure to phenol or ethyl chloride spray, and premenstrual flares.

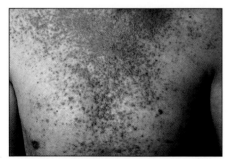

Typical appearance of intensely pruritic eruption due to Darier's disease.

Chrysalyne Delling Schmults and Irwin M. Freedberg

Treatment

Diet and lifestyle

• Minimize or eliminate predisposing factors.

• Recommended: use of absorbent powders and cool cotton clothing in warm weather to minimize moisture and friction, air conditioning to control humidity, and sun screens to avoid flare-ups related to ultraviolet light.

Pharmacological treatment

Topical

• Moisturizers containing 6% salicylic acid or lactic acid help to reduce scale (avoid using on excoriated areas).

• Topical retinoids (tretinoin, tazarotene) decrease hyperkeratosis, but irritation limits usefulness. Topical corticosteroids may be used concomitantly with retinoids to decrease irritation. Treatment should be initiated on alternate days, then advanced to daily application.

• Antibacterial solutions (chlorhexidine) or ointments to control bacterial colonization (usually with *Staphylococcus aureus*).

Systemic

• Oral retinoids are the mainstay of treatment. Acitretin is begun at 25 mg/d and dosage is increased until disease is controlled (0.6 mg/kg is generally the maximum). Dosages as low as 10 mg/d may be sufficient, and medication can sometimes be discontinued without relapse. Maximal effect is reached in 2–3 months. Women must avoid pregnancy during and for 2 years after therapy. Isotretinoin, 0.5–1.5 mg/kg/d is especially useful for women of childbearing age because pregnancy is safe 2 months after discontinuation of therapy.

• Oral antibiotics (antistaphylococcal) are useful for control of bacterial superinfection. Long-term low-dose antibiotic prophylaxis may be needed to prevent infections that result in disease flares.

• Herpes antivirals may be used if herpes virus infection is suspected

• Oral contraceptives may reduce premenstrual disease flares.

Nonpharmacological treatment

• Surgical excision has been used to debulk hypertrophic lesions.

• CO_2 and YAG laser ablation and electrodesiccation have been used to treat refractory lesions; lesion resolution has been reported.

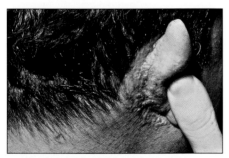

Hyperkeratotic, greasy-looking papules become confluent into excoriated, crusted, warty, lichenified plaques in the postauricular area, of a man with Darier's disease.

Treatment aims

To control disease and promote remission.

Special therapeutic considerations

Bullous or erosive forms of Darier's disease may be very difficult to manage and may require hospitalization for careful monitoring of fluid balance and electrolytes and for aggressive treatment of infections.
Control pruritus with antipruritic lotions and antihistamines to prevent koebnerization.

Prognosis

The disease is chronic, with multiple flares and remissions. Severity varies widely between patients and within cases.

Follow-up and management

Patients should be followed at regular intervals, particularly if they are receiving topical or oral retinoid therapy.

Support organizations

F.I.R.S.T.—Foundation for Ichthyosis and Related Skin Types, P.O. Box 669, Ardmore, PA 19003, Phone: 610-789-3995 or 800-545-3286, fax: 610-789-4366, e-mail: ichthyosis@aol.com, Internet: http://www.libertynet.org/ichthyos.

General references

Sakuntabhai A, *et al*.: Mutations in ATP2A, encoding a CA2+ pump, cause Darier disease. *Nature Genet* 1999, **21**:271–277.

Burge S: Management of Darier's disease. *Clin Exp Dermatol* 1999, **24**:53–56.

Telfer NR, *et al*.: Vesiculo-bullous Darier's disease. *Br J Dermatol* 1990, **122**:831–834.

Burge SM, *et al*.: Darier-White disease: a review of the clinical features in 163 patients. *J Am Acad Dermatol* 1992, **27**:40–50.

Diagnosis

Keratosis pilaris (KP) is a common disorder in which orthokeratotic plugs dilate follicular infundibula. In addition to classic KP, there are three rare, related disorders: **keratosis pilaris atrophicans faciei (ulerythema ophryogenes; KPAF), keratosis follicularis spinulosa decalvans (ichthyosis follicularis; KFSD),** and **atrophoderma vermiculatum (AV).** A similar disorder, **folliculitis decalvans (FD),** which may be infectious in etiology, also occurs.

Signs

KP: Gray-to-white keratotic papules in follicular distribution, often with perifollicular erythema. If erythema is prominent, condition is termed keratosis pilaris rubra. Most commonly affected sites are extensor surfaces of upper arms (92%), upper lateral thighs (59%), and buttocks (30%).

KPAF: KP present, but face is also involved. Lateral third of the eyebrow is affected first, often during infancy. Gradual hair loss becomes evident during childhood. Cheeks and neck may also be involved, and perifollicular erythema is prominent.

KFSD: Follicular keratotic papules on scalp and eyebrows present in early childhood, followed by progressive scarring alopecia. Face, neck, and body (KP) also often involved. Eyelashes often grow in different directions. Axillary and pubic hair may be thin.

AV: Follicular plugging involving cheeks and preauricular areas. Atrophic scarring is more severe than in the other atrophic forms of KP, resulting in pit-like scars in a reticulate or honeycomb pattern.

FD: Follicular keratotic plugging of scalp, with prominent inflammation and pustules. As disease progresses, scarring occurs, with tufts of surviving follicles present within lesions.

Symptoms

KP and **KPAF** are generally asymptomatic but pruritus may occur.

KFSD: Photophobia often occurs.

Investigations

- Diagnosis is generally made by clinical appearance.
- Skin biopsy in both KP and KPAF shows a superficial perivascular and sometimes perifollicular lymphohistiocytic inflammatory infiltrate. In KPAF, giant cells and atrophic hair bulbs are seen in later stages of disease; hair bulbs may be absent. A foreign-body reaction may lead to the atrophy and sclerosis seen in end-stage disease.
- Immunofluorescence is negative.
- Electron microscopy shows increased numbers of abnormal keratohyalin granules and delayed desmosomal dissolution.

Complications

KP: Association with atopy, ichthyosis vulgaris, renal insufficiency, vitamin B_2 and C deficiencies, Cushing's disease, hypothyroidism, prolidase deficiency, systemic adrenocorticotropic hormone administration, Noonan syndrome, cardiofaciocutaneous syndrome, Down syndrome, Fairbanks syndrome, Olmstead syndrome, and ectodermal dysplasia.

KPAF: Association with monosomy 18p, ectodermal defects, Noonan syndrome, and multiple congenital abnormalities.

KFSD: Corneal dystrophy, which generally does not affect vision. Cicatricial alopecia can also be prominent. KFSD has been reported to occur in Noonan syndrome and aminoaciduria.

AV: Pit-like scarring, which can occur in patients with Down syndrome, epidermal cysts, folliculitis decalvans, Rombosyndrome, and intraauricular septal defect.

Differential diagnosis

KP: Lichen spinulosus, pityriasis rubra pilaris, phrynoderma.

KPAF: Seborrheic dermatitis (in early KPAF).

KFSD: Atopic dermatitis, follicular ichthyosis, KID syndrome (keratitis, ichthyosis, and deafness), atrichia.

AV: Acne infantum, acne scarring in adults.

Etiology

All: Initial event is considered to be abnormal keratinization of follicular infundibulum, resulting in dilation of infundibular orifice by a keratotic plug.

KP: Increased incidence in puberty and in hyperandrogenetic obese women; hormonal influence has been suggested. Inheritance appears to be autosomal dominant, but an X-linked recessive form may also exist. Three reports have documented 18p deletions.

KPAF is thought to be autosomal dominant.

KFSD: X-linked recessive disorder mapped to Xp21.13-22.2 in most pedigrees analyzed.

AV: Probably an autosomal dominant disease, but recessive inheritance has also been proposed.

Epidemiology

KP: Incidence is estimated to be 40% in adults, 50%–80% in adolescents (girls less often than boys). Begins during the first decade in 51%, second decade in 35%, third decade in 12%.

KPAF: Most common of the atrophic keratosis pilaris, but incidence is unknown.

KFSD and **AV**: Very rare. AV begins later than other atrophic keratosis pilaris diseases (at 5–12 years in most cases).

Chrysalyne Delling Schmults and Cynthia Loomis

Treatment

Pharmacological treatment

Topical
- Urea, 10% to 40%, cream or lotion.
- Salicylic acid, 5% to 10%, compounded in an emollient or in propylene glycol; ammonium lactate, 12% cream or lotion.
- Peels: Salicylic acid, 20% or 30%, and trichloroacetic acid, 15% to 50%, for recalcitrant KP.
- Glycolic acid lotions or peels (with or without Jessner solution).
- Tretinoin 0.1% cream or gel (avoid irritation).
- Corticosteroids: For inflamed disease and to avoid irritation from topical retinoids and keratolytics.

Systemic
- Isotretinoin, 0.1–1.5 mg/kg/d.
- Acitretin, up to 0.6 mg/kg/d (25–50 mg/d).

Surgery

KFSD: Scalp reduction and hair transplantation may be helpful in burned-out cicatricial alopecia.

AV: Dermabrasion and collagen implants have been used successfully to treat pitted scars. Laser resurfacing may be helpful.

Special considerations

KP: There is little justification for prolonged use of oral retinoids.

KPAF: Topical retinoids, corticosteroids, and keratolytics have been disappointing, but isotretinoin has been reported to be beneficial in individual cases of AV.

KFSD: Reports on the efficacy of oral retinoids have been contradictory.

FD: There are anecdotal reports of improvement with prolonged courses of topical and/or systemic antibiotics (fusidic acid with zinc or rifampin).

Treatment aims

KP: Can generally be controlled with a variety of exfoliating agents, but follicular dilatation remains in most cases.

Atrophic forms of KP: Generally refractory to treatment.

Prognosis

KP: Generally improves and sometimes remits with age. It usually worsens in winter and improves in summer.

KPAF: Disease progression halts after puberty.

General references

Lateef A, Schwartz RA, Janniger CK: Keratosis pilaris. *Cutis* 1999, **63**:205–207.

Oosterwijk JC, *et al.*: Molecular genetic analysis of two families with keratosis follicularis spinulosa decalvans: refinement of gene localization and evidence for genetic heterogeneity. *Human Genet* 1997, **100**:520–524.

Nazarenko SA, *et al.*: Keratosis pilaris and ulerythema ophryogenes associated with an 18p deletion caused by a Y/18 translocation. *Am J Med Genet* 1999, **85**:179–182.

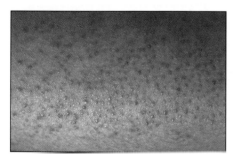

Hyperkeratotic follicular pink and skin-colored papules on the lateral arms in keratosis pilaris

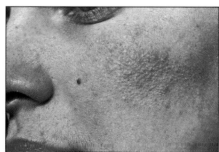

Atrophoderma vermiculata: follicular papules, keratotic plugs, milia and pitlike depressed scars; over time, a reticulate "honeycomb-like" pattern develops.

Lichen planus, lichen planopilaris, lichen nitidus

Diagnosis

Signs

Lichen planus (LP): Erythematous to violaceous, flat-topped, polygonal papules; fine whitish reticulated scale networks (Wickham striae). Symmetrical, bilateral on extremities, especially flexor surfaces of wrists, arms, legs. Also on male genitalia (25% of cases, usually as annular plaque on glans penis), oral mucosal (60% to 70%; sole manifestation in 20% to 30% of all cases, usually with white, reticulated patches, erosions), nails (10% to 15%, usually with thinning, longitudinal ridging, distal splitting of nail plate; characteristic—pterygium [forward growth of eponychium], adherence to proximal nail plate). Clinical variants: Hypertrophic lichen planus (thickened, hyperkeratotic, purplish plaques on shins, interphalangeal joints); lichen planus pemphigoides (blisters arising from papules and normal skin, usually on extremities); lichen planus actinicus or pigmentosus (annular lesions, pigmented centers on sun-exposed areas); erosive lichen planus (erosions and ulcers, usually on feet). Linear plaques develop after scratching, trauma (Koebnerization).

Lichen planopilaris (LPP): Follicular papules, perifollicular erythema and acuminate keratotic plugs on scalp, which coalesce to form patches that eventuate in scarring alopecia.

Lichen nitidus (LN): Multiple, discrete, small, smooth, flat, round, flesh-colored to hypopigmented papules. Anywhere, but common on flexor surfaces of arms, wrists; lower abdomen; breast; penile glans, shaft; genitals.

Symptoms

LP: Degree of pruritus correlates with disease extent; more intense pruritus associated with generalized disease. Hypertrophic LP is extremely pruritic. Erosive oral LP produces burning, pain.

LPP: Generally pruritic; end-stage usually symptomatic.

LN: Generally asymptomatic.

Investigations

LP: The "five P's" of LP—purple, polygonal, planar, pruritic, papules. Skin biopsy—hyperkeratosis, focal hypergranulosis, irregular acanthosis, colloid bodies, liquefaction degeneration of basal-cell layer, band-like mononuclear dermal infiltrate.

LPP: Biopsy—band-like mononuclear dermal infiltrate surrounding hair follicles; keratotic plugs, damaging dermal hair papillae.

LN: Circumscribed mononuclear infiltrate (occasional epithelioid, multinucleated giant cells), extends into overlying flattened epidermis. Lateral rete ridges may enclose infiltrate. Hydropic degeneration of basal-cell layer and parakeratosis in stratum corneum.

Complications

• Squamous-cell carcinoma develops in 0.5% to 5% of patients with oral LP. Malignant transformation risk factors include long-standing disease, erosive lesions, tobacco use.

Differential diagnosis

LP: In skin—hypertrophic-lichen simplex chronicus, prurigo nodularis, lichen amyloidosis. In mouth—leukokeratosis, candidiasis, lupus erythematosus, mucous patches of secondary syphilis. **LPP**: Lupus erythematosus, alopecia areata, cicatricial pemphigoid of Brunsting-Perry, pseudopelade. **LN**: Verruca plana, keratosis pilaris, lichen spinulosus, papular eczema, lichen scrofulosorum.

Etiology

Cause of these diseases is unknown.

Epidemiology

LP: Prevalence—worldwide, 0.14% to 0.8%; US, 0.44%. Women affected after age 50; men somewhat earlier. Rare in very young and elderly. **LPP**: More common in women than men. **LN**: Predilection for blacks, children, young adults, males. Incidence is about 3 in 10,000 population.

Violaceous, polygonal, planar papules with reticulated scaling (Wickham striae) characteristic of lichen planus.

Jonathan Dosik and Jerome Shupack

Treatment

Diet and lifestyle

•Advise patients to avoid oral, cutaneous trauma, to limit Koebner reactions. Oral LP: Encourage good oral hygiene, regular dental care; may respond dramatically to replacement of amalgam or gold dental restorations with composite materials, even without evidence of relevant patch test results.

Pharmacological treatment

Topical

LP: Class I–II corticosteroid (clobetasol propionate 0.05%) ointment. Flurandrenolone tape often effective in hypertrophic lesions. Oral lesions: super-high-potency corticosteroids (clobetasol propionate 0.05%) in gels or in an occlusive oral base. Cyclosporine (500 mg/5 mL) rinses useful for oral lesions; may be injected (0.5 mL/lesion). Rectal and vaginal cortisone suppositories for mucosal lesions. Intralesional triamcinolone acetonide: 2.5–10 mg/mL for oral, nail, cutaneous lesions; 10–20 mg/mL for hypertrophic lesions.

LPP: Intralesional or high-potency topical corticosteroids in combination with oral agents.

LN: Medium- to high-potency topical corticosteroids (mometasone, fluticasone).

Systemic

LP: Acitretin, 25–50 mg/d for 8 weeks, significantly improves cutaneous and mucosal lesions. Oral corticosteroids (prednisone, 30–60 mg/d for 4–6 weeks, with subsequent taper over 4–6 weeks) may be useful for acute cutaneous or oral flares. However, relapse may follow withdrawal of prednisone. Cyclosporine, 2–5 mg/kg/d (for recalcitrant LP). Oral antipruritic agents, *eg*, antihistamines, may relieve symptoms.

LPP: Prednisone, 30–40 mg/d for 3 months in conjunction with intralesional triamcinolone acetonide and high-potency topical corticosteroids. High relapse rates after cessation.

•Griseofulvin, hydroxychloroquine, thalidomide, dapsone: Anecdotal success in LP, LPP.

Nonpharmacological treatment

Supportive methods

•Oral LP: Topical anesthetics (viscous Lidocaine, Dyclonine, Maalox-Benadryl-Lidocaine 1:1:1) mouthwash to ease eating, chewing pain.

Physical modalities

•Psoralen and ultraviolet A photochemotherapy and ultraviolet B phototherapy may be useful in cutaneous LP and LN.

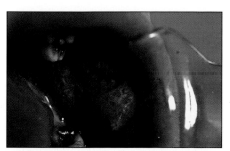

Macerated, white, reticular patches on buccal mucosa are most common oral lichen planus finding. Oral involvement is sole manifestation in 15% to 25% of cases.

Treatment aims

To control symptoms and achieve remission of disease. Treatment choices should be assessed in terms of risks and benefits and tailored to the severity and extent of disease. LN is generally asymptomatic and self-limiting and requires no intervention in most patients.

Prognosis

LP: Generally persists, perhaps for years; chronic, relapsing course over many years possible. Duration depends on extent and site of involvement. Hypertrophic lesions also follow protracted course. Purely mucosal disease generally more chronic than cutaneous mucosal disease, which, in turn, is more chronic than purely cutaneous disease. Generalized cutaneous eruptions often heal faster than limited disease. Relapse: approximately 15% to 20% of cases.

LPP: Generally results in irreversible scarring alopecia. Malignancy rare.

LN: Usually resolves spontaneously after months to a year; rarely, lesions may persist indefinitely.

Follow-up and management

Frequency of follow-up is based on severity of disease and treatment. Systemic therapy requires close follow-up to monitor adverse effects.

General references

Cribier B, *et al.*: Treatment of lichen planus: an evidence based medicine analysis of efficacy. *Arch Dermatol* 1998, **134**:1521–1530.

Daoud MS, Pittelkow MR: Lichen planus and lichen nitidus. In *Dermatology in General Medicine*, edn 5. Edited by Freedberg IM, *et al.* New York: McGraw-Hill; 1998:561–581.

Laurberg G, *et al.*: Treatment of lichen planus with acitretin: a double-blind, placebo-controlled study in 65 patients. *J Am Acad Dermatol* 1991, **24**:434–437.

Diagnosis

Signs

Linear IgA dermatosis (LIGAD): Tense blisters or vesicles; heal without scarring; extensor surfaces of extremities, trunk, mucosal surfaces, perioral area. Mucous membranes involved in approximately one third of patients. Variant: *chronic bullous dermatosis of childhood (CBDC)*, characterized by annular and configurate erythema, blisters; predominantly in flexural areas of lower trunk, thigh, groin. Tense blisters adjacent to crusted erosions: "crown of jewels."

Dermatitis herpetiformis (DH): Erythematous papules, vesicles, erosions with crusts (often, only excoriated erosions), usually symmetrically distributed over extensor surfaces (knees, elbows, sacrum, scalp).

Symptoms

LIGAD: Lesions may be pruritic or painful.

DH: Intense pruritus, often described as stinging or burning itch; antedates blister formation.

Investigations

LIGAD: Histology: subepidermal blisters, predominance of neutrophils or eosinophils in dermis. Direct immunofluorescence: linear band of IgA along basement membrane. Indirect immunofluorescence: in > 50%: low-titer circulating IgA that binds to epidermal or dermal side of 1-mol salt split skin.

DH: Histology: blisters with collection of neutrophils in papillary tips of dermis. Direct immunofluorescence: granular IgA deposits within papillary tips. Indirect immunofluorescence does not reveal circulating antibodies, although patients often have circulating antireticulin and antiendomysial antibodies.

Complications

LIGAD: Superficial infection of lesions; ocular involvement may lead to visual loss.

DH: Pyoderma due to excoriations. In 60% to 70%: asymptomatic gluten-sensitive enteropathy; typical gastrointestinal symptoms in 10%. Increased association with gastric atrophy, hypochlorhydria, thyroid abnormalities, diabetes mellitus, other autoimmune diseases. Bowel malignancy reported in 6% to 7%.

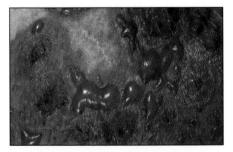

The presence of pruritic, grouped vesicles and bullae at the periphery of circinate, erythematous plaques is characteristic of linear IgA dermatosis. The lesions are most commonly located on extensor surfaces, including elbows, knees, and buttocks.

Differential diagnosis

LIGAD: Bullous pemphigoid, dermatitis herpetiformis; difficult to distinguish. Also exclude bullous erythema multiforme, bullous lupus erythematosus. Mucosal lesions may resemble cicatricial pemphigoid, lupus erythematosus.

DH: Erythema multiforme, herpes gestationis, bullous pemphigoid, LIGAD, transient acantholytic dermatitis, papular urticaria, scabies, bug bites, neurotic excoriations.

Etiology

LIGAD: Circulating IgA antibodies bind to LAD-1 antigen, a component of BPAG2 (BP 180).

DH: Target antigens unknown, but electron microscopy shows IgA bound to superficial dermis.

Epidemiology

LIGAD: Usually begins after age 60. (CBDC more prevalent among preschool-age children). Associated with autoimmune diseases, gastrointestinal diseases, malignancies, infections, medications.

DH: Presents in second, third decade. Anglo-Saxon, Scandinavian populations more affected than Asians and blacks; probably due to strong associations with HLA-B8, DR3, DQw-2 haplotypes.

Jeanie Chung-Leddon and M. Joyce Rico

Treatment

Diet and lifestyle

DH: Strict adherence to gluten-free diet improves cutaneous, gastrointestinal disease. At least 5 months may be needed before dosage of dapsone can be reduced; over a year before dapsone can be discontinued in approximately 80% of patients. Compliance difficult because gluten is in wheat, rye, oat, barley. Corn, rice contain no gluten; education by dietitian is encouraged to identify appropriate foods.

Pharmacological treatment

Topical

•Topical wound care to prevent infection of erosions.

Systemic

Dapsone: 1–2 mg/kg/d (50 mg initially; increase dosage weekly until symptoms controlled). Usual dosage, 100 mg/d; should not exceed 3–4 mg/kg/d. Closely monitor patients for side effects from dapsone, including hemolysis, methemoglobinemia, peripheral neuropathy. Before dapsone therapy, assess glucose 6-phosphate dehydrogenase enzyme deficiency.

Sulfapyridine: 500–2000 mg/d. Less severe toxicity; can be used if dapsone is not tolerated. During sulfapyridine, hydration important to avoid renal calculi formation; regular urinalysis.

Prednisone: 10–40 mg/d, for refractory cases.

Cyclosporine: 3–5 mg/kg; may be useful in severe disease if no response to dapsone.

Colchicine: 0.6–0.9 mg, t.i.d., if sulfone not tolerated.

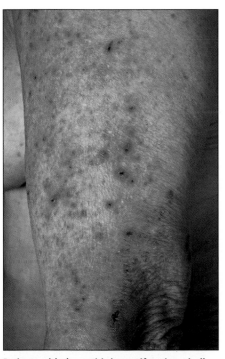

Patients with dermatitis herpetiformis typically develop grouped vesicles symmetrically distributed on the extensor surfaces of the extremities, buttocks, shoulders, and sacral areas, but because the lesions are intensely pruritic, only excoriations and crusted erosions may be present at the time of examination.

Treatment aims

To prevent the formation of new blisters, allow healing of lesions, and control pruritus.

Special therapeutic considerations

Oral, topical antipruritics offer little relief of itching in DH. Regular urinalysis should be performed.

Prognosis

Most patients respond to dapsone or sulfapyridine within in 48 to 72 hours; disease may persist (intermittent remissions, exacerbations), but tends to resolve within 3–5 years.

CBDC: Rarely persists past adolescence.

DH: Chronic; symptoms wax, wane. Not definite that gluten-free diet reduces risk of small-bowel lymphoma.

Follow-up and management

Treatment with dapsone or sulfapyridine requires close monitoring for side effects. Once the disease is controlled, attempt tapering of medication to assess spontaneous clinical remission. Ophthalmologist should follow ocular involvement.

Support organizations

Dermatitis Herpetiformis American Celiac Society, 58 Musano Court, West Orange, NJ 07052. Phone: 973-325-8837; fax: 973-669-8808.

Gluten Intolerance Group of North America, 15110 10th Avenue, SW, Seattle, WA 98166. Phone: 206-246-6652; fax: 206-246-6531, Web site. http://www.gluten.net.

General references

Hall RP, Rico MJ, Murray JC: Autoimmune skin disease. In *Clinical Immunology*. Edited by Rich RR, Fleisher TA, Schwartz BD, Shearer WT, Strober W. St. Louis: Mosby; 1996:1316–1342.

Gawkrodger DJ, Blackwell JN, Gilmour HM, *et al.*: Dermatitis herpetiformis: diagnosis, diet and dermography. *Gut* 1994, **25**:151.1.

Lipodystrophy, atrophoderma, and anetoderma

Diagnosis

Signs

Lipodystrophy: Absence of fat over part or all of the body, without superficial skin changes. Findings: cachetic facies; lost buccal fat pads; prominence of chin, zygomas; sunken eyes; prematurely aged appearance; hypertrophied appearance of muscle, veins; excessive fat deposition over hips, thighs. Two major groups (partial, generalized) based on distribution: **Partial**: More common form; gradual loss of fat; demarcated, symmetric distribution begins on face, progresses downward. At onset, fever , constitutional symptoms possible. **Generalized**: Lack of extracutaneous, subcutaneous fat. Associated findings in both congenital (Seip-Lawrence syndrome) and acquired (Berardinelli-Seip syndrome) forms: acanthosis nigricans, hypertrichosis, generalized hyperpigmentation, thick, curly scalp hair, visible hepatosplenomegaly in infancy. Moderate mental retardation often present in congenital form. HIV-associated lipodystrophy found in patients on antiretroviral treatment, with and without protease inhibitors. Wasting similar to partial lipodystrophy; increased fat, deposited in dorsocervical ("buffalo hump") area, abdomen, and breasts.

Lipoatrophy: Localized areas of fat loss.

Atrophodermas: Atrophic depressions in the skin. Distribution depends on type. **Follicular artophoderma**: Presents as dimple-like depressions at hair follicles, mostly on hands, feet; begins at birth or early life. **Linear atrophoderma of Moulin**: Hyperpigmented atrophoderma, with good prognosis; follows lines of Blaschko; usually develops during childhood, adolescence. **Vermiculate atrophoderma**: Reticulate type of atrophy found around horny follicular plugs on cheek. **Atrophoderma of Pasini and Pierini**: Round or oval depressed patches—usually on back, chest, abdomen—smooth, often slate-colored; atrophic areas progress over years, then remain static indefinitely.

Anetoderma: Rare; soft, saclike circumscribed, herniated areas protruding above skin surface; may start as urticarial or pink patches.

Symptoms

•All are disfiguring, but otherwise asymptomatic.

Investigations

Biopsy shows significant loss of subcutaneous fat, without inflammation. Lipid profile and fasting glucose to detect metabolic abnormalities. C3 serum complement is diminished in 70% of partial lipodystrophy patients. C3 nephritic factor, a C3 inhibitor, is present and may be toxic to adipocytes. **Abdominal CT** to distinguish generalized form by detecting reduced amounts of fat around viscera, increased fat accumulation in liver. **HIV testing**.

In atrophoderma, histopathologic changes are subtle, limited to reduction in dermal thickness.

In anetoderma, elastic fibers are fragmented or destroyed by mononuclear infiltrate.

Atrophoderma elastolytica discreta: Unique; skin lesions simulate atrophoderma of Pasini-Pierini but histopathologic changes of anetoderma.

Complications

Lipodystrophy: Hyperlipidemia and insulin-resistance diabetes develop in almost all patients; may be associated with glomerulonephritis, with or without hypocomplementemia. Hepatomegaly and subsequent cirrhosis from fatty liver can be found in generalized form. Partial immunosuppresion due to C3 deficiency in partial lipodystrophy. Patients with HIV-associated lipodystrophy also have insulin resistance, lipidemia. Follicular atrophoderma rarely associated with basal cell carcinomas, hypotrichosis (Bazex-Dupre-Christol syndrome).

Differential diagnosis

Generalized lipodystrophy differentiated from partial lipodystrophy by extent of involvement, extracutaneous manifestations. Differentiating various forms of atrophoderma depends mostly on distribution, associated conditions. Follicular atrophoderma associated with several syndromes, conditions, including calcifying chondrodysplasia (Conradi syndrome), Basex-Dupre-Christol syndrome, palmoplantar hyperkeratosis, follicular keratosis. Vermiculate atrophoderma considered part of keratosis pilaris syndrome. Atrophoderma of Pasini and Pierini clinically similar to morphea.

Etiology

No genetic factor reliably identified for **lipodystrophies, atrophodermas**; familial cases described. HIV-associated lipodystrophy syndrome thought to be caused by either metabolic effects of protease inhibitors alone or combined with direct effects of HIV on adipocyte apoptosis and differentiation. Lipoatrophy usually due to injection into fat (insulin, penicillin) or panniculitis.

Anetodermas may be primary (idiopathic) or associated with drugs (penicillamine), trauma, cutis laxa, infectious or inflammatory skin diseases (acrodermatitis chronica atrophicans, acne, varicella, lupus, syphilis, cuaneous T-cell lymphoma)

Epidemiology

About 80% of patients with partial lipodystrophy are female. Onset usually before age 15. HIV-associated lipodystrophy in 8%-50% of infected persons.

Paul Frank and Cheryl Thellman

Treatment

Diet and lifestyle

•A strict diabetic diet may help control associated insulin resistance and the increased metabolic rate associated with generalized lipodystrophies.

Pharmacological treatment

Lipodystrophy: No primary treatment. Antilipid and diabetic medications are used to control complications. Lipoatrophy may improve with administration of human insulin by jet injector or continuous subcutaneous infusion. Changing antiretrovirals (*eg*, from protease inhibitor to nonnucleoside reverse-transcriptase inhibitors) may improve HIV-lipodystrophy. Androgens may produce improvement. Improvement during treatment with growth hormone has been reported.

Atrophoderma: No effective treatment documented for atrophoderma of Pasini-Pierini.

Atrophoderma vermiculata: Responded to long-term treatment with isotretinoin in one reported case.

Surgery

Lipodystrophy: Fat transplanted to areas of atrophy or adipofascial flaps for facial contour reconstruction; results may be temporary, due to the progression of the disease.

Liposuction to areas of relative fat excess improves cosmetic appearance. Renal transplantation in cases with progressive uremia.

Atrophoderma: Psoralen and UVA beneficial in some patients.

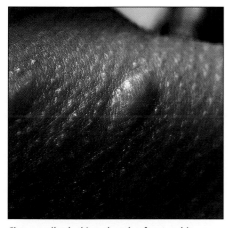

Circumscribed, skin-colored soft, atrophic outpouchings of skin due to loss of elastic tissue (anetoderma).

Treatment aims

To control associated complications and improve cosmetic appearance.

Prognosis

Lipodystrophy and atrophoderma are progressive and chronic in all forms. Emotional support and psychological counseling should be provided when needed.

Follow up and management

Lipodystrophy patients require close follow-up to monitor and manage complications. Patients with atrophoderma should be observed during follow-up due to its association with other conditions.

General references

Ketterings C: Lipodystrophy and its treatment. *Ann Plast Surg* 1988, **21**:536.

Beuscher SA, Rufli T. Atrophoderma of Pasini and Pierini. *J Am Acad Dermatol* 1994, **30**:441–446.

Braun RP, Borradori L, Chavaz P, *et al*.: Treatment of primary anetoderma with colchicine. *J Am Acad Dermatol* 1998, **38**:1002–1003.

Carr A, Samaras K, Thorisdottir A, *et al*.: Diagnosis, prediction, and natural course of HIV-1 protease-inhibitor-associated lipodystrophy, hyperlipidaemia, and diabetes mellitus: a cohort study. *Lancet* 1999, **353**:2093–2099.

Diagnosis

Signs

• Lipomas are soft, mobile, deeply palpable nodules or plaques (2 to 10 cm, rarely larger) that are either solitary or multiple.

• Sites of predilection are neck and trunk, but they can develop on any subcutaneous area.

• Benign lesions usually have no surface abnormalities.

Symptoms

• Usually asymptomatic. Pain is an intrinsic symptom of the angiolipoma variant, but any lipoma can cause pain by mass effect.

• Asymmetric protrusions, particularly on the head and neck, may be considered disfiguring by patients.

Investigations

• Usually can be diagnosed clinically by inspection and palpation.

• Biopsy confirms diagnosis, distinguishes variants, and excludes potential malignancy and other subcutaneous tissue disorders.

• Lipomas are aggregations of mature fatty cells. The neoplasms are encapsulated by a delicate fibrous capsule or have smooth lobulated margins.

• Malignant lesions, which are rare, tend to be more affixed to the skin and have superficial skin changes.

Complications

• Trauma and ischemia can cause necrosis within lesions.

• Pseudocysts may form as a consequence of resorbed necrotic adipocytes.

• Fibrosis and dystrophic calcification can be late sequelae.

• Rarely can grow to "giant" sizes.

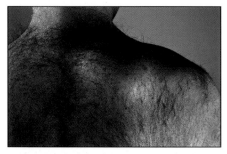

Rubbery, compressible, well-demarcated subcutaneous nodules consistent with lipomas on a man's upper back.

Differential diagnosis

Most common: Pilar cysts, which are usually firmer. Most lipoma variants clinically identical. Solitary lipomas can contain other mesenchymal elements differentiated only by histology (angiolipomas, chondroid lipomas, myolipomas, fibrolipomas, myxolipomas); other variants: spindle-cell, pleomorphic lipomas.

Hibernomas: Fatty tumors; differ from typical lipomas by histologic resemblance to embryonic brown fat. Typically, tan to reddish brown, reside in interscapular, lower cervical, axillary regions of young adults.

Patients with numerous lipomas may have one of many familial and sporadic multiple lipoma syndromes. **Familial multiple lipomas:** Transmitted in autosomal dominant fashion; become apparent in third decade of life; lesions disseminated, but most pronounced on extremities.

Benign symmetric lipomatosis (Madelung's disease): Sporadic disorder; numerous, symmetrically distributed, poorly encapsulated fatty tumors situated mostly around shoulders, suboccipital region, neck, upper arms. **Adiposis dolorosa (Dercum's disease):** Sporadic; found in middle-aged, obese people, primarily in menopausal women. Many slow growing, exquisitely tender lipomas on extremities, trunk. **Congenital diffuse lipomatosis:** Can be seen during first few months of life; may be manifestation of Proteus syndrome; found mostly on chest; can infiltrate skeletal muscle. **Lipoblastomas** appear within first 3 years of life; solitary, diffuse forms; ill defined; mature adipocytes, embryonic white fat cells. **Liposarcomas:** Arise de novo rather than in preexisting lipoma; usually in elderly; rapidly enlarging masses; can involve skin, compress local tissue, infiltrate nerves.

Etiology

Unknown. Tumors have been found to demonstrate chromosomal aberrations.

Epidemiology

Most common mesenchymal neoplasms in humans. Angiolipomas represent 5% of fatty tumors. Malignant fatty tumors are rare, occur in elderly.

Treatment

Diet and lifestyle

• Lipomas are associated with obesity, but diet has no known effect on the clinical course.

Nonpharmacological treatment

Surgery

• Surgical excision is the standard treatment. Lesions typically "shell out" because of a sharply circumscribed rim of fibrous tissue.

• Liposarcomas require wide and deep excision with adjuvant local radiation and/or chemotherapy.

Physical modalities

• Liposuction with local anesthesia can be used for larger and more ill-defined fatty collections and tumors with excision of the remaining fibrous tissue through a small incisional opening.

Special therapeutic considerations

• Recurrence of lipomas is minimized by completely excising tumors within their fibrous capsule.

Treatment aims

When small, solitary, and benign, treatment is cosmetic for all variants. Larger, infiltrating, or multiple fatty tumors are treated to ease pain and prevent consequences of mass effect. Liposarcomas are treated to prevent metastasis.

Prognosis

Most fatty tumors are slow-growing and benign. Malignant lesions are rapidly progressive. Well-differentiated tumors have a lesser chance of metastasis than poorly differentiated ones; but they are often locally recurrent.

Follow up and management

Liposarcomas require close follow-up for local recurrence and metastasis.

General references

Martinez-Escribano JA; Gonzalez R, et al.: Efficacy of lipectomy and liposuction in the treatment of multiple symmetric lipomatosis. Int J Dermatol 1999, 38:551–554.

Collins PC, Narins RS, et al.: Liposuction surgery and autologous fat transplantation. Clin Dermatol 1992, 10:365–372.

Allen PW, Strungs I, MacCormac LB: Atypical subcutaneous fatty tumors: a review of 37 referred cases. Pathology 1998, 30:123–135.

Diagnosis

Signs

• Skin disease is the second most common clinical manifestation of lupus, after joint inflammation.

• Arthritis, myositis, pleuropericarditis, lymphadenopathy, peritonitis, seizures, psychosis, peripheral neuropathy, proteinuria, hematuria, elevated creatinine level, renal failure, nephrotic syndrome, anemia, leukopenia.

Investigations

• Complete blood count with differential (for anemia, leukopenia); erythrocyte sedimentation rate; renal function studies; complement levels (C3, C4, CH50); antinuclear antibody; rheumatoid factor; anti–double-stranded DNA antibody; skin biopsy, direct immunofluorescence; lupus band test comparing nonlesional photoexposed to photoprotected skin (not diagnostic, but prognostic); anti-SSA (Ro) antibody (subacute, acute, neonatal); anti-SSB (La) antibody (subacute, acute, neonatal), anti-Sm (acute) antibody; anti–nuclear ribonuclearprotein antibody (neonatal; mixed connective tissue disease); anti-histone antibody (drug); Venereal Disease Research Laboratory test or rapid plasma reagin test; prothrombin time/partial thromboplastin time (lupus anticoagulant); urinalysis; C reactive protein.

Complications

• Scarring hair loss, skin lesions, hypertension, renal failure; cardiovascular disease, myocardial infarction, coronary artery disease, congestive heart failure, pericarditis, central nervous system and parasympathetic nervous system disease, chronic arthritis.

Differential diagnosis

Photocontact dermatitis, polymorphous light eruption, drug eruption, rosacea.

Etiology

Multisystem autoimmune disease. Neonatal: Transplacental passage of maternal IgG anti-SSA (Ro), anti-SSB (La), and/or anti-U1 ribonucleoprotein antibodies. Drug: Procainamide, hydralazine, isoniazid (systemic lupus erythematosus; SLE), hydrochlorothiazide, estrogen (subacute cutaneous LE, SCLE).

Epidemiology

Chronic cutaneous LE (CCLE): Female predeliction, 6:5 ratio; peak incidence, fourth decade. **Subacute cutaneous LE (SCLE)** Female predeliction. **Acute cutaneous LE (ACLE):** Female predeliction, 8:1 to 10:1 ratio. **Neonatal:** Occurs in 2% of anti-Ro–, anti-La–, or anti-U1 ribonucleoprotein–positive mothers. Skin lesions occur in half of affected infants within first month, heal by 6 months without scarring. Congenital heart block occurs in 50% of affected infants and is permanent. Drug: Slow acetylators at higher risk.

Macrene Alexiades-Armenakas and Andrew Franks, Jr.

e

Treatment

Diet and lifestyle

• Recommend avoiding sunbathing (natural or artificial), unshielded fluorescent light (advise plastic covering), sunlight (at midday, at high altitudes, around reflective surfaces), alfalfa and photosensitizing foods; recommend wearing broad-brimmed hat, tightly woven clothing; special sun-protective clothing, using sunblock, camouflage cosmetics.

Pharmacological treatment

Topical

Sunscreen (broad-spectrum ultraviolet A/ultraviolet B). **Corticosteroids**: Creams, ointments, gels.
Triamcinolone acetonide intralesional injection, 3–5 mg/mL (facial), 5–10 mg/mL (elsewhere) every 2–4 weeks during induction phase and every month until resolution.

Systemic (first-line)

Antimalarial agents for at least 6 weeks. Follow with baseline and periodic ophthalmologic examinations for retinopathy, laboratory evaluations for hematologic, hepatic, renal toxicity.
Hydroxychloroquine: 200 mg/d orally initially, up to 200 mg twice a day maximum; or 200 mg orally twice daily initially for 6–8 weeks, then decrease to 200 mg orally.
Chloroquine: 250 mg orally daily initially, up to 500 mg daily maximum.
Quinacrine: 100 mg orally daily (often in combination with hydroxychloroquine).
Corticosteroids during induction phase to prevent imminent disfigurement or organ system involvement.
Prednisone: 1 mg/kg/d orally tapered over 6–8 weeks.

Systemic (second-line)

Diaminodiphenylsulfone (dapsone): 100–200 mg orally daily for G6PD-positive patients unresponsive to antimalarial agents; drug of choice for bullous LE. **Retinoids** for discoid LE (DLE). **Isotretinoin**: 0.6–1.5 mg/kg (usual dose is 1 mg/kg) orally daily. **Acitretin**: 0.5–2.0 mg/kg orally daily. **Colchicine**: 0.6 mg orally once to three times daily for cutaneous vasculitis.

Systemic (third line)

Methylprednisolone i.v., pulse dose.
Azathioprine: 1–2 mg/kg orally daily.
Methotrexate: 7.5–25 mg orally or i.m. once a week.
Cyclophosphamide: 1–2 mg/kg orally daily.
Cyclosporine: 1–3 mg/kg orally daily.
Clofazamine: 100–300 mg orally daily.
Interferon-α2a: 1 million U subcutaneously 3–5 times a week.
Thalidomide: 50–200 mg orally daily.

Surgery

• Hematopoietic stem-cell transplantation. Pulsed-dye laser, 565 nm, or Dialite laser, 532 nm for vascular lesions. CO_2 resurfacing for scars.

Special therapeutic considerations

• Avoid photosensitizing drugs, exogenous estrogens.

Treatment aims

To prevent scarring; induce remission.

Prognosis

ACLE: follows pattern of underlying SLE exacerbations and remissions. **SLE**: Approximately 25% of patients with SLE develop discord LE (DLE) (a good prognostic sign). **Lupus profundus**: About 50% develop SLE, which is less severe. **CCLE**: Indolent progression of cutaneous scarring if untreated. Squamous-cell carcinoma may develop. Five percent of patients with DLE develop SLE; risk factors: diffuse nonscarring alopecia; generalized lymphadenopathy; periungual telangiectasia; Raynaud's phenomenon; coexistence of acute or subcutaneous lupus lesions; vasculitis; anemia; leukopenia; false-positive result on rapid plasma reagin test; high-titer results on antinuclear antibody assay; anti–single-stranded DNA antibody; and erythrocyte sedimentation rate > 50 mm/h).

Follow-up and management

Monitor closely for evolution into systemic disease, opportunistic infections, and disease-associated and iatrogenic complications.

Support organizations

The Lupus Foundation of America, 4 Research Place, Suite 180, Rockville, MD 20850-3226; phone: 800-558-0121, 301-670-9292.

General references

Cooper GS, Dooley MA, Treadwell EL, *et al*.: Hormonal, environmental, and infectious risk factors for developing systemic lupus erythematosus. *Arthritis Rheum* 1998, **41**:1714–1724.

Soter NA, Franks AG Jr: The Skin. In Kelley's Textbook of Rheumatology edn 6. Edited by Ruddy S, Harris ED Jr, Sledge CB. Philadelphia: WB Saunders; 2001:401–416.

Swaak AJG *et al*.: Systemic lupus erythematosus: clinical features in patients with a disease duration of over 10 years, first evaluation. *Rheumatology* 1999, **38**:953–958.

Macrene Alexiades-Armenakas and Andrew Franks, Jr.

Diagnosis

Signs

Erythema migrans: Between 4 days and several weeks after bite, erythematous plaque, rarely tender or pruritic, usually at bite site. Thigh, popliteal fossa, groin, nape of neck, axillae commonly affected. Expands slowly over days; gradual central clearing; resolves spontaneously in 3–5 weeks. Difficult to detect if dark skin. In 30%, bull's-eye appearance; may go unnoticed. Only 30% recall bite. May be bullous, ulcerated, or necrotic center; generalized aching, headache, regional lymphadenopathy.

Dissemination (stage II) in days to weeks; multiple lesions in 10%; flulike symptoms independent of presence of skin lesions. Also malar eruption, conjunctivitis, "evanescent" lesions, lymphoctoma, rarely diffuse urticaria. Absence of nasal congestion helps differentiate from viral syndromes. Complications: Meningitis with seventh cranial nerve involvement, temporary facial paralysis; spinal nerve involvement, radiculopathies resolve in weeks; usually reversible heart block.

Late (stage III) disease months to years after initial infection. Manifestations usually neurologic and musculoskeletal: arthritis (usually one or two large joints), almost always reversible but often relapsing. Also memory loss, mood changes, sleep disorders, numbness, tingling, confusion, disorientation, abnormal sensitivity to light.

Acrodermatitis chronica atrophicans: Violaceous patches or plaques become atrophic or sclerotic.

Investigations

• Physical examination for skin lesions, facial asymmetry.

• IgG or IgM enzyme-linked immunosorbent assay (ELISA) titer; confirm positive or unequivocal result by Western blot.

• Serologic tests do not produce positive result until several weeks after bite. No antibiotics for at least 6 weeks before testing.

• Negative ELISA test results in suspect patients should be repeated in 2–4 weeks. Results from polymerase chain reaction (PCR) specific but not sensitive for diagnosis in blood, more sensitive in joint fluid, cerebrospinal fluid (CSF), tissue specimens produced during biopsy.

• CSF analysis of patients with pronounced neurologic manifestations, if seronegative, or are still have significant neurologic symptoms after completion of treatment.

Differential diagnosis

Erythema multiforme, eczema, cellulitis, erythema annulare centrifugum, subacute lupus erythematosus, granuloma annulare.

Etiology

Borrelia burgdorferi, which replicates every 12 to 24 hours, is transmitted through tickbite, *Ixodes dammini* (Northeast, Midwest US), *Ixodes pacificus* (Western US), *Ixodes ricinus* (Europe), *Ixodes persulcatus* (Asia). Between 10% and 50% of Ixodes ticks in New York and Connecticut are infected. Tick must be attached at least 24 hours. Incubation period: 3–32 days. Mice and deer commonest vectors.

Epidemiology

First described in Old Lyme, Connecticut in 1975. In 1996, more than 16,000 cases reported; more than 90% from Connecticut, Rhode Island, New York, New Jersey, Pennsylvania, Delaware, Maryland, Wisconsin; most others from elsewhere in upper Midwest, Pacific Coast (but reported in all US states, Europe, Asia).

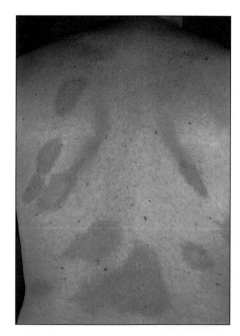

Elliptical, erythematous, blotchy patches with central clearing on the back of a man with Lyme Borreliosis.

Miguel Sanchez

Treatment

Pharmacological treatment

• Early disease, facial palsy, or first-degree atrioventricular (AV) block: Doxycycline, 100 mg, orally, twice daily, 20 to 30 days, adults. Amoxicillin, 500 mg, orally, three times daily, 20 to 30 days (with or without probenecid, 500 mg, orally, three times daily); children: 250 mg daily, if older than 8 years; 20 mg/kg/d, three divided doses, if younger adult. Cefuroxime axetil, 500 mg, twice daily, 20 to 30 days, adult; children: 125 mg, twice daily. Erythromycin, 250 mg, four times daily, 20 to 30 days, adult; children: 250 mg, three times daily.

• Arthritis: Doxycycline, 100 mg, twice daily, 30 to 60 days, adults; Penicillin, G, 20 million units, i.v., daily, four doses, every 6 hours, 14 to 30 days.

• Neurologic disease or high-degree AV block: Ceftriaxone, 2 g, i.v., 14 to 30 days; penicillin G, 20 million IU, i.v., daily, four doses, q. 6h, 14–30 days; doxycycline, 100 mg, three times daily, for 14–30 days, adults.

Other therapeutic considerations

• Nonsteroidal antiinflammatory drugs and hydroxychloroquine for arthritis.

• Sulbactam/ampicillin, imipenem, vancomycin if cephalosporin treatment failure.

• Symptoms may flare in four-week cycle; minimum treatment duration of 4 weeks.

• Symptoms may worsen during the last week of treatment. Azithromycin, clarithromycin, for adults.

Nonpharmacological treatment

• Physical therapy, rehabilitation, a graded exercise program (arthritis).

Special considerations

• Protection from ticks: Light-colored clothing; limiting exposure; careful tick checks after possible exposure; frequent pet examinations for ticks.

• Removal of tick by pulling firmly with tweezers, not by using heat or chemicals, or by grasping by the body.

• Pest control: Focus on mice.

• Repellants: Permethrin-containing repellants sprayed on clothing before wearing, but not directly on the skin. Other repellants for application to skin.

• Heat: Treating clothing in dryer for a few minutes after being outdoors in an infested area kills any ticks attached to clothing.

• Prophyllactic antibiotics are not recommended before a tick bite and are discouraged after a tick bite because the risk of infection from a tick bite, even in areas with very high Lyme disease prevalence, is only 1% to 3%. No evidence shows that antibiotics after a tick bite prevent Lyme disease and no studies suggest dosage or treatment duration.

• Prescribe antibiotics based on disease stages and manifestations.

• Chronic Lyme disease may resemble chronic fatigue syndrome but should respond to treatment, unless misdiagnosed.

• There is no evidence that Lyme disease is more harmful in preganacy to woman or fetus.

• Vaccination: Adults at high risk for Lyme disease should consider vaccination. Protection declines over time and revaccination may be necessary after several years. Three doses are given initially, during the first month, and at 12 months after the first dose. Vaccination decreases Lyme disease by 75% to 90%. The need for booster doses still needs to be determined. The vaccine is not recommended for the elderly or children.

Treatment aims

To eliminate the infection and prevent complications.

Prognosis

If diagnosed in early stages, the disease is curable with antibiotics. Untreated, rheumatologic, cardiac and neurologic, complications can occur. Arthritis may occasionally fail to respond to treatment, but other symptoms improve.

In some cases, multiple courses of either oral or IV (depending on symptoms) antibiotics may be indicated. However, IV treatment courses for longer than the recommended 4–6 weeks are not usually advised due to possible adverse side effects. Anecdotally, longer courses may be more effective. Symptoms may persist due to an immunologic response that may trigger fibromylagia and/or chronic fatigue syndrome; or due to emotional factors related to incorrect fears about Lyme disease. Persistent symptoms are rarely due to the failure of therapy and usually do not respond to a second treatment course.

The immuncompromised are at greater risk for disseminated borrelial infection before treatment and treatment failure (defined as the onset of severe, minor or major manifestations of Lyme borreliosis, persistence of *B. burgdorferi* in the skin and/or persistence of EM after treatment). Retreatment may be required in 20%. However, the short-term outcome of Lyme disease is excellent.

General references

Nadelman RB, Wormser GP: Lyme borreliosis. *Lancet* 1998, **352**:557–565.

Berger BW: Current aspects of Lyme disease and other *Borrelia burgdorferi* infections [review]. *Dermatol Clin* 1997, **15**:247–255.

Hulshof MM, Vandenbroucke JP, Nohlmans LM, *et al.*: Long-term prognosis in patients treated for erythema chronicum migrans and acrodermatitis chronica atrophicans. *Arch Dermatol* 1997, **133**:33–37.

Weber K: Treatment failure in erythema migrans–a review. *Infection* 1996, **24**:73–75.

Diagnosis

Signs

Lymphoid papulosis (LyP): Polymorphic eruption with erythematous, smooth papules or nodules that occur in crops on the trunk and extremities. Central necrosis, scaling, and resolution with scarring are common. Regression and then recurrence of eruption within weeks are a hallmark of LyP.

Pseudolymphoma (PsL): Solitary or multiple papules, plaques, or nodules with a smooth surface and a firm consistency. Erythematous to violaceous in color, these lesions are commonly found on the head, neck, and extremities.

Symptoms

LyP: Lesions are usually asymptomatic, but pruritus, tenderness, and pain have been reported.

PsL: Lesions are asymptomatic. When PsL is caused by drug reaction, fever and lymphadenopathy may occur.

Investigations

LyP: Skin biopsy may reveal one of three pathologic patterns: type A, with Reed-Sternberg–like cells, as seen in Hodgkin's disease; type B, with large atypical epidermotropic lymphocytes similar to mycosis fungoides; and type C, with aggregates of large atypical CD30+ T cells mimicking CD30+ large T-cell lymphoma. Immunohistochemistry reveals CD30+T cells. T-cell receptor gene rearrangement studies may show clonality in up to 60% of patients.

PsL: Thorough history, including drug intake, to identify culprit oral medication; review of systems to recognize concomitant symptoms, such as fever, weight loss, and night sweats. Physical examination, including palpation of lymph nodes, liver, and spleen. Routine blood tests (*ie*, complete blood count with differential) and chest radiography. Deep skin biopsy should be performed; typical finding is a "top-heavy" lymphocytic infiltrate but no epidermotropism or Pautrier abscesses. If pathological features of malignant lymphoma are present, immunohistochemical studies should be done. If skin biopsy results are not conclusive, systemic work-up should be considered, such as CT and bone marrow biopsy.

Complications

LyP: Associated with malignant lymphoma in 10% to 20% of cases, most frequently mycosis fungoides, Hodgkin's disease, or CD30-positive large-cell lymphoma. Patients also have an increased risk for nonlymphoid malignancies.

PsL: Some experts believe that patients with PsL are at a higher risk for developing malignant lymphoma. This could reflect an initial misdiagnosis in a patient who had malignant lymphoma at the onset.

Differential diagnosis

LyP: Pityriasis lichenoides et varioliformis acuta (PLEVA), acute lymphoma, large-cell anaplastic T-cell lymphoma, mycosis fungoides, histiocytosis X, cutaneous Hodgkin's disease, scabies, arthropod-bite reaction, drug eruption, papular urticaria.

PsL: Cutaneous lymphoma.

Etiology

The etiology is unknown. Experts consider both LyP and PsL benign extremes of a lymphoproliferative disease spectrum that terminates in malignant lymphoma. In some cases, PsL is a benign lymphoproliferative response to a systemic drug, such as anticonvulsants, analgesics, and antihistamines.

Epidemiology

LyP: Affects all ages, with median age at onset of 40–50 years. No sex or inheritance pattern predominates. History of lymphoproliferative disorder, radiation therapy, or exuberant response to mosquito bite are common.

PsL: Affects all ages and affects women more commonly than men.

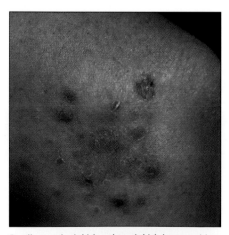

Small, round, pinkish red to pinkish brown, shiny, smooth clustered papules on the lateral aspect of a knee. Histological diagnosis is lymphomatoid papillomatosis. Lesions usually resolve spontaneously, but some may ulcerate and scar.

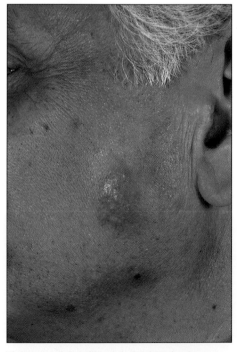

Violaceous pink, infiltrated, slowly-enlarging, smooth plaque on the face which histologically shows the changes of pseudolymphoma.

Jeremy Rothfleisch and Jo-Ann Latkowski

Treatment

Pharmacological treatment

Topical

• Corticosteroids (for LyP or PsL) of intermediate to high potency (class I to III) applied to affected area twice a day. If needed for the face, groin, or axilla, these corticosteroids should be used for a maximum of 1 week. Side effects occur with prolonged use and include striae and atrophy of the skin.

• Nitrogen mustard (for LyP), 10 mg dissolved in 60 mL of water and applied daily to the entire body. Most common side effect is contact dermatitis.

• Carmustine (for LyP) applied to skin daily at a dose of 10 mg in dilute ethanol.

• Intralesional triamcinolone (for PsL) at a concentration of 5–40 mg/mL, depending on the thickness of the lesions.

Systemic

• Methotrexate (for LyP) administered at a low dose of 5–15 mg per week. Complete blood count and liver function test should be determined before the administration of weekly dose, initially every week and then monthly (once dose is stable). Liver biopsy may be necessary for prolonged use.

Side effects: Nausea, vomiting, bone marrow suppression, liver toxicity.

Contraindications: Pregnancy, active infectious disease, renal or hepatic disease, alcohol use.

Drug interactions: Salicylates, sulfonamide.

Corticosteroids (for LyP) at a dosage of 20–60 mg/d, tapering with resolution of disease.

Side effects: Hypertension, Cushing's disease, diabetes, osteoporosis.

Contraindications: Active infectious disease, hypertension, peptic ulcer disease.

Drug interactions: Warfarin, salicylates, oral contraceptive pills.

• Cyclosporine (for LyP) at a dosage of 3–5 mg/kg per day. Before use, blood pressure and renal function (*ie*, creatinine clearance) should be checked.

Side effects: Renal toxicity, hypertension, electrolyte imbalance (potassium, magnesium), nausea, vomiting, hypertrichosis, increased risk of malignancy

Drug interactions: Any drug metabolized through the hepatic P450 enzyme system.

• Antibiotics at standard doses (tetracycline, erythromycin, and sulfones for LyP; penicillin for PsL).

• Discontinuation of therapy with offending oral agent (for PsL).

Nonpharmacological treatment

• Ultraviolet B phototherapy (for LyP).

• Psoralen with ultraviolet A phototherapy (PUVA) (for LyP).

• Local radiation therapy (for PsL) for limited disease. **Not recommended for children.**

• Cryotherapy (for PsL) with liquid nitrogen.

Treatment aims

LyP: If patient has few lesions, goals are observation and reassurance. For more diffuse disease, decrease the number of new lesions and slow the progression of disease.

PsL: To rule out malignant lymphoma and eradicate disease.

Prognosis

Clinical course varies from chronic, recurrent course, lasting months to years, to spontaneous remission. These patients are at a higher risk for malignant lymphoma and, in the case of LyP, nonlymphoid malignancies.

Follow-up and management

Patients must have regular clinical follow-up. Given the increased risk for malignancy, a systemic work-up may be indicated.

General references

Orchard GE: Lymphomatoid papulosis: a low-grade T-cell lymphoma? *Br J Biomed Sci* 1996, **53**:162–169.

Ploysangam T, Breneman DL, Mutasim DF: Cutaneous pseudolymphomas. *J Am Acad Dermatol* 1998, **38**: 877–895.

Rijlaarsdam JU, *et al.*: Cutaneous pseudo T cell lymphoma. *Cancer* 1992, **69**:717–724.

Wang HH, *et al.*: Increased risk of lymphoid and nonlymphoid malignances in patients with lymphomatoid papulosis. *Cancer* 1999, **86**:1240–1245.

Diagnosis

Signs

Classification
• Most common to least common: Indolent (cutaneous disease, syncope, ulcers, malabsorption, bone marrow involvement, skeletal disease, hepatosplenomegaly, lymphadenopathy); associated hematologic abnormalities (myeloproliferative or myelodysplastic); aggressive (lymphadenopathic mastocytosis and eosinophilia); associated mast-cell leukemia.

Skin manifestations
Urticaria pigmentosa (UP), diffuse cutaneous mastocytosis (DCM), solitary mastocytoma (M), telangiectasia macularis eruptiva perstans (TMEP).

Lesions
UP: Multiple small, yellow-tan to reddish-brown macules or slightly elevated papules; may coalesce to form cobblestone plaques. Young children may develop hemorrhagic bullae. **DCM**: Yellow-brown, diffuse thickening of entire skin, without discrete lesions; may also have fine papules (like grain leather); young children may develop bullae. **M**: Macules, papules, or nodules 5–60 mm. **TMEP**: Tan to brown macules and patchy erythema; telangiectases.

Systemic manifestations
• Diarrhea, vomiting, tachycardia, palpitations, flushing, hypotension, syncope.

Distribution
UP: Scattered diffusely over the body; may spare palms, soles, face, scalp. **DCM**: Diffuse infiltration of entire skin. **M**: Isolated or generalized, especially at trunk and extremities. **TMEP**: Widespread; may involve face. **SM**: Skeletal, hematopoietic, reticuloendothelial, gastrointestinal, cardiovascular, central nervous system.

Symptoms

Skin: Pruritus.

Systemic mastocytosis (SM): Abdominal pain, nausea, bone pain, dizziness, headache, affective and cognitive abnormalities.

Investigations

• **Darier's sign**: Urtication and erythema, elicited by rubbing or other minor trauma (due to mast-cell degranulation); patients with UP, DCM and solitary mastocytoma are positive for this sign.

• **Biopsy**: Increased numbers of dermal mast cells that may be subtle or marked.

• **Plasma histamine and 24-hour urine** for histamine, N-methylhistamine, and prostaglandin-2 metabolites.

• **Additional studies:** Complete blood count, blood chemistry profile with liver function tests; at times, bone marrow biopsy or aspirate, bone scan, gastrointestinal studies (upper gastrointestinal series, small-bowel radiography, computed tomography, endoscopy), neuropsychiatric assessment.

Complications

• Vascular collapse; intense flushing and telangiectases.

• Gastrointestinal: Peptic ulcer disease.

• Hepatic/splenic: Fibrosis, portal hypertension, ascites.

• Bone/fractures.

• Hemarologic: Poncytopenia, mast-cell leukemia, other abnormalities.

Differential diagnosis
Flushing disorders, lentigines, café-au-lait spot, neurofibroma, xanthogranuloma, eruptive xanthoma, Langerhans-cell histiocytosis, telangiectases (eg, essential, dermatoheliosis, rosacea), blistering disorders in neonates.

Etiology
Mutations in factors that regulate mast-cell number and differentiation (eg, point mutations in the receptor for stem-cell factor, c-kit). Increases in mast-cell number and excess release of mast-cell mediators (eg, histamine, certain leukotrienes and cytokines) have local and systemic effects.

Epidemiology
Peak incidence in children, especially those < 6 months of age; second peak in young adults; all races; male predominance (1.5:1). **UP**: Most common skin lesion; seen in >90% with indolent disease. **DCM**: Rare; usually occurs in patients < 3 years of age. **Solitary mastocytoma**: Onset usually < 6 months of age. **TMEP**: Rare; almost exclusively in adults. **SM**: Usually in adults.

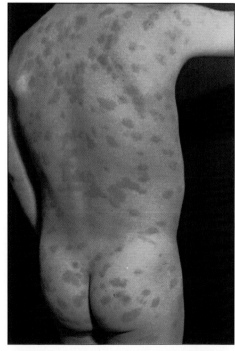

Reddish brown, irregular plaques that urticate upon rubbing (Darier's sign) in a patient with urticaria pigmentosa.

Treatment

Diet and lifestyle

• Avoid exacerbating factors (*eg*, hot beverages and spicy foods in patients with UP).

• Take anaphylaxis precautions—medical alert bracelet, subcutaneous epinephrine, awareness of increased risk for adverse reactions with certain general anesthetic agents—with extensive involvement or severe cardiovascular symptoms.

Pharmacological treatment

Systemic

Antihistamines: H_1 are useful in reducing pruritus, flushing, and tachycardia; may add H_2-antihistamines, which are particularly useful for hyperchlorhydria.

Disodium cromoglycate are especially useful for gastrointestinal symptoms; 200 mg, orally, four times daily (adults); 100 mg, orally, four times daily (ages 2–12); 20–40 mg/kg in four divided doses (< 2 years old); may take for 4-6 weeks, for maximum clinical response.

Topical glucocorticoids *eg*, betamethasone dipropionate ointment 0.05%, under occlusion, 8 hours per day for 8-12 weeks) for extensive UP or DCM; condition recurs after discontinuation of therapy.

• Systemic glucocorticoids and interferon-α may be beneficial in severe mastocytosis (especially to control severe skin disease, malabsorption, ascites).

Nonpharmacological treatment

Physical modalities

Photochemotherapy: Psoralen and ultraviolet A radiation (PUVA) for extensive cutaneous disease unresponsive to other therapies; may relieve pruritus after 1-2 months; benefits are temporary.

Surgery

Surgical excision of solitary mastocytomas; rarely indicated, except if patient has severe cardiovascular or respiratory symptoms; splenectomy may be beneficial in selected cases of SM.

Treatment aims

To control mast-cell mediator–induced signs and symptoms and reduce number of mast cells.

Prognosis

Indolent: Including most children; good prognosis, especially if only skin involvement. **Aggressive:** Worse prognosis; mean survival for lymphadenopathic mastocytosis and eosinophilia is 2–4 years without therapy. Mast-cell leukemia: mean survival < 6 months. **Associated hematologic disorder:** Hematologic disorder determines overall prognosis.

UP in children: More than 50% of cases clear by adulthood, and most of the remainder have only residual, lightly pigmented asymptomatic macules; in adults, the condition usually gradually progresses to systemic disease, rarely to hematologic disease. **DCM after age 5:** Usually associated with indolent systemic disease. **M:** Most cases involute spontaneously.

Variables associated with poor prognosis: Older age, constitutional symptoms, anemia, thrombocytopenia, hepatosplenomegaly, lymphadenopathy, abnormal liver function test results, lobated mast-cell nucleus, low percentage of fat cells in bone marrow biopsy specimen, associated hematologic disorder or mast-cell leukemia.

Follow-up and management

Individualize, depending on type; hematologic abnormalities may develop.

General references

Alto WA, Clarcq L: Cutaneous and systemic manifestations of mastocytosis. *Am Fam Phys* 1999, **59**:3047–3054.

Golkar L, Bernhard JD: Mastocytosis. *Lancet* 1997, **349**:1379–1385.

Diagnosis

Signs

•Quasi-symmetric, uniformly, irregular, sharply-demarcated tan-brown to grey macules and patches on face and less on anterior chest, upper back and photoexposed sides of arms. Three main facial variants: centrofacial type involves forehead, nose, cheeks, upper lip (mustache area), chin; malar type predominantly affects cheeks, nose; mandibular type primarily involves ramus of mandible.

Symptoms

•Pigmentation produces no symptoms, but may be associated with psychological tendencies to dysmorphia as well as cultural and social stigmatization.

Investigations

•Wood's light examination helps determine location of pigment. If pigmentation is epidermal, pigment contrast with normal skin is increased, but no significant contrast appears if pigmentation is dermal or mixed (epidermodermal).

•Skin biopsy, usually not indicated, shows increased melanin deposition in basal and suprabasal layers and increased numbers of highly dendritic, hyperactive melanocytes that anastamose with each other in the epidermal type; and melanin-filled macrophages (melanophages) throughout superficial dermis with no inflammatory infiltrate in dermal type. These changes are more prominent with dihydroxyphenylalanine staining; potassium hydroxide examination if tinea versicolor suspected.

Complications

•Mostly psychosocial (especially low self-esteem, confidence lack from poor self-image); hyperpigmentaion, leukoderma, scarring from treatment.

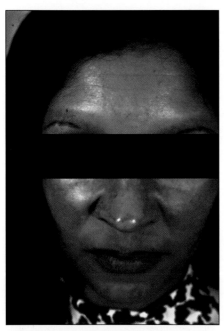

Irregular brown patches in a centrofacial distribution in a woman with melasma.

Differential diagnosis

Most important condition to differentiate is postinflammatory hyperpigmentation due to inflammatory cutaneous diseases (> *eg*, contact dermatitis, seborrheic dermatitis, acute lupus malar eruption). Other lesions and pigmentary diseases include lentigines, ephelides, fixed drug eruption, photosensitizing chemical reactions, drug-induced pigmentation (clofazimine), photosensitizing drug eruption, exogenous ochronosis, use of mercury contain creams, facial erythema *ab igne* (usually in cooks), chronic actinic dermatitis, actinic lichen planus, acquired bilateral nevus-of-Ota-like macules, late onset dermal melanosis (upper lip and back), and friction hypermelanosis.

Etiology

Multifactorial, mostly related to pregnancy, oral contraceptive use, ultraviolet light exposure; also genetics, endocrine or hepatic dysfunction, medications (phenytoin, isotretinoin). Male hormones do not precipitate melasma, but increased circulating LH levels, decreased testosterone levels possible.

Epidemiology

Approximately 90% of cases are women of child-bearing age, 10% men and older women, with increased incidence in Hispanics, Asians, Caribbeans. Anyone may be affected, but predominates in those with skin types IV–VI. Family history present in 50% to 70% of cases.

Treatment

Diet and lifestyle

• Mandatory: aggressive sun avoidance; compulsive use of UVA- and UVB-blocking sunscreens (SPF 15 to 30); discontinuation of oral contraceptives. If oral contraceptives must be maintained, reduce to lowest possible estrogen dose or switch to progesterone-only contraceptives.

Pharmacological treatment

Topical

• Hydroquinone: Once daily, initially; twice daily, after tolerance established; 2% to 5%; concentrations up to 10%; concentrations above 5% increase incidence of side effects, especially paradoxical hyperpigmentation. Available in 3% solution; 4% cream (alone or with sunblock, sunscreen). Tachyphylaxis may require temporary discontinuation. Faster, better results when combined with other agents; hydroquinone, tretinoin synergistic. Kligman formula: hydroquinone 5%, tretinoin 0.01%, dexamethasone 0.1%, in hydrophilic ointment. Pathak recommendation: 2% hydroquinone, 0.05 to 0.1% tretinoin, no corticosteroids, in cream or lotion. Imperative to have pharmacist experienced in compounding make formulation. May apply each agent separately (eg:hydroquinone, morning; corticosteroids, afternoon; tretinoin, night), to better control patient intolerance. Available: hydroquinone 4% with glycolic acid,with or without sunscreen.

• Monobenzyl ether of hydroquinone causes irreversible depigmentation, confetti-like depigmentation; never use for melasma.

• Tretinoin 0.1% cream, nightly, for facial melasma; clinical effect may not be apparent until after 24 to 40 weeks; gel more irritating than cream. Stinging, peeling, irritation may produce dermatitis causing hyperpigmentation. At 0.025% or .05%, applied every 2 to 3 days, as tolerated. Photosensitivity may occur.

• Azelaic acid 20% cream, twice daily: progressively but slowly effective over a 5 to 8 months. Stinging, itching usually transient, but irritation may be significant.

• Corticosteroid creams produce hypopigmentation directly related to potency of agent. Clobetasol propionate, used alone, reduces pigmentation in 6 to 8 weeks; carefully monitor for atrophy, acne telangiectasia. Low-potency (hydrocortisone, dexamethasone, aclometasone) or fourth-generation (fluticasone, mometasone) corticosteroid creams may also reduce inflammatory effects of other depigmenting agents.

• Glycolic acid most effective in peel; in lotion, cream, washes, may improve efficacy of other bleaching agents. Other α-hydroxy acids for melasma: lactic acid, citric acid, malic acid, tartaric acid.

• Kojic acid (cream, lotion), most beneficial combined with other bleaching agents.

• Arbutin well tolerated; little scientific experience to recommend it.

Nonpharmacological treatment

Physical modalities

• Chemical peels (chemabrasion), with glycolic acid 20% to 70% or trichloracetic acid 15% to 25%, hasten effect of topical therapy. During healing stage, topical corticosteroid creams or emollients. Once healing occurs, treatment between peels—hydroquinone (preferably) or tretinoin or azeleic acid—is essential. Also beneficial: kojic acid, salicylic acid (20% to 30%), Jessner peels.

• Spot chemoabrasion with trichloroacetic acid, 15% to 25% may be necessary.

• Microdermabrasion: Effect similar to peels, but postinflammatory pigmentation can occur, if used alone.

Surgery

• Lasers (eg, Nd:Yag, Erbium:YAG, Alexandrite, Q-switched ruby): results in melasma unimpressive; risks outweigh benefits. Hyperpigmention may develop, requiring extensive treatment; melasma can return.

Treatment aims

Consistent, prolonged decrease in pigmentation. Complete remission, cure unrealistic; expect 6 to 12 months of treatment before significant benefit visible.

Prognosis

Melasma is chronic; usually improves in winter, but pigmentation often recurs after exposure to ultraviolet light or precipitating agent. In general, melasma of recent onset responds to treatment better than does long-standing pigmentation. Epidermal melasma is easier to bleach than the dermal or mixed types.

Follow-up and management

Except severest cases, manage with some combination of bleaching agents, α-hydroxy acids or tretinoin and, if needed, corticosteroids. Key to success: patience, sun avoidance.

General references

Goldberg DJ: Laser treatment of pigmented lesions. *Dermatol Clin* 1997, **15**:397–407.

Piamphongsant T: Treatment of melasma: a review with personal experience. *Intern J Dermatol* 1998, **37**:897–903.

Kauh YC, Zachian TF: Melasma. *Adv Exp Med Biol* 1999, **455**:491–459.

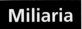

Diagnosis

Signs

The appearance of the eruption is different for each of the four types:

• **Miliaria crystallina:** Fine, tiny vesicles, no erythema on the head, neck, upper trunk

• **Miliaria rubra:** Diffuse erythema with small vesicles and papules on the neck, groin, axillae, and antecubital and popliteal fossae.

• **Miliaria pustulosa:** Resembles folliculitis of the intertriginous areas because pustules are found there, but lesions are not associated with hair follicles

• **Miliaria profunda:** Cobblestone non-erythematous papules with a widespread distribution, but sparing hands, feet, face, and axillae.

Symptoms

• Vary from none for mild cases to severe itching or burning, which is often described as intense prickling. In miliaria profunda, sweating is decreased or absent; malaise and fever are possible.

Investigations

• Skin biopsy reveals obstruction of the sweat ducts with formation of vesicles. The level of blockage corresponds to the type of miliaria (biopsy is not usually done because diagnosis is clinically apparent).

• Cultures may be needed to rule out staphylococcal folliculitis or *Candida* infection

Complications

• Secondary bacterial or fungal infection may develop in miliaria crystallina, rubra, or pustulosa. Widespread miliaria profunda may cause weakness, fever and malaise.

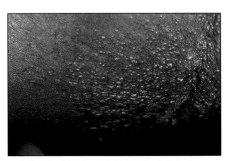

Grouped, pinpoint, papulovesicles and pink papules at the opening of the eccrine glands, resulting in a prickly appearance (miliaria rubra).

Differential diagnosis

Folliculitis, periporitis, contact dermatitis, erythema neonatorum, viral exanthem, herpes simplex, and candidiasis.

Etiology

The cause has been reported to be an alteration of epidermis by high heat and humidity with subsequent blockage and rupture of sweat duct. More recently, it has been suggested that an extracellular polysaccharide substance produced by *S. epidermis* and other bacteria is responsible for duct occlusion. Others believe that the lesions are caused by disruption rather than blockage of the sweat ducts.

Miliaria may follow a previous skin rash such as contact dermatitis, lichen simplex, or intertrigo. This eruption can be reproduced by occlusion of skin with polyethylene wrap.

Epidemiology with patient profile

Miliaria is more common among whites living or visiting hot, humid tropical climates.

Miliaria crystallina: Febrile patients, infants, and after sunburn

Miliaria rubra: Children

Miliaria pustulosa: Following another skin disorder

Miliaria profunda: Workers or military personnel in tropical climates

Special

Commonly called prickly heat

Bruce Burgreen

Treatment

Diet and lifestyle
• Affected patients should avoid occlusive clothing or topical preparations in hot humid environments and should restrict activities during periods of extreme heat and humidity.

Pharmacological treatment

Topical
• Talc-based powders, such as talcum (contains magnesium silicate), ZeaSORB(microporous cellulose provides greatest absorption), Gordomatic (antipruritic because it contains menthol, camphor, thymus, eucalyptus, and potassium alum), Every Step (antibacterial because it contains triclosan and chlorhexidine) and Gold Bond (salicylic acid, methyl salicylate, zinc oxide, and eucalyptol).

• Shake lotions, such as Calamine (zinc oxide, calamine), Caladryl (calamine, pramoxine, camphor) and Caladryl Clear (zinc acetate, pramoxine, camphor).

• 4% Salicylic acid tincture (keratolytic).

• Low potency topical corticosteroids.

• Antipruritics to relieve itching, such as 5% doxepin (Zonalon) and any lotions containing menthol, camphor, phenol, pramoxine, or lidocaine.

Systemic
• Antihistamines as needed for itching.

• Vitamin C, 1 g daily, has been anecdotally reported to improve some cases.

• Isotretinoin (for disabling miliaria profunda) (anecdotal indication).

Nonpharmacological treatment

Supportive methods
• Affected individuals should be placed in an air-conditioned (low heat, humidity) environment.

Physical modalities
• Cool baths.

• Cold compresses with tap water or aluminum acetate.

• Air-conditioned room and loose, porous clothing.

Special therapeutic considerations
• Use of powders in infants is discouraged.

Treatment aims
To remove causative factors (heat, humidity), reduce symptoms.

Prognosis
Eruption spontaneously improves within a week due to the natural epidermal turnover and complete recovery is usual within 2–3 weeks. In cases of continuous exposure to heat and humidity, miliaria profunda may develop, which can have severe complications.

General references
Kirk JF, Wilson BB, Chun W, *et al.*: Miliaria profunda [review]. *J Am Acad Dermatol* 1996, 35:854–856.

Feng E, Janniger CK: Miliaria [review]. *Cutis* 1995, 55:213–216.

DiBeneditto JP, Worobec SM: Exposure to hot environments can cause dermatological problems. *Occup Health Saf* 1985, 54:35–38.

Diagnosis

Signs

• Smooth, round, dome-shaped, often umbilicated, gray-white to flesh-colored papules, usually 2–5 mm; scattered, grouped, often symmetrical crops. Firm, gray-white core can be expressed. Erythema common at papule border. Ususally on face, less common on neck, trunk, axillae, extremities; rarely lips, oral mucosa.

•In healthy adults, usually sexually acquired; mainly genitals; less common on pubic area, groin, upper thighs, perineum, lower abdomen, buttocks. Usually fewer than 20 lesions; if immunosuppression, atopic dermatitis, more than 100 possible. Lesions may grow to 3.0 cm. or become confluent into plaques.

Symptoms

• Molluscum contagiosum (MC) is usually asymptomatic; occasionally pruritic, especially in genital, body-fold areas. May be tenderness or erythema 1 week before regression of lesions.

Investigations

Diagnosis: Visual inspection. **Confirmation**: Shave biopsy or crush prep. Lesion punctured, core expressed, crushed between glass slides, air-dried specimen, Giemsa or Wright stained, microscopically (10-times power lens) examined for Henderson-Paterson bodies. **Histopathology**: Lobules of enlarged epidermal cells; intracytoplasmic, faintly basophilic inclusion bodies containing viral particles. **Serum antibodies**: Not useful for diagnosis.

Complications

•Children, immunocompetent: Benign, usually self-limited. Lesions may ulcerate, crust. Secondary bacterial abscesses, impetigo possible in affected area. In 10%, perilesional eczema. Post-inflammatory hypopigmentation or hyperpigmentation may remain after healing. Conjunctivitis, keratitis may complicate eyelid lesions.

Differential diagnosis

Most frequent misdiagnoses: Genitals—human papillomavirus infection; follicular lesions—folliculitis; facial lesions—comedonal acne.

In HIV infection, confirm MC diagnosis to exclude similar skin lesions produced by opportunistic infections. MC can be misdiagnosed as lichen planus, sebaceous hyperplasia, trichoepitheliomas, syringomas, nodular basal-cell carcinomas, keratoacanthomas, papillomas, neurilemmomas, other neoplasms.

Etiology

Poxvirus; replicates in human keratinocyte cytoplasm. Strains: MC virus (MCV)-1, MCV-2. Morphologically, anatomically identical. MCV-1 causes 75% to 92% of infections.

Epidemiology

Incubation: 2–7 weeks after close skin-to-skin contact. Common in childhood; second incidence peak in young adulthood, from sexual transmission.

Risk factors: Immunodeficiency, atopic dermatitis, sarcoidosis.

HIV: MC may be initial manifestation of HIV infection; usually with CD4 counts below 100 cells/mm³; 9% to 18% of AIDS patients develop lesions.

Contact-sport athletes vulnerable.

Self-inoculation via scratching, shaving can spread infection.

Can be acquired from masseurs, medical personnel, hairstylists, cosmeticians, possibly gymnasium machines, electrolysis needles, shared towels, sponges, swimming pools, saunas, bathing facilities.

Adults: Sexual transmission increasing.

Children: Genital lesions common, but thoroughly evaluate for potential sexual abuse.

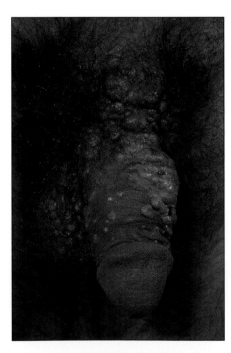

Grouped, pearly pink, discrete, smooth, papules with central umbilication are scattered throughout the penis, scrotum, and perigenital pubis in this man with molluscum contagiosum.

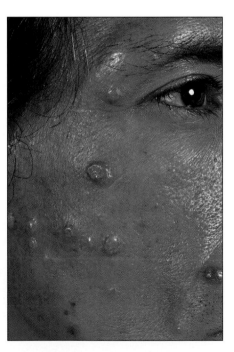

Large molluscum contagiosum lesions on the face of an immunocompromised patient.

Judith Shapiro and Miguel Sanchez

Treatment

Diet and lifestyle
•Condoms protect only shielded areas. No dietary intervention or nutritional supplementation alters course. No alternative treatment proven efficacious.

Pharmacological treatment

Topical
• Tricloroacetic acid (TCA), 35% to 90%, directly on lesions with small, calcium alginate swab until surface whitens. Petroleum jelly to avoid burning surrounding skin. Puncturing lesion may increase efficacy. Preferred method for pregnant women; little or no scarring, pigmentation usually returns within days to weeks.

• TCA peels, 25% to 35%, every 2 weeks (15 peels), in severe cases associated with HIV.

• Podophyllin resin, 25% to 50%, directly on lesions with cotton-swab applicator, washed off in 4-6 hours. Dusting powder aids drying, helps prevent smearing. Used after TCA, may enhance effect.

• Podophyllotoxin, 0.5% solution or gel, twice daily, 3 consecutive days (main adverse effects: tolerable pruritus, erythema).

• Tretinoin cream: Lower concentrations (0.025%) to prevent new lesions; higher concentrations (0.1% twice daily) to resolve lesions.

• 5-fluorouracil cream, 5%: every day or every other day to prevent; once to twice daily, to resolve.

• Cantharidin solution, 0.7%, effective, painless (unavailable in US). Post-treatment pruritus, burning, erythema, crusting, ulceration (well tolerated). **Cantharidin**, 0.9%, with **salicylic acid, podophyllin** in acetone, flexible collodion—more potent, well tolerated.

• Salicylic acid, 17%, in polyacrylic solution or karaya gum daily.

Imiquimod cream, 1%, 3-5 days/week, 4 weeks.

• Cidofovir gel, daily; also compounded in 3% concentration in combination vehicle, daily. Iirritating but highly effective.

• Other: Repeated applications of potassium hydroxide (twice daily for 30 days), silver nitrate, benzoyl peroxide gel, 10% tincture of iodine (alone or with 40% salicylic acid plaster), puncturing lesion with toothpick dipped in phenol.

Systemic
• Cimetidine, 40 mg/kg/d, three divided doses, 2 months. **Interferon**-α: Subcutaneous injections, for severe MC in immunodeficient children.

Nonpharmacological treatment
Electron beam, single application. **Light electrodesiccation**: 0.4-1.0 W for small lesions, with or without curettage. **Curettage**, then 25% aluminum chloride or Monsel's solution. Ethyl chloride spray may decrease pain, facilitate curettage. **Incision** of lesion surface with 19-gauge needle or sharp-end scalpel blade, expression of viral load with comedone extractor. **Shave excision** with rounded scalpel. **CO₂ laser**. **Pulsed-dye laser**, 585-nm, flashlamp pumped, single treatment, in HIV-infected, immunocompromised patients; no recurrence after 4 months. **Pinpoint cryotherapy** with liquid nitrogen, -196 °C, either by spray or soaked cotton swab. Duration of application depends on size of lesion, force of spray. Keep each lesion frozen for at least 7 seconds. Repeat twice for lesions larger than 4 mm. Use petrolatum to protect surrounding skin. Dimethyl ether propane cryogenic spray (-56 °C) also effective.

Supportive methods
•Application to lesions of lidocaine/prilocaine cream under occlusion or 5% lidocaine in liposomal-based cream for 60 minutes decreases pain during treatment.

Treatment aims
To treat lesions, to cease spread of infection to patient, and to prevent transmission to other persons.

Special therapeutic considerations
AIDS cases: Highly active antiretroviral therapy often works within 6 months. Sexually acquired **MC**: Evaluate for other sexually transmitted diseases. New lesions may erupt for weeks, months. Prophylaxis of affected skin with imiquimod, tretinoin, fluorouracil advocated by some. Response depends on size, number of lesions. Avoid scarring; in children, healthy adults, lesions regress spontaneously. More aggressive treatment if immunocompromised. Recommendations hampered by lack of large, well-designed, controlled studies. Multiple therapy may be necessary.

Prognosis
Even without treatment, lesions usually heal without scarring in 6–9 months, but may remain for years. Infection spreads easily to others; lesions unsightly. Sexually acquired MC: shame, discrimination.

General references
Waugh MA: Molluscum contagiosum. *Dermatol Clin* 1998, **16**:839–841.

Lewis EJ, Lam M, Crutchfield CE: An update on molluscum contagiosum. *Cutis* 1997, **60**:29–34.

Gottlieb SL, Myskowski PL: Molluscum contagiosum. *Int J Dermatol* 1994, **33**:453–461.

Diagnosis

Signs

Onychomycosis (O)

Distal lateral subunguial (DLSO): Begins as focal onycholysis, progresses to yellow-brown discoloration, hyperkeratosis of nail bed (subungual debris).

White superficial (WSO): Chalky-white areas on dorsal surface of nail plate; gradually coalesce, cover entire nail plate; eventually, entire nail becomes crumbly.

Proximal subungual (PSO): Whitish-brown discoloration of proximal nail plate; may proceed to involve entire nail; subungual hyperkeratosis may develop.

Candidal (CO): Rough, thickened, furrowed nail plate becomes hyperkeratotic, brittle, crumbly, dystrophic.

Paronychia (P)

Candidal (CP): Erythema, edema, inflammation, swelling; most common: proximal nail fold; retracted in chronic cases. Creamy exudate possible if nail fold is pressed. Onycholysis, discoloration, ridging possible in nails of affected fingers.

Bacterial (BP): Usually due to *Staphylococcus aureus*; exquisite tenderness, abscess formation of proximal or lateral nail fold. Infection spreads to eponychium, eventually to opposite nail fold or pad of finger (felon).

***Pseudomonas* nail infection (PNI):** green discoloration.

Investigations

•Microscopic examination: Chalazion curette to remove subungual debris Avulse unattached nail plate, remove scales from nail bed at most proximal areas of involvement. Most hyphae found proximally.

WSO: Scrape nail-plate surface.

P: Scrape nail. Mix specimen in glass slide with potassium hydroxide, 10% to 20%; examine microscopically. Chlorazol black E selectively stains hyphae, helps identify fungal elements. Potassium hydroxide: most sensitive diagnostic procedure.

•Culture: Crushed nail clippings in appropriate media; allows identification of causative organism. Cycloheximide-containing media: identify dermatophytes (*eg*, mycologic culture). Sabouraud's glucose agar to identify nondermatophyte infections.

•Histopathologic examination: Examine avulsed or biopsied nail plate fragment for fungi after periodic acid-Schiff staining.

•Gram stain, bacterial culture for BP, nail infection.

Complications

•Spread of infection to other nails or areas of skin. Infected nail may be reservoir for recurrent fungal infections. Dystrophy, nail loss. Cellulitis more common in onychomycosis patients, especially those with diabetes, impaired peripheral circulation.

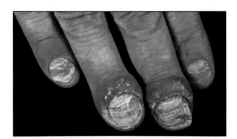

Crescent-shaped erythema, induration, edema of proximal nail folds of a woman with chronic paronychia; candidal onychomycois on fingernails.

Differential diagnosis

O: Psoriasis, lichen planus, eczema, alopecia areata, trauma.
P: Psoriasis, eczema.

Etiology

O: Most cases (91%) caused by dermatophytes, most commonly *Trichophyton rubrum,,* then *Trichophyton mentagrophytes* and *Epidermophyton floccosum. T. mentagrophytes* usually causes WSO in immunocompetent persons, but if AIDS, *T. rubrum. Candida albicans* causes 5.5% of cases (usually in persons with chronic CP). Pathogenic molds (< 3%) can cause DLSO.
P: Acute usually caused by *Staphylococcus aureus*; chronic usually begins as irritant dermatitis that becomes superinfected with *Candida* species or bacteria.
PNI: Begins with onycholysis, which permits bacterial entrance.

Epidemiology

O: Estimated to occur in 8.9% of population; may affect up to 20% of persons 40–60 years. Toenails affected four times more often than fingernails. More common in men than women. Rare in prepubertal children. High incidence in elderly persons. Predisposing factors: diabetes mellitus, immunosuppression, hyperhidrosis, trauma, poor peripheral circulation.
P: Common in homemakers, workers who frequently immerse hands in water (bartenders, nurses, bakers), resulting in drying, irritation, subsequent infection of nail fold. Manicures with retracted cuticles may also predispose to P.

Erick Mafong and Paul Kechijian

Treatment

Diet and lifestyle
• Prophylaxis using antifungal foot powder; prevention of overhydration by avoidance of occlusive footwear, prolonged contact with water, trauma.

• Persons prone to P should avoid predisposing conditions, such as moist environments (by using gloves), aggressive manicures, irritants.

Pharmacological treatment

Topical
• Antifungal creams (ketoconazole, oxiconazole, miconazole, clotrimazole, ciclopirox, terbinafine, butenafine) effective in CP and may prevent relapses of treated O. SWO can initially be treated with debridement of superficial fungi, followed by topical antifungals. 2% miconazole tincture is approved for CP, but may have improved nail penetration. Miconazole-undecylenic acid-urea-tea tree oil cream reportedly better results.

Systemic
Terbinafine (fungicidal allylamine), 250 mg/d; 6 weeks, fingernails; 12 weeks, toenails. Cure rate: 70%, toenails; 79%, fingernails. Also effective against some nondermatophytes. Neutropenia, agranulocytosis (especially in immunodeficient patients); increased liver enzyme levels if administered for more than 6 weeks.

Itraconazole: *Continuous therapy*: 200 mg/d, with food, 6 weeks for fingernails, 12 weeks for toenails; *pulse therapy*: 400 mg/d; 1 week per month for 2 months, fingernails; 3–4 months, toenails. Cure rate: 64%, toenails, either regimen. Reversible hepatitis (< 1 in 800 patients); multiple drug interactions.

Fluconazole: 300 mg, once weekly; 4 months, fingernails; 8 months, toenails. Cure rate: 70% to 80% (slightly lower if 150 mg/week dosage).

Griseofulvin: 500 mg, b.i.d, 6–9 months, fingernails; 12–18 months, toenails.

Relapse rate is 80%.

BP: Use antibiotics that cover *S. aureus* and to which cultured organism is sensitive.

Nonpharmacological treatment

Surgery
• If few nails involved, nail avulsion followed by topical antifungal therapy; improves cure rate in O. Incision, drainage of purulent, bulging infected nail folds.

Other
• Adjuvant treatments for P used in conjunction with antifungals: warm soaks with saline or aluminum acetate, applications of 3% thymol in 70% isopropyl alcohol or 50% povidone-iodine solution–50% isopropyl alcohol, and topical corticosteroids for 1–2 weeks.

• Oral antifungals for recalcitrant CP; Fluconazole most active against *Candida*.

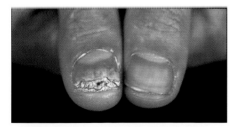

Subungual hyperkeratosis of distal nail bed, breakage of distal nail plate in patient with distal subungual onychomycosis; early involvement of hyponychium, distal nail bed visible on other side.

Treatment aims
To treat infection, prevent recurrence, eliminate predisposing factors.

Prognosis
Recurrences (as high as 50%) common in O, unless precautions taken after treatment. P prone to recur unless predisposing factors removed. Some patients, especially those with candidal endocrinopathy, tend to develop candidal infection.

Follow-up and management
Before treatment with systemic agents, verify fungal infection using potassium hydroxide preparation, culture, histology.

General references
Baran R, Hay R, Haneke E, *et al.*: Onychomycosis. The Current Approach to Diagnosis and Therapy. London: Martin Dunitz; 1999.

Roberts DT: Oral therapeutic agents in fungal nail disease. *J Am Acad Dermatol* 1994, **31**:578–581.

Elewski BE, Charif MA, Daniel CR: Onychomycosis. In *Nails: Therapy, Diagnosis, Surgery*. Edited by Scher RK, Daniel RC. Philadelphia: WB Saunders; 1997:151–162.

Diagnosis

Signs

- Skin lesions that are present in the newborn, have resolved or started to resolve by 30 days of age, and require minimal or no intervention are considered transient.

Milia: Multiple 1- to 2-mm whitish or yellow papules distributed over the forehead, cheeks and nose.

Epstein's pearls: Milia in the oral cavity, usually on the gingiva and palate.

Miliaria crystallina: Clear, thin-walled, easily ruptured; generalized distribution, with increased lesions in intertriginous areas. Lesions resemble water droplets.

Miliaria rubra: Small, red papules or papulovesicles, often grouped. Face, neck trunk most often involved in neonates.

Sebaceous gland hyperplasia (SGH): Tiny, 1-mm yellow macules or papules at orifice of pilosebaceous follicles on nose, cheeks.

Erythema toxicum neonatorum (ETN): Blotchy, 1- to 3-cm erythematous macules with central vesicle or pustule; on trunk, genitalia, proximal extremities; palms, soles spared. Lesions resemble flea bites.

Transient neonatal pustulosis (melanosis) (TNP): Vesicles, pustules; may be ruptured. Surrounding collarette of scale. Most common on neck, trunk, extremities. Lesions often heal with residual brown macules.

Neonatal cephalic pustulosis (NCP): Monomorphic erythematous papulopustules on face, neck, scalp.

Acne neonatorum (AN): Inflammatory papules, pustules, open and closed comedones; primarily on face, also chest, back, groin.

Symptoms

- Lesions asymptomatic.

Investigations

- Essential to differentiate transient, benign dermatoses in newborn from more serious lesions caused by infection and requiring prompt treatment. Diagnostic tests strongly advised if diagnosis is questionable.

- Evaluation of pustules, vesicles, blisters in neonate by Gram stain; Wright–Giemsa stain; Tzank preparation; potassium hydroxide preparation; viral, bacterial, and fungal culture; direct fluorescent antibody detection (for viral studies); biopsy of skin lesions for histopathologic examination and for immunofluorescence.

Other studies: Complete blood count with differential, peripheral blood and cerebrospinal fluid culture, as indicated.

ETN: Wright stain of a smear prepared from a central vesicle or pustule shows numerous eosinophils.

TNP: Wright stain of a smear prepared from a vesicle or pustule shows numerous neutrophils.

NCP: Giemsa stain of a smear prepared from a pustule shows *Malassezia* yeast with a predominance of neutrophils and occasional eosinophils, basophils, lymphocytes, and epithelial cells.

Differential diagnosis

Bacterial sepsis, *Pityosporum* folliculitis, herpes neonatorum, congenital herpes simplex, congenital rubella, congenital candidiasis, congenital syphilis, infantile acropustulosis, nevus comedonicus, pustular psoriasis, neonatal varicella, impetigo.

Etiology

Milia: Cystic retention of keratin in the papillary dermis.

SGH: Overgrowth of sebaceous glands secondary to stimulation by maternal androgens.

ETN: Unknown.

TNP: Unknown.

NCP: Inflammatory reaction against colonization by yeasts of the genus *Malassezia*.

AN: Stimulation of sebaceous glands by maternal and infant androgens.

Epidemiology

Milia: Cutaneous lesions seen in up to 40% of newborns; oral cavity lesions in up to 64%.

SGH: Seen in 50% of newborns.

ETN: Seen in 30%–50% of newborns, but rarely in premature newborns.

TNP: Present at birth. Seen in approximately 5% of black and 0.5% of white newborns.

NCP: Age at onset: 1–3 weeks.

AN: Seen in up to 50% of infants. Rarely seen before 2–4 weeks of age.

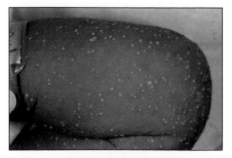

Erythema toxicum on the leg of a newborn presenting with tiny sterile pustules

Sara L. Tarsis and Samuel Weinberg

Treatment

Pharmacological treatment

Topical

AN: Severe cases can be treated with topical 2.5% benzoyl peroxide gel or lotion.

NCP: Can be treated with 2% ketoconazole cream, usually for 1 week.

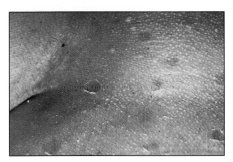

Transient neonatal pustulosis with superficial vesicles and pustules that rupture leaving pink macules surrounded by collarettes of scale.

Treatment aims

These conditions are mild and self-limiting and require no or minimal treatment. Reassurance of the parents or caregivers is important.

Proper diagnosis is essential. Lesions due to infectious causes that present in the neonate can lead to significant morbidity and death if not treated appropriately in a timely manner.

No treatments are needed for milia, SGH, ETN, and TNP.

Prognosis

Milia: Self-resolving, with spontaneous rupture and exfoliation at several weeks of age.

SGH: Self-resolves by 4 months of age.

ETN: Lesions usually begin at 24–48 hours of life and self-resolve in 4–5 days. New lesions may be observed up to day 10 of life; all lesions are resolved by age 2 weeks.

TNP: Vesicles and pustules last 48–72 hours; residual hyperpigmented macules fade over 3 weeks to 3 months.

NCP Resolves after 1 week of treatment and may resolve spontaneously.

AN: Usually self-resolves, can persist for the first few months of life.

General references

Treadwell PA: Dermatoses in newborns. *Am Fam Phys* 1997, **56**:443–450.

Van Praag MCG, *et al.*: Diagnosis and treatment of pustular disorders in the neonate. *Pediatr Dermatol* 1997, **14**:131–143.

Rapelanoro R, *et al.*: Neonatal *Malassezia furfur* pustulosis. *Arch Dermatol* 1996, **132**:190–193.

Frieden IJ: Blisters and Pustules in the Newborn. Yale University/Glaxo Dermatology Lectureship Series, 1999.

Diagnosis

Signs

Postherpetic neuralgia (PHN): Involved skin may show pigmentary changes, discrete scars. Generally limited to area of skin innervated by a single sensory ganglion (dermatomal distribution).

Peripheral neuropathy (PN): No specific cutaneous findings; skin may be dry, hyperpigmented, lichenified, erythematous, scaly. Often in stocking-glove, urogenital, perianal, or distal extremity distribution.

Notalgia paraesthetica (NP): May be hyperpigmented patch above or below scapula, close to medial border.

Symptoms

PHN: Pain that persists or appears after lesions have healed or 30 days after onset of eruption. Symptoms: deep aching or burning pain (dysesthesia), altered sensitivity to touch (paresthesia), exaggerated responses to stimuli (hyperesthesia), electric shock–like pains, pain provoked by otherwise trivial stimuli (allodynia). Motor paralysis in 1% to 5% of patients with herpes zoster (HZ).

PN: Dysesthesia, paresthesia, hyperesthesia, electric shock–like pains, allodynia, anhydrosis.

NP: Episodes of localized pruritus or skin pain.

Investigations

• Dermatopathology is not helpful in any of these conditions.

Complications

PHN and **PN**: Depression (correlates with pain severity, duration), neuropathic ulcers, irritant dermatitis (from loss of bladder control), arthropathy.

Differential diagnosis

PHN: Peripheral neuropathy, herpes simplex with neuralgia.
PN: Psychological disease.
NP: Macular or lichen amyloidosus, lichen simplex chronicus, post-inflammatory pigmentation, fixed drug eruption, Hansen's disease.

Etiology

PHN: Herpes simplex virus–related damage of nerve cells. PN: Systemic disease (diabetes mellitus, sarcoid, Hansen's disease, HIV infection, neurologic disease), medications (dapsone, thalidomide, chemotherapeutic agents, tacrolimus), nutrition deficiencies (vitamin B_{12}, beriberi), idiopathic.
NP: Unknown

Epidemiology

PHN: Of patients with untreated zoster, approximately 50% of those older than 60 and 75% of those older than 75 will develop PHN, which may persist for months or years. Incidence is closely linked to increasing age.
PN and **NP**: Unknown

Steven Natow and Allen Natow

Treatment

Diet and lifestyle

• There is no support for vitamin B_{12} supplementation or a diet high in calcium citrate and low in oxalate.

Pharmacological treatment

Topical

Capsaicin, 0.025% or 0.075% cream, t.i.d. to q.i.d.; worsening of initial pain is due to release of substance P. **Intralesional corticosteriods**, 2.5–5.0 mg/mL, up to a maximum of 12 treatments. **"Tumescent" mixture** of 500 mL saline, 60 mg triamcinalone acetonide, 50 mL 1% Xylocaine, with 1:1,000,000 epinephrine: **Force** injected with 20-gauge lumbar puncture needle into deep fat, subcutaneous tissue, and dermis until entire affected area is indurated; variable success. **Ketamine, gabapentin, clonidine, ketoprofen have been compounded for topical use**

Systemic

Antidepressants, such as amitriptyline, 10 mg, increased daily for 5–7 days until reasonable relief is achieved (usually at 75 mg), effective in 75% of patients who begin receiving regimen within 6 months after HZ. Continue treatment for 3–6 months after relief is achieved. Nortriptyline, desipramine, paroxetine, venlafaxine also reportedly improve neuralgia. Tricyclic antidepressants appear to have better efficacy than serotonin inhibitors.

Anticonvulsants, such as phenytoin (usual dosage, 150 mg, b.i.d.); divalproex sodium, 15 mg/kg/d, 2 divided doses, gradually increased up to 60 mg/kg/d; carbamazepine, 100 mg, twice daily, gradually increased up to 1200 mg/d, if needed. Gabapentin promising: 300 mg/d (day 1); 300 mg, b.i.d. (day 2); 300 mg, t.i.d. daily (day 3); then increasing gradually up to 600 mg, t.i.d. (up to 2400 mg/d).

Pimozide, 2 mg, t.i.d., reported successful within 3 weeks, but phenoziazines neither improve PHN nor augment the effect of tricyclic antidepressants.

Nonpharmacological treatment

Supportive methods

For pain: Topical anesthetics (*eg*, 10% lidocaine gel); doxepin 5% cream, t.i.d.; compounded piroxicam, 0.5% gel, or ketoprofen, 2.5% gel; oral acetaminophen or salicylates; nonsteroidal anti-inflammatory drugs (NSAIDs): celecoxib, 100 mg, q.d. to b.i.d.; rofecoxib, 12.5–25 mg/d; ketoprofen, 50–100 mg, t.i.d.; tramadol, 50–100 mg, every 4–6 hours, up to 400 mg/d. **Narcotic analgesics** containing codeine, hydrocodone, or oxycodone; meperidine; and, for recalcitrant cases, oral morphine or fentanyl patches.

Physical modalities

Cold packs. Splinting. Acupuncture. Ultrasound or vibration (with a vibromassager). **Transcutaneous electrical nerve stimulation** (TENS), and other methods directed at preventing affected area from being touched, may provide temporary relief. **Nerve blocks**: peripheral, regional, epidural, or subarachnoid. **Psychotherapy** or **hypnosis**.

Surgery

Implantation of nerve-block stimulator. **Cordotomy, rhizotomy, sympathectomy** are treatments of last resort, carrying substantial risk for prolonged hemiparesis, sensory deficits; they are not advocated.

Special therapeutic considerations

NP is treated with injections of triamcinolone acetonide, with or without lidocaine; topical medications; oral analgesics.

Early treatment of HZ with antiviral agents (acyclovir, valacyclovir, famciclovir) benefits quality of life, may decrease neuralgia risk, but may not alter pain. **Systemic corticosteroid therapy** can decrease pain during HZ infection; effect in preventing neuralgia controversial, unproven. **HZ vaccination for those at high risk for neuralgia: studies underway.**

Treatment aims

To prevent complications, eliminate pain, restore nerve integrity, prevent progression.

Prognosis

PHN usually resolves within 12 months, but may persist for years. PN is difficult to treat and may ultimately be refractory to treatment.

Support organizations

American Pain Society; phone: 708-966-5595. Varicella-Zoster Virus Research Foundation; phone: 212-472-3181.

General references

Gerson AA: Epidemiology and management of postherpetic neuralgia. *Semin Dermatol* 1996, **15**:8–13.

Wood AJ: Postherpetic neuralgia: pathogenesis, treatment, and prevention. *N Engl J Med* 1996, **335**:32–42.

Portenoy RK: Acute herpetic and postherpetic neuralgia: clinical review and current management. *Ann Neurol* 1986, **20**:651–662.

Weber PJ, *et al*.: Notalgia paresthetica. *J Am Acad Dermatol* 1988, **18**:25–30.

Archer CB: The skin and the nervous system. In:. *Rook/Wilkinson/Ebling Textbook of Dermatology*, edn 6. Edited by Champion RH, *et al*. London: Blackwell Science; 1998:2773–2783.

Diagnosis

Signs

Brittle nails (BN): Increased longitudinal ridging, horizontal layering, roughening of surface, distal splitting of nail, nail edge.

Onycholysis (OL): Distal separation of nail plate from nail bed. Areas of separation may appear white or yellow due to air, debris trapped beneath nail plate.

Onychodystrophies (OD): Longitudinal melanonychia (LM): Tan, brown, or black pigmented band from proximal nail fold to free edge of nail plate. Hutchinson's sign may suggest malignancy (*ie*, subungual melanoma; SM). Benign lesions often associated with multiple nail involvement, childhood onset. Color not a critical factor. SMs associated with older age, nail dystrophy, recent change in color or width, blurred margins; more common on larger digits.

Symptoms

BN, and **melanonychia** : Asymptomatic, but cosmetic embarrassment possible.

OL, and **OD** may become irritated, painful.

Investigations

OL: Culture to rule out dermatophytosis, secondary bacterial infection; nail biopsy.

LM: Photographic documentation of change in appearance; punch biopsy of nail matrix (not of nail bed).

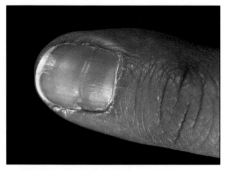

Horizontal ridge of the nail plate, due to an episode of slower nail growth (Beau's line) in a patient with chronic hand dermatitis.

Differential diagnosis

BN: Koilonychia (spoon nails; associated with anemia and collagen vascular disease), nail crescents (associated with chronic illness), Mees' lines (associated with arsenic poisoning, Hodgkin's disease, renal failure, pneumonia), Muehrcke's lines (associated with albumin ≤ 2.2 g/dL), yellow nails (associated with chronic bronchitis, cancer, lymphedema).

OL: Psoriasis, infection (bacterial, fungal, yeast), trauma, idiopathic drug induced, maceration, hyperthyroidism, hypothyroidism.

Hyperpigmentation of nail plate (HNP): Benign melanocytic conditions, SM, subungual hematoma, drug, pregnancy, Addison's disease, racial variations.

Etiology

BN: Exogenous factors that dehydrate the nail plate; associated with repeated cycles of immersion in water, particularly alkaline substances (*eg*, detergents, solvents, nail polish remover). Endogenous factors: iron deficiency, avitaminosis, poor peripheral circulation.

OL: Overhydration, use of nail enamel or nail wraps, occupational or recreational trauma (*eg*, piano playing), trauma in long fingernails, onychomycosis, allergic contact dermatitis, drug reactions; more prevalent with diabetes, thyroid abnormalities, pregnancy, peripheral vascular disease.

HNP: Release of pigment from nail matrix into nail plate by normal or malignant proliferation of melanocytes.

Epidemiology

BN: More common in elderly and those doing cleaning, housework.

OL: More common in workers whose hands are often immersed in water (bartenders, dishwashers, those doing cleaning, housework.

LM: More common in darker-skinned persons, usually multiple digits, can be secondary to medications (*eg*, minocycline, zidovudine, antimalarials). Highest incidence of SM: Caribbeans of African descent. Higher suspicion for melanoma in older individuals with a single new band.

Treatment

Diet and lifestyle

BN: Avoid unnecessary contact with water, detergents, other alkaline solvents, irritants; use nonacetone-based nail remover.

OL: Keep nails trimmed short; avoid trauma, water immersion.

Pharmacological treatment

Topical

OL: If caused by infection, apply 1:1 mixture of iodide tincture and isopropyl alcohol twice a day to the nail plates or 3% thymol in 70% isopropyl alcohol, followed by antifungal lotion or cream. Medium-potency topical corticosteroids may help, if inflammed.

Systemic

BN: Oral biotin is controversial.

Nonpharmacological treatment

BN: Eliminate exacerbating factors. Rehydrate nail plate with petrolatum, mineral oil, special nail oils, nail emollients, emollients containing lactic acid or urea cream applied frequently, especially after wetting hands. Cut nails after bathing when they are soft and file down and remove any irregularities in the distal edge of the nail plate to avoid trauma. Nail enamel may serve to strengthen the nail plate but its removal with acetone may lead to further dehydration.

OL: Removal of unattached nail, to allow nail bed to dry, and to facilitate application of antimicrobials.

HNP: Treatment of SM is amputation of digit. Smaller lesions may be locally excised. Isolated limb perfusion chemotherapy does not improve survival.

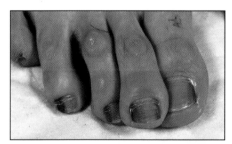

Longitudinal pigmented nail bands in a man treated with zidovudine.

Treatment aims

BN: To improve appearance and lessen brittleness.

OL: To facilitate attachment.

LM: To differentiate between benign and malignant causes.

Prognosis

BN and **OL**: Tend to be chronic, unless causative factors are identified, removed, or treated.

Follow-up and management

BN and **OL**: Monitor improvement and encourage lifestyle changes.

HNP: Monitor for clinical change in LM. SM requires metastatic evaluation. Evaluate every 3–6 months in first year to assess for lymph node involvement, metastases, local recurrence.

General references

Baran R, Kechijian P: Longitudinal melanonychia (melanonychia striata): Diagnosis and management. *J Am Acad Dermatol* 1989, **21**:1165.

Kechijian P. Onycholysis of the fingernails: Evaluation and management. *J Am Acad Dermatol* 1985, 12:552–560.

Kechijian P. Brittle fingernails. *Dermatol Clin* 1985, **3**:421–429.

Diagnosis

Definition

• Many types of hair loss are classified as nonscarring alopecias. These diagnoses differ in etiology, morphology and prognosis.

Diffuse global hair-loss: Congenital hypotrichosis/atrichia, alopecia areata, telogen effluvium, anagen effluvium, loose anagen syndrome, secondary syphilis, primary hair-shaft abnormality (*ie*, acquired trichorrhexis nodosa).

Focal hair loss: Alopecia areata, androgenetic alopecia, tinea capitis, traction alopecia, triangular alopecia, trichotillomania, secondary syphilis, primary or acquired hair shaft abnormality.

Signs

• Various degrees of increased hair shedding or breakage.

• Hair loss can be sudden, gradual, or variable in onset.

• Congenital triangular alopecia is present at birth but usually not discovered until early childhood.

Sudden onset: Alopecia areata, telogen effluvium, anagen effluvium, trichotillomania.

Gradual onset: Androgenetic alopecia, traction alopecia, trichotillomania, acquired trichorrhexis nodosa.

Variable onset: Tinea capitis, loose anagen syndrome, secondary syphilis

Investigations

• Careful medical history (including medications), hair-pull test, hair-pluck test, hair-shaft evaluation, scalp biopsy, fungal culture, serologies.

Androgenetic alopecia: Physical examination: Male-pattern characterized by bitemporal recession and/or vertex thinning; female-pattern characterized by slight frontal recession and diffuse thinning of postfrontal region extending gradually to entire crown; normal blood tests; positive family history (polygenic inheritance). Scalp biopsy rarely indicated.

Telogen effluvium: Abnormal hair-pull test. Increased hair shedding (100–400/day) precipitating cause generally 2–4 months prior to onset.

Alopecia areata: Excessive shedding. Physical examination: exclamation-point hairs in the periphery and total absence of hair or variable amounts of spontaneous/fine hair regrowth in the center; atypically faint erythema with associated itching/burning; nail changes, pitting: scalp usually appears normal; biopsy generally unnecessary for diagnosis.

Anagen effluvium: Variable degree of hair shedding, usually due to chemotherapy.

Traction alopecia: Variable patterns dictated by tight hairstyles secondary to prolonged pulling on hair shafts, resulting in chronic low-grade inflammation/ischemia on scalp biopsy.

Trichotillomania: No shedding. Physical examination: widespread or focal patches of short hairs of variable length; scalp biopsy confirms diagnosis. Prove diagnosis by occluding a small area of scalp for several weeks to allow normal hair growth to occur.

Acquired trichorrhexis nodosa: No shedding. Pattern of hair loss consistent with type of external damage/ physical examination: Periodic tiny white "nodes" that look like two opposing broom heads "stuck together" under light microscopy; hair shafts vary in length.

Secondary syphilis: Physical examination: "moth eaten" pattern, associated with lateral loss of eyebrows; confirmed by findings of *Treponema pallidum* infection on serologic testing.

Tinea capitis: No shedding. Physical examination: varying degrees of scaling, erythema, crusting, pustules; hair shafts break off close to scalp or positive test result to Wood's light; if *Microsporum canis*, diagnosis confirmed by microscopic examination of plucked hairs, culture, and/or scalp biopsy.

Loose anagen syndrome: Increased shedding. Hair-pull test yields anagen hair shafts.

Congenital triangular alopecia: Present at birth. Physical examination: may contain vellus hairs; scalp biopsy to distinguish from alopecia areata.

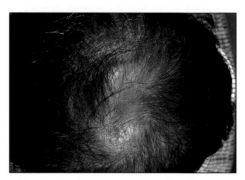

Androgenetic alopecia, most common type of hair loss: Man with triangular frontotemporal regression, thinning; eventually, complete loss of hair on vertex (Norwood-Hamilton classification tanner III vertex).

Lesley Clark-Loeser, Ken Washenik, and Michael Reed

Treatment

Pharmacological treatment

•Drug-based treatment directed against etiology (*eg*, infection, hormonal, drug-induced).

Topical

High to ultrapotent corticosteroids: Alopecia areata, low efficacy.

Minoxidil solution: Androgenetic alopecia, 2% or 5%; alopecia areata 5%; telogen effluvium, 2% or 5%.

Anthralin: 0.1% to 1%, used as a short contact therapy, 20–60 minutes, (alopecia areata).

Intralesional

Corticosteroids: Alopecia areata: 5–10-mL triamcinolone acetonide or mixture of 4-mL triamcinolone acetonide with 5-mL triamcinolone hexacetonide.

Systemic

Antifungal: Tinea capitis—griseofulvin, 10 mg/lb, divided, twice daily dose, for 4–6 weeks, or itraconazole, 2.5mg/lb, daily, or terbinafine, <20 kg, 62.5 mg/d, 20–40 kg, 125mg/d, >40 kg, 250mg/d.

Corticosteroids: Alopecia areata—restricted to short duration for severe disease; start with 40–60mg/d and taper over 1 month.

Hormonal: Androgenetic alopecia—finasteride, 1 mg/d; may be increased to 5 mg/d.

Antibiotics: Secondary syphilis—benzathine penicillin, 2.4 million units, intramuscularly, 2 weekly doses.

Nonpharmacological treatment

•Hair transplantation, follicular unit graft (androgenetic alopecia, congenital triangular alopecia); scalp reduction (androgenetic alopecia, congenital triangular alopecia).

Physical modalities

•Hair prosthesis (wig, hairpiece); change of hair style to camouflage hair loss; behavior modification to accept appearance.

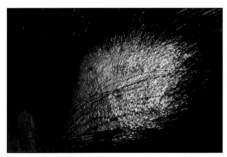

Sharply-circumscribed patch of nonscarring hairloss in a woman with alopecia areata. Exclamation-point hairs present at periphery of patch.

Prognosis

Androgenetic alopecia: Can be slowed or partially reversed in most cases, if treated early.

Telogen effluvium: Acutely self-limited, resolves in several months.

Alopecia areata: Variable, usually temporary in mild cases with localized hair loss; can unpredictably progress to alopecia totalis or universalis; prognosis for regrowth is poor if present longer than 2 years.

Anagen effluvium: Resolves with regrowth after removal of offending agent.

Traction alopecia: Hair can regrow if traction is removed early in course. Becomes permanent (*ie*, scarring) with prolonged course.

Trichotillomania: Resolves if behavior modification is successful.

Acquired trichorrhexis nodosa: Reversible with cessation of causative process.

Syphilis: Regrowth with treatment of underlying disease.

Tinea capitis: Regrowth with antifungal therapy.

Loose anagen syndrome: May improve with age.

Congenital triangular alopecia: Usually permanent, but some improvement possible with minoxidil therapy.

Support organizations

National Alopecia Areata Foundation: PO Box 150760, San Rafael, CA 94915-0760; 415-456-4644; http://www.alopeciaareta.com.

General references

Price V: Treatment of hair loss. *N Engl J Med* 1999, **341**:964–973.

Olsen E, Hordinsky M, McDonald-Hull S, *et al.*: Alopecia areata investigational assessment guidelines. National Alopecia Areata Foundation. *J Am Acad Dermatol* 1999, **40**:242–246.

Diagnosis

Signs

Facticious ulcer (F): Often, bizarre, geometric shapes; linear patterns common.

Basal-cell carcinoma ulcer (BCC): Rolled borders typical; translucency, telangiectasias common.

Squamous-cell carcinoma ulcer (SCC): Firm, hyperkeratotic, elevated margins.

Radiation ulcer (R): Sharp borders; blistering possible; diffuse involvement of irradiated area.

Drug ulcer (D): Solitary lesion; may be bulla that develops into ulceration.

Infectious ulcer (I): *Aspergillus*, *Cryptococcus*, *Histoplasma*, and *Blastomyces* species may cause ulcerated, inflammatory plaques with erythema, edema, fibrosis. Primary infection with *Mycobacterium tuberculosis* starts as papule, then becomes tuberculous chancre (ulcer up to 4–5 cm in diameter) with shallow granular base. *Mycobacretium ulcerans*: very large ulcers; clean base, undermined margins; *Mycobacterium marinum*: verrucous papules, plaques; can ulcerate. Long-standing, untreated syphilis: gummatous lesions; plaques, nodules can ulcerate in center.

Insect bite ulcer (B): Brown recluse spider bites may cause ulceration.

Vasculitis (V): Palpable purpura most common clinical finding; if severe inflammation, hemorrhagic blisters develop, necrose, ulcerate.

Distribution

F: Ulcers occur within reach of patient; face usually spared.

Neoplastic (N): BCC most common on nasolabial folds; medial, lateral canthi. SCC most common on sun-exposed areas.

R: Any irradiated site.

D: Genital, oral mucosa.

I: Deep fungal infections (DF): face, extremities, trunk most common; *M. tuberculosis* primary infection: usually exposed skin at minor-injury sites; *M. marinum*: elbows, fingers, knees. *M. ulcerans*: usually legs; gummatous syphilis: usually arms, face, back.

V: Lower extremities most common.

Symptoms

• Pain may occur with any ulcer, and is more common in ulcers caused by pyoderma gangrenosum, vasculitis, insect bite, radiation, and ulcerated drug eruptions.

Investigations

• Depends on suspected disease: rapid plasma reagin test if syphilis suspected; tissue culture biopsy if fungal, mycobacterial cause suspected. Biopsy to confirm diagnosis.

Complications

• Vary according to cause. Monitor for dissemination of fungal infection. Invasive carcinomas, especially SCC, must be excluded. V can involve kidneys, muscles, joints, gastrointestinal tract, peripheral nerves. SCC may develop in chronic radiation dermatitis. Superinfection may occur in any of these ulcers.

Differential diagnosis

Pressure and vascular causes (arterial and venous).

Epidemiology

D: Most common: phenolphthalein, sulfon-amides, nonsteroidal anti-inflammatories, barbiturates, oral contraceptives, quinine.
I: deep fungal, herpes simplex virus ulcers more common in immunosuppressed host and the very elderly. *M. marinum*: Around water, fish tanks. *M. ulcerans*: Endemic to Africa, Australia.

Leonard Kim, Michael Cohen, and Miriam Pomeranz

Treatment

Diet and lifestyle

BCC and **SCC**: Sun avoidance; daily use of sunscreens.

D: Avoidance of offending agent(s); sulfa drugs have many cross-reactants.

Pharmacological treatment

D: Identify and discontinue therapy with causative drug; most frequent: sulfonamides, tetracycline, nonsteroidal anti-inflammatory drugs, phenolphthalein, barbiturates; bacitracin, silvadene may be applied to ulcerative areas.

DF: Skin infections: fluconazole (400–600 mg/d), itraconazole (400 mg/d); systemic infections: amphotericin B, 120–150 mg/week; amphotericin B against *Aspergillus fumigates*, *Candida albicans*, *Coccidioides immitis*, *Cryptococcus neoformans*. *M. tuberculosis* infections: at least two antituberculous drugs. Isoniazid and rifampin for at least 9 months can be combined with ethambutol, streptomycin, or pyrazinamide. If four drugs are used in first 2 months, treatment may be shortened to 6 months. *M. marinum*: minocycline, 100 mg twice daily; bactrim. In infections resistant to these antibiotics: rifampin, ethambutol. *M. ulcerans*: Trimethoprim-sulfamethoxazole, rifampin, minocycline usually do not work.

Gummatous syphilis: Benzathine penicillin G, 2.4 million U, i.m., in 3 doses, 1 week apart; pregnant or allergic to penicillin: doxycycline, 100 mg orally twice daily, 4 weeks, or tetracycline, 500 mg orally four times daily, 4 weeks.

V: If associated with precipitating event, treat infection or withdraw medication. Early stages: H_1 antihistamines with nonsteroidal anti-inflammatories; afterward, colchicine or hydroxychloroquine . If disease progresses, systemic therapy with oral corticosteroids, azathioprine, cyclophosphamide, or methotrexate.

Nonpharmacological treatment

F: Consultation, management with psychiatrist.

BCC and **SCC**: Surgical excision with primary closure, skin flaps, or grafts. If close to cosmetic site (*eg*, eyes), Mohs surgery may be indicated.

R: Often require surgical treatment. SCC may develop; BCC in patients treated with x-rays for acne.

DF: *M. ulcerans* infection heals faster with application of heat. Surgical grafting usually required.

B: Antisera against *Loxosceles lata* in South America (10 species of *Loxosceles* exist). Cold compresses, analgesics alleviate pain; delay surgical debridement until necrosis clearly delineated.

Special therapeutic considerations

F: Physician must gain patient's trust, so appropriate treatment or referral be accomplished.

Treatment aims

To treat the underlying cause of skin ulceration.

Prognosis

F: Related to severity of psychopathology. Less severely affected patients may be able to improve with support and empathy. If pathology and abuse are severe, the prognosis is poor. **BCC** almost never metastasizes. **SCC** has an overall metastatic rate of 3% to 4%. Metastatic rate higher if lesion occurs in setting of chronic osteomyelitis, burn scars, chronic radiation dermatitis. **R**: Chronic radiation dermatitis can be progressive, irreversible; SCC may develop in affected areas and carry a poor prognosis. **D**: After discontinuing offending agent, lesion should resolve. **I**: If limited to skin, oral antifungal therapy leads to good prognosis. Disseminated infections have a high mortality rate. *Mycobacterium* infections have good response to oral regimens. Syphilis is very responsive to benzathine penicillin. **B**: If not carefully monitored, insect bite can extend, cause large areas of necrosis, disseminated intravascular coagulation. **V**: Depends on underlying disease. Idiopathic variant can have self-limited course or recur for years. Kidney involvement is most serious long-term consequence; monitor frequently.

Follow-up and management

Patients must be followed very closely for development and complications. Neoplasms need to observed for recurrence or spread. Radiation ulcers should be monitored for SCC. Infections need to be followed through complete resolution, and patients with syphilis require periodic blood tests to ensure remission. Patients with vasculitis should be watched for systemic symptoms, and renal function should be followed closely.

General references

King LE Jr: Spider bites. *Arch Dermatol* 1987, **123**:98–104.

Jennette JC: Nomenclature of systemic vasculitides: proposal of an international consensus conference. *Arthritis Rheum* 1994, **37**:187–192.

Chow RK: Treatment of pyoderma gangrenosum. *J Am Acad Dermatol* 1996, **34**:1047–1060.

Leonard Kim, Michael Cohen, and Miriam Pomeranz

Diagnosis

Signs

Structure

Nonallergic contact urticaria (NCU): Erythematous, edematous papules, plaques; no scale. **Chemical burns (CB)**: Range: tender, warm, erythematous patches (vesiculation possible) to ulceration, necrosis. Severe lesions may involve subcutaneous fat, muscles, tendons. **Acne of external chemical origin ("acne venenata;" AV)**: Chloracne; large comedones, straw-colored cysts. **"Oil acne" (OA)**: follicularly based papules, pustules. **Chemical leukoderma (CL)**: Depigmented or hypopigmented macules, patches.

Distribution

Contact dermatitis (CD): Depends on contact site; usually exposed skin; in 80% to 90% of occupational CD, hands affected, sometimes exclusively. **CU**: Contact site. **CB**: Exposure site. **AV**: Chloracne preferentially involves malar and pre- and retroauricular regions of face, scrotum. **OA**: Sites of greatest exposure to oil (arms, thighs), oil-soaked clothes. **CL**: Contact site, often dorsa of hands.

Symptoms

NCU; allergic contact urticaria (ACU): Pruritus; systemic symptoms (rhinitis, swollen mucous membranes, shortness of breath). **CB**: Pain, stinging. **AV**: Cosmetic disfigurement, occasionally painful cysts. **CL**: Cosmetic loss of pigment.

Investigations

• Find out personal, occupational, environmental exposures. Distribution may suggest cause but insufficient to identify causative agent. Workplace site visit may be necessary; for every chemical produced or used in US workplace, chemical manufacturer, importer, distributor must provide Material Safety Data Sheet.

CD: Patch testing for allergic CD (ACD); there is no standardized test for irritant CD (ICD); histopathologic evaluation of skin biopsy specimen does not differentiate between ACD and ICD. **NCU**: Test for dermatographism, provocative skin challenges. **ACU**: Test for dermatographism; patch or prick testing. Test for immediate-type hypersensitivity in presence of trained medical personnel with resuscitation equipment; radioallergosorbent test (RAST) for specific allergen-directed IgE safer than challenge test (*eg*, prick test, use test), especially if history of severe reactions. **AV**: Physical examination. **CL**: Wood's lamp examination, physical examination. Biopsy may help exclude other depigmenting diseases.

Complications

ACU: Widespread urticaria, conjunctivitis, rhinitis, oropharyngeal edema, bronchoconstriction, anaphylaxis, death. **CB**: Necrosis; infection; fluid, electrolyte imbalances; scarring; functional limitation from contractures; post-inflammatory pigment change; neoplasia. Chemical absorption may cause systemic toxicity. **AV**: Scarring, post-inflammatory hyperpigmentation; hypertrichosis, conjunctivitis, systemic symptoms sporadically reported with chloracne.

Differential diagnosis

NCU, ACU: Idiopathic, physical, autoimmune, or complement system–mediated urticaria (*eg*, necrotizing venulitis, infections); urticaria due to specific antigens (*eg*, foods, medications, therapeutic agents, aeroallergens). **AV**: Acne vulgaris, rosacea, folliculitis. **CL**: Acquired hypomelanosis due to endocrine disease, vitiligo, infection, post-inflammatory hypopigmentation, idiopathic guttate hypomelanosis.

Etiology

Common irritants include alkalis (*ie*, soaps, detergents, lye), acids, and organic solvents. **NCU**: Sensitization not required; causes: preservatives, additives used in food, pharmaceuticals (benzoic acid, cinnamic acid, cinnamic aldehyde, alcohol, balsam of Peru), arthropods, caterpillar hair, moths, nettles. **ACU**: Requires prior sensitization; mediated by type I (immediate) hypersensitivity (IgE antibodies to protein peptides); common causes: latex proteins (may become airborne allergens), chemicals (acrylic monomers, epoxy resins, formaldehyde resin), raw foods (potato, meat [especially liver], fish). **CB**: Acids, alkalis, phosphorus, phenol, bitumen, hot asphalt, wet cement. **AV**: Halogenated aromatic hydrocarbons, *eg*, polychlorinated biphenyls, dioxins, dibenzofuranes (chloracne), insoluble (neat) cutting oils (oil acne), crude petroleum, heavy coal-tar distillates, asbestos. **CL**: Phenols/catechols (including hydroquinones).

Epidemiology

Dermatoses: 20% to 70% of all occupational diseases. CD: 70% to 90% of occupational dermatoses; 4% to 7% of all dermatologic consultations. Irritant CD more common than ACD, and is most common form of occupational skin disease. Increased incidence of ACD in certain occupational groups (*eg*, hairdressers; nurses; metal, chemical workers). NCU more prevalent than ACU; affects gardeners, chefs, medical personnel. ACU: Occupational risk group dominated by biomedical workers; increased prevalence because of implementation of universal precautions; increased incidence in atopic patients. Up to 83% of chemical burns are work related.

Joshua P. Fogelman and David E. Cohen

Treatment

Diet and lifestyle

•Allergen avoidance may necessitate changes in clothing, personal products, hobbies. Recommend gloves with cotton liners, for avoidance of irritants.

Pharmacological treatment

Topical

CD: Emollients, topical corticosteroids (ointment based), wet compresses with saline or aluminum sulfate/calcium acetate for weeping areas; avoid topical antihistamines. **CB**: Topical antibiotic with nonstick gauze; specific remedies available for only a few chemicals; buffered phosphate solution for acid, alkali burns. **AV**: Topical tretinoin, topical antibiotics.

Systemic

Severe acute or generalized CD: Oral corticosteroid therapy (prednisone, 1 mg/kg, tapered over 10-21 days, or 60 mg orally every morning for 3 days for acute flares). **Chronic CD**: Cyclosporine (requires careful monitoring of blood pressure, electrolytes, renal function), azathioprine. **CU**: Antihistamines. **CB**: Antibiotics; antifungal medication; fluid, electrolyte support, as indicated. **AV**: Isotretinoin, 0.5-2.0 mg/kg for approximately 20–30 weeks, antibiotics.

Nonpharmacological treatment

Physical modalities, surgery

CB: Irrigation with copious amounts of water (except for metallic potassium and sodium, which ignite); debridement, skin grafting as indicated. **CD**: Bullae may be drained; leave bulla roof intact. **Chronic CD**: Grenz ray radiation therapy, ultraviolet B phototherapy, topical or systemic psoralen plus ultraviolet A (PUVA) photochemotherapy. **CL**: PUVA photochemotherapy.

Supportive methods

•Latex-safe environment; strict avoidance of offending agent(s); regulation of potential irritants, allergens in workplace. Personal protective equipment. Barrier creams for plant resins. Patient education: stress examination of labels for offending substances, cross-reactants; provide guidelines for substitutions; teach personal, environmental hygiene.

CB: Removal of contaminated clothing; analgesia; cold applications for minor burns. **CB**. **CL**: Psychological support for patients with cosmetic disfigurement. **CL**: Cosmetics to blend altered pigmentation.

Special therapeutic considerations

CD, ACU: May complicate an underlying dermatosis because of a compromised epidermal barrier. **ACU**: Anaphylaxis treatment may be necessary; epinephrine pen for potential inadvertent exposures.

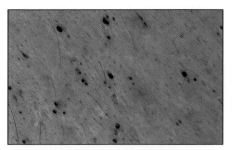

Numerous open and closed comedones, as well as inflammatory cysts, due to chloracne.

Treatment aims

Identify and avoid offending agent(s); provide education on substitution of nonprovocative agents.

Prognosis

CD: Resolves with proper treatment and avoidance of allergen or irritant, may resolve. Untreated, progresses to chronic CD. **CU**: Excellent prognosis with avoidance of stimulus. NCU remains localized; ACU patients may develop systemic manifestations (conjunctivitis, rhinitis, oropharyngeal edema, bronchoconstriction, anaphylaxis). **CB**: Severity of burn, depth of necrosis depend on chemical properties of agent, concentration, duration of contact. **AV**: Responds poorly to treatment; after exposure is stopped, resolution occurs slowly over months, maybe years. **CL**: Hypopigmented/depigmented areas may enlarge, spread, even without contact with agent; may or may not repigment; PUVA therapy usually ineffective.

Follow-up and management

Prevention: Avoidance of offending agent(s); use of physical barriers if complete avoidance cannot be achieved.

Support organizations

U.S. Department of Labor, Occupational Safety and Health Administration (OSHA), Office of Public Affairs, Room N3647, 200 Constitution Avenue, Washington, DC 20210; emergency telephone: 800-321-OSHA (6742); telephone: 202-693-1999; Internet: http://www.osha-slc.gov.

General references

Brandt CP, Fratianne RB: Diagnosis and management of common industrial burns. *Dermatol Clin* 1994, **12**:469–475.

Hogan DJ, Tanglertsampan C: The less common occupational dermatoses. *Occup Med* 1992, **7**:385–401.

Diagnosis

Signs

Kaposi's sarcoma (KS): Pink, violaceous, or deep purple macules, plaques, or nodules (brown in dark-skinned persons); distribution often symmetrical, usually on head (tip of nose, periorbital area, ears, scalp), trunk, penis, legs, palms, soles, mucous membranes. Visceral involvement nears 80%. Gastrointestinal tract (75%), lymph nodes (30%), pulmonary, liver, urogenital tract, and kidneys are more commonly affected.

Oral hairy leukoplakia (OHL): White or grayish, well-demarcated plaques; finely corrugated, villous surface, typical on lateral, inferior tongue surfaces; rarely on buccal mucosa, soft palate.

Bacillary angiomatosis (BA): Red to purple; 1 mm papules to nodules measuring several centimeters. Usually on skin, spleen, liver (peliosis hepatis); may affect any organ system.

Symptoms

KS: Edema, ulceration, pain, secondary infection. Pulmonary involvement may be symptomatic; high mortality if untreated. Gastrointestinal lesions rarely symptomatic.

OHL: Rarely symptomatic.

BA: Lesions sometimes painful, usually because of ulceration or secondary infection. Visceral involvement can cause nausea, vomiting, diarrhea, fever, chills.

Investigations

KS: Biopsy—proliferation of small, irregular, jagged endothelial-lined spaces lined by cytologically bland, spindled cells surrounding normal dermal vessels and adnexal structures. Histologic stages: patch, plaque, nodular. Immunohistochemical analysis with CD31, CD34 helpful, but variable with Ulex europaeus agglutinin-I .

OHL: Clinical diagnosis; confirmation by biopsy showing acanthotic epithelium with hyperkeratosis, hairlike projections of keratin,.

BA: On biopsy, lobular vascular proliferations of plump "epithelioid" cells. Neutrophils scattered through lesion, especially around eosinophilic granular aggregates (masses of bacteria visualized by silver staining). Culture unnecessary, difficult to process. *Bartonella* DNA from tissue can be amplified via polymerase chain reaction, if diagnosis still uncertain.

Complications

KS: Chronic lymphedema on lower-extremity lesions. Nodules can ulcerate, become secondarily infected. Internal lesions can cause obstruction, gastrointestinal hemorrhage.

OHL: Rarely, dysphagia from exuberant overgrowth.

BA: Obstruction from oropharyngeal involvement; death from peliosis hepatis; *Bartonella* bacteremic syndrome.

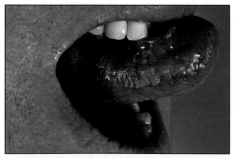

White, band-like plaques with corrugated surfaces on tongue due to oral hairy leukoplakia.

Differential diagnosis

KS: Bacillary angiomatosis, pyogenic granuloma, hemangioma, melanocytic nevus, purpura, granuloma annulare, insect bite reactions, dermatofibroma, stasis dermatitis, acral angiodermatitis, ecchymosis, granuloma faciale. **OHL**: Hyperplastic oral candidiasis, condyloma acuminatum, geographic or migratory glossitis, oral lichen planus, other leukoplakias, syphilitic mucous patch, squamous-cell carcinoma. **BA**: Kaposi's sarcoma, pyogenic granuloma, hemangioma, dermatofibroma.

Etiology

KS: Human herpesvirus type 8. **OHL**: Epstein-Barr virus. **BA**: *Bartonella henselae* or *B. quintana*. **All**: Infectivity/incubation period unknown.

Epidemiology

KS: Early 1980s: 50% of HIV-infected men; 95% of cases in homosexual men. By 1991, 15% of HIV-infected homosexual men, 3% of HIV-seropositive heterosexual patients, 1% of HIV-infected women. With highly active antiretroviral therapy (HAART), new cases rare. **OHL**: As common in men as in women; 48% develop symptomatic full-blown AIDS within 16 months of diagnosis. **BA**: Has almost disappeared.

Clinical staging

National Institutes of Health–sponsored AIDS Clinical Trials Group staging for KS: **Good risk**: Tumor confined to skin, lymph nodes, oral cavity (few non-nodular lesions); CD4 cell count ≥ 200 cells/mm³; no history of opportunistic infections, thrush, symptoms (fever, night sweats); Karnofsky performance status ≥ 70. **Poor risk** (any of the following): Skin tumor associated with edema, ulceration; nodular or extensive oral involvement or involvement of gastrointestinal tract or other viscera; CD4 cell count <200 cells/mm³; opportunistic infection, thrush; > 10% involuntary weight loss or diarrhea persisting > 2 weeks; Karnofsky performance status < 70; other HIV-related opportunistic infection.

Treatment

Diet and lifestyle

•Disfigurement can lead to social isolation, depression, stigmatization, severe anxiety, requiring counseling.

Pharmacological treatment

Topical

KS: Alitretinoin for patch-stage lesions results in 34% overall response rate, low morbidity; irritating, expensive.

Intralesional cytotoxic chemotherapy: Vinblastine, 0.1 mg/cm². Overall response rate: 88%; side effects: mild to severe local inflammation, ulceration, pain, pigmentation.

OHL: Resolves spontaneously with HAART. Topical tretinoin gel and single application podophyllin 25% resin (total amount limited to one cotton swab) reported effective, few side effects.

Systemic

KS: Systemic chemotherapy (for extensive, disabling, or life-threatening disease), with liposomal doxorubicin, or liposomal daunorubicin, or paclitaxel. Paclitaxel may offer best benefit to side-effects profile; may be first choice in debilitated patients. Vinblastine or vincristine has been used with success. Interferon-α rarely used because of 4–6-month delay in maximum response.

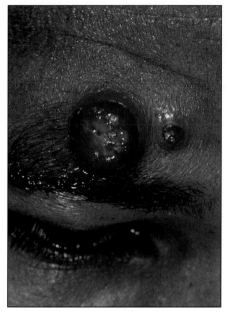

Bright red, firm, friable, exophytic nodules in a man with bacillary angiomatosis.

OHL: Acyclovir, 200–800 mg five times daily, anecdotally successful. Lesions disappear with HAART.

BA: First-line treatment: oral erythromycin, 500 mg four times daily for 8–12 weeks, or doxycycline, 100 mg twice daily. Alternatives: ciprofloxacin, 750 mg twice daily; azithromycin, 500 mg daily; clarithromycin, 500 mg twice daily. Rifampin, 300 mg twice daily, can be added in severe cases.

Nonpharmacological treatment

KS: **Superficial radiation therapy** for large skin lesions unresponsive to other treatment; extensive use can cause postradiation vessel fibrosis, consequent chronic lymphedema. Complete response rate: 70%–80%. High local morbidity in lower extremities. Avoid in mucous membranes because of severe mucositis.

Cryosurgery: Duration of thaw time depending on lesion depth. Overall response rate: 87%. Cosmetic improvement, but KS can persist in deep reticular dermis.

Electrosurgery, especially for ulcerated, bleeding nodular lesions; wounds heal slowly.

Laser surgery (argon; pulsed-dye) effective, but concern (despite lack of supporting evidence) for aerosolization of HIV or human herpesvirus 8.

Excisional surgery effective for selected small lesions.

Treatment aims

HAART is most important therapeutic intervention for all HIV-related opportunistic infections.

KS: For most KS cases, start with HAART; if no resolution in 3–6 months, consider topical or systemic therapy.

OHL: Resolves after immunologic state improves.

BA: Treat with antibiotics.

Prognosis

KS: Lesions may resolve spontaneously but usually become increasingly widespread as immunity deteriorates.

BA: Fatal if untreated.

OHL: May resolve spontaneously with improvement of immunity.

Support organizations

National HIV/AIDS Hotline, Center for Disease Control and Prevention, Phone: 800-342-AIDS.

Gay Men's Health Crisis, New York, NY, Phone: 212-807-6655.

Pediatric AIDS Foundation, Santa Monica, CA, Phone: 310-395-9051.

General references

Porras B, *et al.*: Update on cutaneous manifestations of HIV infection. *Med Clin North Am* 1998, **28**:1033–1077.

Friedman-Kien AE, Mitsyasy RT, eds. *Redefining Clinical Unmet Needs in the Treatment of Kaposi's Sarcoma*. Newtown, PA: Oxford Institute for Continuing Education; 1999.

Signs

Recurrent aphthous stomatitis (RAS): (Mikulicz's aphthae, periadenitis mucosa necrotica recurrens. Sutton's disease, canker sores): Round or oval; painful, tender, 2–10 mm, well demarcated; yellow-gray slough, marginal erythema, predominantly on oral mucosa. Classification: *minor*: 80% of cases; 1–5 ulcers; less painful; heal in 7–10 days; *major*: 12%; often larger than 1 cm in size; 1 or 2 ulcers; side of tongue, fauces, palate, rarely lips; painful; persists for 2 weeks to several months; *herpetiform*: 8%; grouped, 5–100; up to 3.0 mm; heal in 1–8 weeks.
Mucoceles (M): Soft, rounded cyst; pearly-blue, translucent; 2–10 mm; usually inside lower lip; also under tongue, in buccal mucosa. Cyst easily ruptures, releasing sticky, straw-colored fluid.
Leukoplakia (L): White patches or plaques; more common in older men; can develop into malignancy, usually on tongue (50%) or floor of mouth (15%).
Erythroplakia: Red patch or plaque of mucus membrane, more likely than L to be associated with cancer; can occur as speckled form with L.

Symptoms

RAS: Localized pain, burning; may be severe. Prodromal tingling or pain before ulceration.
M: Asymptomatic unless traumatized. **L:** Burning, especially if candidal superinfection.

Investigations

RAS: Skin biopsy shows nonspecific ulcer changes. Bacterial and viral cultures can exclude other causes of oral ulcers.
M: Skin biopsy shows central space containing mucin and inflammatory cells; bordered by vascular and cellular granulation tissue.
L: Skin biopsy to exclude squamous cell carcinoma (SCC), candidiasis.

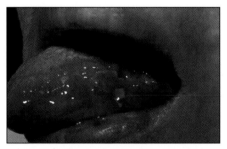

Discrete, painful, aphthous ulcer covered by yellow-gray pseudomembrane and surrounded by an erythematous halo on the lateral aspect of the tongue.

Differential diagnosis

Warts, pyogenic granulomas, smoker's melanosis, fibrous hyperplasia, epulides, granular cell myoblastomas, necrotizing gingivitis, Fordyce's granules (present in over 75% of adults), nicotinic stomatitis, scrotal tongue, median rhomboid glossitis, (in 1% of the population, three times more often in men), benign migratory glossitis, black hairy tongue, hemangiomas, lingual varices, tori palatinus, granular cell tumor, pleomorphic adenoma, papillary cystadenoma lymphomatosum (Warthin's tumor), mucoepidermoid carcinoma, adenoid cystic carcinoma, necrotizing sialometaplasia. **RAS:** herpes simplex infection, Vincent's angina, SCC, paracoccidioidomycosis, pemphigus vulgaris, paraneoplastic pemphigus, erosive Candidiasis, cytomegalovirus infection; ulcers in Behçet's syndrome, Reiter's disease clinically and pathologically indistinguishable from RAS.

Etiology

RAS: Unknown. Autoimmune or hypersensitivity reaction proposed. Minor local trauma may precipitate lesions. More frequent in patients with iron, folate, or vitamin B12 deficiencies, Crohn's disease, Reiter's disease, Behçet's syndrome, gluten enteropathy, neutropenia and immunodeficient states, especially HIV infection.
M: Traumatic blockage and subsequent rupture of salivary gland ducts, with extravasation of sialomucin into the submucosa. **L:** Tobacco, ultraviolet irradiation, immunosuppression. Certain types of human papillomavirus can cause leukoplakic changes.

Epidemiology

RAS in 10%–25% of the population; may be even more common among higher socioeconomic groups, women. **M** in 2.5/100 people. **Other common lesions:** torus palatinus (27/1000), fibromas (12/1000); hemangiomas (5.5/1000); papillomas (4.6/1000), epulis fissuratum (4.1/1000). **L:** Common among tobacco users.

Miguel Sanchez

Treatment

Diet and lifetyle

• Slow eating to avoid trauma with utensils. Avoidance of acidic fruits and juices, salty, very hot and spicy foods, and crunchy foods with rough texture. Brush teeth gently with extra soft brush and SLS-free toothpaste. Avoidance of irritating mouth rinses.

Pharmacological treatment

Topical

RAS: Triancinolone, 0.1% acetonide in Orabase, or hydrocortisone, 2.5 mg pellets, or clobetasol gel or ointment, applied directly to ulcers three times a day; beclomethasone dipropionate aerosol 2 100-mug puffs, up to 8 puffs per day. Triamcinolone acetonide, 5 to 10 mg/mL intralesionally. Antiseptic oral rinses. benzydamine hydrochloride 0.15% or chlorhexidine gluconate 0.2%. Tetracycline, 250mg capsules dissolved in 10-mL water, held in mouth 3 minutes and expectorated; for herpetiform ulcers. Anesthetics (such as lidocaine 2% gel or 10% spray), for pain. Mylanta, lidocaine, and benadryl elixer, mixed in 3:1:2 ratio, as needed, for relief. Bioadhesive films for pain relief. Baking soda and salt rinse, half a teaspoon each in 8 ounces of water, for pain relief. Phylorinol, 1 tsp, rinse for 2–4 minutes then expectorated, for small ulcers. 5% Amlexanox oral paste. ORA (Copper sulfate and iodine), applied for 2 minutes, three to four times daily, for pain and to improve healing. DEBACTEROL (Northern Research Laboratories, Minneapolis) cauterizing agent.

Geographic tongue: Corticosteroids, anesthetics.

Systemic

RAS: Colchicine, 0.6 mg, two or three times daily. Patients with frequent episodes may require daily prophylactic treatment with one to three tablets. Cortosteroids: 0.05–1.0 mg/kg, tapered gradually over 2–4 weeks. Prednisolone, 40 mg for 5 days, reducing by 5 mg every 2 days to 5 mg, then reducing by 1 mg per day, or small alternate-day doses. Azothiaprine, 50–100 mg daily (steroid-sparing or single agent); Thalidomide,200 mg at night, if HIV infection.

L: In challenging cases, 13-cis retinoic acid, 1 mg/kg/d. Beta-carotene, 30 mg/d.

Nonpharmacological treatment

RAS:Cautery with silver nitrate or trichloroacetic acid. Laser cautery. Nicotine chewing gum may prevent recurrence. Anecdotal: benzocaine and 2-deoxy-D-glucose; L-lysine, 1000–1500 mg, three times a day with meals during acute episodes and then 500 mg once to three times daily as prophylaxis; mouthwash; benzoic acid-iodine liquid; Night guard dental fittings to prevent ulcers on lateral aspects of tongue.

M: Incision and drainage; recurrence possible. Surgical excision of lesion and contributing salivary gland is curative.

L: Complete surgical excision of lesion or complete destruction with laser (CO_2 most common), cryosurgery or photodynamic therapy.

Black hairy tongue: brushing with soft brush, with or without anticandidal agents.

General references

Garewal HS, Schantz S: Emerging role of β-carotene and antioxidant nutrients in prevention of oral cancer. *Arch Otolaryngol Head Neck Surg* 1995, **121**:141–144.

Popovsky JL, Camisa C: New and emerging therapies for diseases of the oral cavity [review]. *Dermatol Clin* 2000, **18**:113–125.

Porter SR, Scully C, Pedersen A: Recurrent aphthous stomatitis [review]. *Crit Rev Oral Biol Med* 1998, **9**:306–321.

Dent CD, Svirsky JA, Kenny KF: Large mucous retention phenomenon (mucocele) of the upper lip. Case report and review of the literature. *Va Dent J* 1997, **74**:8–9.

Diagnosis

Signs

Mixed connective tissue disease (MCTD): Raynaud's phenomenon, hand edema, arthritis, synovitis, myositis, dyspnea, dysphagia, fever, sclerodactyly, calcinosis cutis, telangiectasias, malar rash, linear extensor erythema (as in dermatomyositis) in a photodistribution. Suggested Criteria for MCTD: Anti-RNP antibody titer >1:1600; at least three of the following: Hand edema, synovitis, myositis, Raynaud's phenomenon, acrosclerosis.

Transfer RNA (tRNA) synthetase overlap syndrome (RSOS): Raynaud's phenomenon, arthritis, myositis, dyspnea, sicca features, dysphagia, calcinosis cutis, dermatomyositis-like eruption, sclerodactyly.

Polymyositis/scleroderma overlap syndrome (PSOS): Raynaud's phenomenon, arthritis, myositis, dyspnea, sicca features, dysphagia, calcinosis cutis, dermatomyositis-like eruption, sclerodactyly.

Systemic lupus erythematosus/Sjögren's syndrome overlap (SSSO): Sicca features, arthritis, Raynaud's phenomenon, dysphagia, calcinosis cutis, dermatomyositis-like rash, sclerodactyly.

Symptoms

MCTD: Arthralgias, heartburn, sicca symptoms, skin tightness over hands.

Investigations

MCTD: Anti-ribonuclear protein (RNP) antibody titer > 1:1600; anti–polymyositis-scleroderma (anti-nucleolar) antibodies; complete blood count, determination of erythrocyte sedimentation rate and rheumatoid factor; negativity for anti-Sm and anti-DNA antibodies. Chest radiographs to monitor for fibrosing alveolitis; bronchioalveolar lavage, if necessary.

RSOS: Anti-histidyl-tRNA synthetase (Jo-1) antibodies; patient is often negative for antinuclear antibody.

PSOS: Anti-polymyositis-1 antibody; anti-scleroderma-70 antibody; positivity for anti-nucleolar antibody.

SSSO: Anti-La (SS-B) antibodies.

Complications

MCTD: Pulmonary hypertension due to fibrosing alveolitis (main cause of death); renal disease (membranous glomerular nephropathy or renal vasculopathy); cerebral disease; myositis.

RSOS: Myositis and fibrosing alveolitis are more common than in MCTD. Erosive deforming arthritis develops.

PSOS: Myositis and fibrosing alveolitis are less frequent than in other overlap syndromes.

SSSO: Myositis and fibrosing alveolitis are less frequent than in other overlap syndromes.

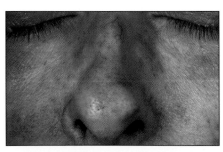

Erythematous plaques in the malar region, facial telangiectasias and heliotrope discoloration of the eyelids in a woman with mixed connective tissue disease.

Differential Diagnosis

MCTD: Lupus erythematosus, polymyositis, scleroderma. **RSOS**: Lupus erythematosus, dermatomyositis, polymyositis, scleroderma, systemic lupus erythematosus. **PSOS**: Polymyositis, scleroderma. **SSSO**: Sjögren's syndrome, systemic lupus erythematosus.

Etiology

MCTD: U1 RNP is involved in messenger RNA splicing. It is composed of eight polypeptides linked to RNA, two of which are epitopes recognized by MCTD sera. Others react with anti-Sm antibodies. Molecular mimicry with viral antigens has been proposed as a trigger to these autoantibodies. It is unclear how autoimmunity to this ubiquitous RNP complex results in the disease manifestations. **RSOS**: Genetic susceptibility with almost 100% association between anti-Jo-1 antibodies and HLA-DR3 alleles. Induction of anti-histidyl tRNA synthetase antibodies by viral triggers is supported by involvement of histidyl tRNA synthetases in the aminoacylation of enteroviruses and of Coxsackie B viruses in polymyositis. One theory: host antiviral antibodies are triggered against the viral RNA at its binding site to host protein and that anti-idiotype antibodies are then generated against the antiviral antibodies; these, in turn, react with host protein at its RNA binding site. **PSOS**: Every patient, to date, has been HLA-DR3 positive. **SSSO**: La antigen (also Sjögren's syndrome B antigen) is involved in RNA pol II transcription and binds to both viral and host RNA. During viral infection, the antigen is translocated from the nucleus to the cytoplasm and cell membrane, theoretically bypassing tolerance by interaction with viral RNA.

Epidemiology

MCTD: Estimated prevalence is 10/100 000. Female:male ratio is 9:1. There is an association with occupational exposure to vinyl chloride.

Macrene Alexiades-Armenakas and Andrew Franks, Jr.

Treatment

Pharmacological treatment

Systemic

- Antimalarials for arthritis and rash.

- Analgesics, nonsteroidal anti-inflammatory drugs for arthralgias.

- Electrically heated gloves, calcium-channel blockers (nifedipine), prostaglandin analogues for Raynaud's phenomenon.

- Hydroxychloroquine for arthritis and extensive skin involvement.

- Low-dose corticosteroids for edema, refractory arthritis, pleuritis, skin eruption.

- High-dose corticosteroids for vasculitis, myositis, fibrosing alveolitis.

- High-dose prednisolone for myositis; 1 mg/kg per day for 6 weeks, then reduce to maintenance level.

- Cyclophosphamide to induce remission: Monitor complete blood count; 1–2 mg/kg per day orally in combination with high-dose corticosteroids; alternatively, pulse therapy as single i.v. infusions of 0.5–1 g every 2–4 weeks or 300 mg orally once weekly to total dose of 3–6 g.

- Azathioprine as a corticosteroid-sparing agent and for arthritis and skin eruption: 2 mg/kg per day after induction with cyclophosphamide.

- Methotrexate for fibrosing alveolitis, although side effect of pulmonary fibrosis poses management difficulties.

SSSO: Tear and saliva substitutes.

Special therapeutic considerations

RSOS: Early usage of immunosuppressants and corticosteroids for fibrosing alveolitis and myositis.

Treatment aims

MCTD: If mild disease, treat symptoms. Treat severe complications with high-dose corticosteroids and immunosuppressants.
RSOS: An aggressive approach is necessary for fibrosing alveolitis.

Prognosis

Up to 75% of cases evolve into systemic lupus erythematosus or scleroderma. Prognosis of patients with polymyositis and fibrosing alveolitis is slightly better for those positive for anti-U1 RNP (mortality at 7 years, 11% and 13% respectively) than for those negative for anti-U1 RNP (mortality at 7 years, 24% and 30% respectively). Pleuritis and pericarditis occur in 60% of patients. Esophageal dysmotility develops in greater than 50% of patients; Sjögren's syndrome, in 50%; and trigeminal neuralgia, 25%. Up to 50% of patients develop renal disease, and cerebral disease occurs in 10%.

Follow-up and management

Monitor closely for development of fibrosing alveolitis, evolution into systemic lupus erythematosus and other complications.

General references

Bibliography: Current world literature on scleroderma and overlap syndromes. *Curr Opin Rheumatol* 1999, **11**:B192–B196.
Kasukawa R: Mixed connective tissue disease. *Intern Med* 1999, **38**:386–393.
Ioannou Y, Sultan S, Isenberg DA: Myositis overlap. *Curr Opin Rheumatol* 1999, **11**:468–474.

Diagnosis

Definition

A group of hereditary and acquired skin diseases that may be part of a more generalized skin disorder or associated with a systemic disease.

Diseases associated with keratodermas

• Basal cell nevus syndrome; congenital bullous ichthyosiform erythroderma; congenital nonbullous ichthyosiform erythroderma; Darier-White disease (keratosis follicularis); epidermodysplasia verruciformis (Lewandowsky-Lutz); epidermolysis bullosa herpetiformis (Dowling-Meara); erythrokeratoderma variabilis (Mendes da Costa), diffuse; ichthyosis vulgaris, autosomal dominant type; incontinentia pigmenti (Nägeli-Franceschetti-Jadassohn type); KID (keratitis, ichthyosis, deafness) syndrome; lamellar ichthyoses, autosomal recessive and dominant types; pachyonychia congenita (Jadassohn-Lewandowsky); pityriasis rubra pilaris, familial type.

Acquired keratoderma

• Keratoderma blenorrhagicum, Norwegian scabies, secondary syphilis, tinea pedis, tuberculosis verrucosa cutis, human papillomavirus infection, arsenical keratoses, calluses, keratoderma climactericum (perimenopausal), corns (clavi), paraneoplastic keratoderma (especially tripe palms), eczema of the hands and feet, lichen planus, psoriasis, pityriasis rubra pilaris, Reiter's syndrome, Sézary's syndrome, mechanical effect of poorly fitted shoes and trauma, pathologic condition of the locomotor apparatus (exostosis, flexion contracture of the toes, amputation stump) or diseases of the peripheral nervous system.

Signs

• Diffuse or localized hyperkeratosis of palms, soles; generally bilateral and symmetrical. Underlying erythema in some types; dorsa of hands, feet may be involved.

Symptoms

• Movement restriction, malodor, itching, pain (rarely), hyperhidrosis, bromidrosis

Investigations

• Physical examination important; can be part of inherited keratinization disorder or acquired systemic/epidermal disease. Family history of hereditary skin disorders must be considered. Skin biopsy, histologic examination; differentiate between diffuse epidermolytic keratoderma (Vorner's) and diffuse orthohyperkeratotic keratoderma (Thost-Unna type)

Complications

• Secondary skin infections, fissuring, pain, movement restriction (especially walking and use of hands, fingers), social embarrassment, possible decrease in self image, disfigurement.

Differential diagnosis

See table 1.

Etiology

Hereditary keratodermas arise from mutations in keratin genes or metabolic or malignant disease.

Epidemiology

Due to multiple underlying causes, palmoplantar keratoderma may affect all ages, but hereditary types usually become evident in infancy or early childhood.

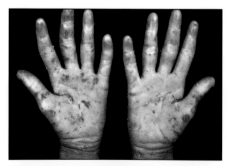

Callous and hyperkeratosis covers the diffusely erythematous skin of the palms and dorsal wrists in this woman with Mal de Meleda keratoderma.

Treatment

Diet and lifestyle
• A diet low in phenylalanine and tyrosine can cure the abnormal keratinization due to tyrosineum type II. Proper footwear and changes in physical activity can ameliorate the symptoms and discomfort of palmoplantar keratoderma.

Pharmacological treatment

Topical
• Keratolytics, preferably under occlusion with plastic gloves, dressings or plastic. These include: salycylic acid 5%–10% compounded in hydrophilic petrolatum or another vehicle; 6% salycyclic acid in propylene glycol (Keralyt, Hydrosilic gel); urea 10% and 20% lotion or 40% cream (Carmol), lactic acid may be compounded with salicyclic acid; and ammonium lactate 12% (Lachydrin, Amlactin) or 10% (Lactinol).

Systemic
• Acitretin (25–75 mg daily) or Isotretinoin (0.5 mg–1.5 mg/kg daily) is often effective, but adverse effects may prevent continuation of treatment.

• After significant improvement, dosage should be decreased to the lowest possible effective amount; however, higher doses are usually needed.

Nonpharmacological treatment

• Keratoderma climactericum may improve with estrogen replacement.

• Spiny keratoderma may improve with 5-fluorouracil 5% cream.

• Careful paring and débridement, dermabrasion, and laser ablation of hyperkeratosis are palliative.

• Surgical intervention to avoid and correct stricture and mutilation.

• Excision and grafting for severe cases.

Treatment aims
To decrease symptoms, prevent disability and improve appearance.

Prognosis
Hereditary types are persistent.

Follow-up and management
Education and occasional medical intervention can help patients live a relatively normal life.

Table 1. Differential diagnosis: hereditary palmoplantar keratoderma

Type	Eponym	Onset (years)	Characteristics
Diffuse orthohyperkeratotic	Unna Thost	2–5	Diffuse, waxy, monepidermolytic keratoderma with transgrediens, significant hyperhidrosis, erythematous borders, "parrot beaking" of nails, cobblestone hyperkeratosis of knuckles.
Diffuse epidermolytic	Vorner	0–3	Erythematous borders, hyperhydrosis, diffuse keratoderma without transgrediens, histological changes of epidermolytic hyperkeratosis.
Focal acral hyperkeratosis	Keratosis punctata (papulosa)	12–30	Verrucous or clavus-like papules; may cause pain.
Striated keratoderma	Siennans	—	Striated hyperkeratosis.
Progressive diffuse keratoderma	Sybert (Greither)	3–8	Progressive involvement of elbows and knees. Rare: Regression during middle age.
Diffuse keratoderma with carcinoma	Howel-Evans	—	Most patients die from esophageal carcinoma.
Mutilating keratoderma	Vohwinkel	Infancy	Transgrediens, hyperhydrosis, erythematous borders, honeycomb palms, starfish dorsal hyperkeratosis, high-tone deafness.
Mutilating keratoderma	Olmsted	Infancy	Diffuse mutilating keratoderma with flexion deformity of digits and constricting bands causing digit autoamputation; progressive perioral, perineal and perianal hyperkeratotic plaques; alopecia; deafness; dental loss.
Keratoderma punctata (spiny)	Music-box- spine keratoderma	12–50	Seen in blacks; umbilicated hyperkeratotic punctate papules at margins of palms, soles, and palmar crease.
Keratoderma palmoplantare	Mal de Meleda	0–3	Diffuse keratoderma with underlying erythema, transgrediens, hyperhidrosis, psoriatic-like plaque on knees and elbows, malodor, common bacterial and fungal colonization, nail changes.
Diffuse keratoderma	Papillon-Lefevre	5–6	Diffuse keratoderma, erythema, hyperhydrosis, fetid odor, dental periodontopathic abnormalities, tooth loss, gingivitis. Similarities with psoriasis and Mal de Meleda.
Circumscribed keratoderma	Richner-Heinhart syndrome	—	Painful circumscribed hyperkeratosis of palms and soles, tyrosenemia type II, photophobia, mental retardation.

Inheritance is autosomal dominant, except for diffuse keratoderma and circumscribed keratoderma, which are autosomal recessive, and mutilating keratoderma (Olmsted), which is usually sporadic.

Diagnosis

Signs

• Persistent urticarial papules that often resemble arthropod bites, usually < 1.0 cm.

• Lesions persist more than 48 hours, develop in symmetrical groups or clusters; may show a central hemorrhagic punctum, or be surmounted by a tiny vesicle.

• Distribution usually involves legs (from ankles to thighs at points where clothing fits snugly, such as the sock line and waistband), forearms, and arms; lower part of trunk and waist may be involved. Characteristically, anogenital area and axillae are spared.

Symptoms

• Intermittent, mild-to-severe pruritus.

Investigations

• Total cutaneous skin examination and history often lead to clinical diagnosis.

• Dermatopathology is not essential for diagnosis. Findings often consistent with insect bite reaction, specifically mild acanthosis, spongiosis with focal exocytosis of lymphocytes, mild to moderate superficial and deep perivascular and interstitial infiltrate of lymphocytes, histiocytes, and eosinophils.

• Bacterial cultures are indicated only if secondary infection is suspected.

Complications

• Secondary bacterial infection.

Differential diagnosis

Allergic contact dermatitis, atopic dermatitis, transient acantholytic dermatitis, urticaria, early varicella, Gianotti-Crosti syndrome, neurotic excoriations, pityriasis lichenoides et varioliformis acuta, lymphomatoid papulosis, dermatitis herpetiformis, delusions of parasitosis.

Etiology

Cases may be due to hypersensitivity reactions to bites of certain insects, although patients are usually not aware of being bitten. Arthropods implicated include dog fleas (*Ctenocephalides canis*), cat fleas (*Ctenocephalides felis*), human fleas (*Pulex* species), fowl fleas (*Ceratophyllidae* species), hedgehog fleas (*Archaeopsylla erinacei*), dog mites (*Sarcoptes scabiei* var. *canis*, *Cheyletiella yasguri*), bird mites (*Dermanyssus gallinae*, *Ceratophyllus gallinae*), cat mites (*Cheyletiella blakei*, *Notoedres cati*), rat mite (*Ornithonyssus bacoti*), snake mite (*Ophionyssus natricis*), and cattle itch mite (*Sarcoptes scabiei* var. *bovis*).

In addition to pets, evaluate patient's contact with environment where rodents may roam (basements, attics, groceries, libraries, construction sites, old carpets) and recreational or occupational activities.

Epidemiology

Any age, but more common in prepubescent period.

Season: Summer in temperate climates.

Steven Natow and Allen Natow

Treatment

Diet and lifestyle

- Modify living environment to reduce exposure to arthropods.
- Reassure patients that they are not contagious and no isolation is needed.

Pharmacological treatment

Topical

- **Insect repellents** containing *N*-diethyl-m-toluamide (Deet) at 10%–30% for backyard or 40%–50% for camping trip.
- **Nonsteroidal antipruritic** lotions containing menthol, camphor, pramoxine, lidocaine, and tar.
- **Colloidal oatmeal baths or cornstarch baths** (1 cup of cornstarch and 1 cup of baking soda to 4 cups of water; make into paste and add to bath water).
- **Steroids**: Potent topical corticosteriods, steroid-impregnated tape (Cordran tape), or intralesional steroids (triamcinolone acetonide, 5 mg/mL) to speed resolution of lesions.
- **Doxepin** 5% cream, applied three times daily.
- **Crotamiton** cream or lotion for antipruritic (not anti-ectoparasitic) effect.
- **Scabicidals**, such as lindane and permethrin, are rarely effective.

Systemic

- **H_1 oral antihistamines**: Long-acting nonsedating antihistamines may be combined with sedating ones at night and as needed to relieve itching. H_2 blockers (cimetidine, ranitidine) may be added if needed.
- **Prednisone or methylprednisolone**, tapered over 5–10 days, for severe flare.
- **Ivermectin**, 6 mg.

Physical modalities

- Ultraviolet B or narrow-band phototherapy if other treatments fail.

Special therapeutic considerations

- Elimination of ectoparasite source is the definitive treatment. Advise patients to avoid contact with cats and dogs, treat flea-infested cats and dogs, spray household with insecticides (eg, fenoxycarb and methoprene). Consultation with commercial pest-control experts useful.
- Veterinary evaluation of possible infested pets if indicated. Consultation with experienced clinical entomologist may be rewarding.

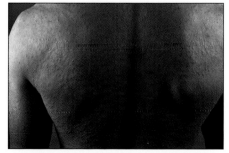

The process is characterized by symmetrically distributed papules that are edematous and extremely pruritic.

Treatment aims

To provide cure, symptom relief, and prevention.

Prognosis

Usually self-limited, but treatment or modification of exposure to arthropods will shorten course.

Follow-up and management

Periodic re-examination of patient is useful to assess response to treatment.

General references

Millikan LE: Papular urticaria. *Semin Dermatol* 1993, **12**:53–56.

Howard H: Papular urticaria in children. *Pediatr Dermatol* 1996, **13**:246–249.

Jordann HF: Papular urticaria: a histopathologic study of 30 patients. *Am J Dermatopathol* 1997, **9**:119–126.

Diagnosis

Signs

Small-plaque parapsoriasis (SPP): Small (< 5 cm), well-defined, oval to round brown patches or macules with fine scale distributed symmetrically on the trunk, proximal extremities, or buttocks. The digitate variant consists of yellow to brown elongated patches or macules that follow the lines of cleavage, usually on the trunk, giving the appearance of fingerprints on the skin.

Large-plaque parapsoriasis (LPP): Large (usually > 5 cm), ill-defined, oval to irregularly shaped, light brown to slightly erythematous patches distributed asymmetrically on the trunk and extremities (especially the flexural areas). Fine scale and cigarette-paper appearance of the patches may be present. The poikilodermatous form consists of slightly atrophic patches with telangiectasias and mottled hypopigmentation or hyperpigmentation.

Symptoms

SPP: Lesions are asymptomatic; patients are in good health.

LPP: Eruption is asymptomatic or mildly pruritic.

Investigations

Both: Skin biopsy.

• If histopathologic features of early mycosis fungoides are present, immunohistologic studies and T-cell receptor gene rearrangement studies on fresh tissue may be necessary to better define the diagnosis.

• Repeated serial biopsies should be performed on patients with progressive eruptions.

Complications

• Many experts consider LPP to be a premalignant or early stage of mycosis fungoides.

LPP: Can progress to full-blown mycosis fungoides.

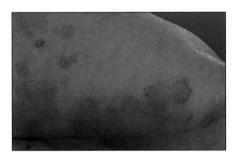

Irregularly-shaped, round light brown-red, thin plaques with fine scaling characteristinc of large plaque parapsoriasis. Older serpiginous lesions blend with the surrounding skin and have developed a tanned, atrophic (cigarette paper) appearance

Differential diagnosis

SPP: Pityriasis lichenoides chronica, pityriasis rosea, secondary syphilis, nummular eczema, LPP, mycosis fungoides.

LPP: SPP, mycosis fungoides, secondary syphilis, lichenoid drug eruption.

Etiology

Unknown.

Epidemiology

SPP: Patients are middle-age or elderly; peak age at onset, 50 years. More common in men; male:female ratio, 3:1.

LPP: Patients are middle-age or elderly. Slightly more common in men.

Jeremy Rothfleisch and Jo-Ann Latkowski

Treatment

Pharmacological treatment

• Emollients (for SPP).

• Corticosteroids (for SPP or LPP) of intermediate to high potency (class I to III) applied to affected area twice a day. If needed for the face, groin, or axilla, these corticosteroids should be used for a maximum of 1 week. Side effects occur with prolonged use and include striae and atrophy of the skin.

• Nitrogen mustard (for LPP), 10 mg dissolved in 60 mL of water and applied daily to the entire body. Most common side effect is contact dermatitis.

• Topical tar preparations (for SPP).

Nonpharmacological treatment

• Psoralen with ultraviolet A phototherapy (PUVA)

• Ultraviolet B phototherapy

Treatment aims

SPP: Reassurance of patients and treatment of symptomatic lesions.

LPP: Relief of pruritus and prevention of possible progression to mycosis fungoides.

Prognosis

SPP: Most patients have a benign, chronic clinical course. Complete resolution is possible. Progression to mycosis fungoides is rare.

LPP: Most patients follow a benign clinical course with either a chronic, persistent eruption or complete resolution. 10% to 30% of patients progress to mycosis fungoides.

Follow-up and management

SPP: As needed for specific treatment.

LPP: Careful cutaneous examination is needed every 3 months for 1 year after initial diagnosis, then every 6 months. Repeated biopsies if eruption progresses or lesions are suspicious for mycosis fungoides.

General references

Hu C-H, Winkelmann RK: Digitate dermatosis: a new look at symmetrical, small plaque parapsoriasis. *Arch Dermatol* 1973, **107**:65–69.

Lindea ML, *et al.*: Poikilodermatous mycosis fungoides and atrophic large-plaque parapsoriasis exhibit similar abnormalities of T-cell antigen expression. *Arch Dermatol* 1988, **124**:366–372.

Zelinckson BD, Peters MS, Muller SA, *et al.*: T-cell receptor gene rearrangement analysis: cutaneous T cell lymphoma, peripheral T cell lymphoma, and premalignant and benign cutaneous lymphoproliferative disorders. *J Am Acad Dermatol* 1991, **25**:787–796.

Kikuchi A, *et al.*: Parapsoriasis en plaques: its potential for progression to malignant lymphoma. *J Am Acad Dermatol* 1993, **29**:419–422.

Haeffner AC, *et al.*: Differentiation and clonality of lesional lymphocytes in small plaque parapsoriasis. *Arch Dermatol* 1995, **131**:321–324.

Burg G, *et al.*: Cutaneous lymphomas consist of a spectrum of nosologically different entities including mycosis fungoides and small plaque parapsoriasis. *Arch Dermatol* 1996, **132**:567–572.

Diagnosis

Signs

Gianotti-Crosti syndrome (GCS): Monomorphous, usually symmetric, flat-topped, 1- to 10-mm flesh-colored to pink-red papules; acrally distributed on cheeks, buttocks, and extensor extremities, especially over elbows and knees. Lesions are generally larger in infants (5–10 mm) and are micropapular in older children (1–2 mm). As the exanthem progresses, lesions may become confluent and form plaques of lichenoid papules.

Hand-foot-and-mouth disease (HFMD): Oral lesions begin as small red macules that evolve into vesicles, 1–3 mm to 2 cm in diameter, on an erythematous base. The vesicles rapidly ulcerate. The distribution is "classic herpangina" enanthem (soft palate, hard palate, uvula, anterior tonsillar pillars) in 30% of cases, and affects the tongue in 44%. The buccal mucosa and gingiva can also be affected. Thin-walled, 3- to 7-mm, superficial vesicles filled with clear fluid, which may be tender or pruritic, appear on dorsal and ventral aspects of hands and feet. Less often, the buttocks, arms, legs, and face are affected.

Vesicles often have characteristic elliptical "football" shape, and may coalesce into bullae.

Unilateral laterothoracic exanthem (ULE): Erythematous macules, papules, or plaques that can have morbilliform, scarlatiniform, or eczematous patterns. Typically, the exanthem begins unilaterally in the axillary region and then spreads centrifugally to a bilateral distribution, retaining a pronounced unilateral predominance.

Symptoms

GCS: The eruption is usually nonpruritic, and constitutional symptoms are absent or mild. An upper respiratory tract infection or low-grade fever may precede the eruption. Occasionally, generalized lymphadenopathy, hepatomegaly, splenomegaly, and acute—usually anicteric—hepatitis may occur.

HFMD: Brief prodrome of low-grade fever, anorexia, sore mouth, malaise, and abdominal pain, diarrhea, arthritis, cervical or submandibular lymphadenopathy (22% of cases).

ULE: Regional axillary or inguinal lymphadenopathy.

Investigations

GCS: Complete blood count, liver function tests, hepatitis B surface antigen test.

HFMD: Viral cultures needed, to rule out herpes simplex virus.

ULE: is usually apparent on initial examination. However, if clinical suspicion exists, individual clinical course should dictate work-up.

Complications

GCS: Hepatitis, leukopenia with increase in monocytes (up to 20%).

HFMD: Rare case reports of myocarditis, pneumonia, meningoencephalitis.

ULE: Complications are exceedingly rare in healthy children.

Differential diagnosis

All: Other viral exanthems.

GCS: Papular urticaria, erythema multiforme, frictional lichenoid dermatitis, drug eruption.

HFMD: Erythema multiforme, dyshidrotic eczema, herpes stomatitis, aphthous ulcers, varicella.

ULE: Contact dermatitis, miliaria, atypical pityriasis rosea, scabies, tinea corporis, scarlet fever.

Etiology

GCS Probably viral etiology. Numerous cases have been associated with hepatitis B, serotype ayw. Epstein-Barr virus, parainfluenza virus, coxsackievirus A16, respiratory syncytial virus, poliovirus vaccine, other enteroviruses, and cytomegalovirus have all been implicated.

HFMD: Coxsackie virus A16 (occasionally A5, A9, A10, A16, B1, B3).

ULE: Unknown. Current theories favor an infectious etiology.

Epidemiology

GCS: Peak incidence in children ages 1–3 years; 85% of affected children are younger than 3 years. Adults have been affected.

HFMD: Infections are more common in late summer and fall. Highly contagious in susceptible populations.

ULE: Seen most commonly in children 2 years of age.

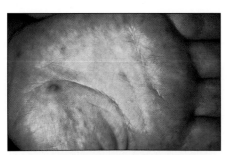

Pink macules become gray-white vesicles on erythematous bases on the palm of a child with hand, foot and mouth disease.

Sara L. Tarsis and Mary W. Chang

Treatment

Diet and lifestyle

HFMD: Encourage oral fluids to avoid dehydration. Avoid hot beverages and soups, which can be painful to oral lesions.

Pharmacological treatment

Topical

GCS: There is no specific treatment for cutaneous lesions. Topical antipruritics or low-potency topical steroids are sometimes useful.

ULE: Administer low-potency topical corticosteroids for pruritus. Moisturizers can be helpful.

Systemic

GCS: Oral antihistamines are sometimes helpful.

HFMD: Rarely, a patient with extensive oral lesions who cannot tolerate oral intake will require intravenous fluid rehydration.

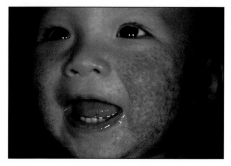

Symmetric, coppery red, lichenoid papules becoming confluent into plaques on the face of a child with Gianotti-Crosti syndrome.

General references

Anthony M: Exanthems in childhood: an update. *Pediatr Ann* 1998, **27**:163–170.

Boeck K, Mempel M, Schmidt T, Abeck D: Gianotti-Crosti syndrome: clinical, serologic and therapeutic data from nine children. *Cutis* 1998, **62**:271–274.

Coxsackie Virus Infection. In: *Clinical Pediatric Dermatology*, edn 2. Edited by Hurwitz S. 1993:359–361.1

McCuaig CC, *et al.*: Unilateral laterothoracic exanthem. *J Am Acad Dermatol* 1996, **34**:979–984.

Sara L. Tarsis and Mary W. Chang

Diagnosis

Signs

Scabies: Burrows or serpiginous tracts (< 10% of cases), erythematous papules, excoriations. May see vesicles on palms, soles in children. Favored sites: finger webs, wrists, axillae, areolas, genitalia, umbilicus; face, scalp generally spared.

Pediculosis capitis (PCa): Head lice; 1-3 mm, reddish brown, wingless insects, nits cemented to hair shafts near scalp; favors occipital, postauricular regions. May see furuncles, local adenopathy.

Pthirus pubis (PP): Pubic lice; 1-3 mm, crab-shaped, wingless insects and nits cemented to hair shafts near skin; adapted to pubic hair, but also axillae, perianal area, eyelids, hairy chest, extremities. Macula cerulaea, blue-gray macules on trunk, thigh.

Pediculosis corporis (PCo): Body lice; 1-3 mm reddish brown insects in seams of clothing. Excoriations, bloody crusts, lymphadenopathy involve neck, trunk.

Symptoms

All: Pruritus. **Scabies (S)**: Pruritus begins 2-6 weeks after infection, can persist several weeks after treatment; worse at night.

Investigations

S: Skin scrapings may show mites, eggs, fecal pellets (scybala); mostly falsely negative; typically only 10-15 mites per patient. **Biopsy** may show mites in stratum corneum.

Complications

All: Secondary infection, usually with *Staphylococcus aureus*.

S: Nodular scabies: 3-5-mm nodules in axillary folds, genital region; persist after treatment; secondary to chronic scratching, immune response.

Crusted ("Norwegian") scabies: Thousands to millions of mites; in neurologically or immunologically impaired patients.

PCo: Linked to *Bartonella quintana* bacteremia, *B. quintana* endocarditis in HIV-positive homeless men.

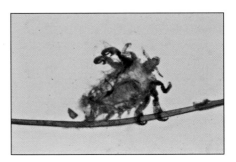

Photograph of a head louse, *pediculus capitis*, perched on a hair.

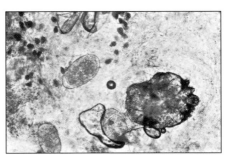

This scraping from the skin a man infested with scabies shows a young itch mite, *Sarcoptes scabiei*, var *humanus*, ova and scybala (fecal pellets).

Etiology

S: *Sarcoptes scabei*, var. *hominis*. Extoparasitic mite confined to humans. Female burrows into stratum corneum, lays 1–3 eggs/day, 30 days, dies. Off host, may live 24–48 hours. Symptoms: delayed hypersensitivity to mites, eggs, scybala. May acquire from animal. Infection self-limited.

PCa: *Pediculus humanus*, var. *capitis*. Female lays 5–10 eggs/day, 30 days. Eggs laid 1–2 days after mating, hatch in 6–10 days; sexual maturity in about. 8 days. Obligate blood feeders; survive up to 55 hours off host; eggs viable to 10 days.

PP: ("Crabs"); etiology similar to that of PCa. **PCo**: *Pediculosis humanus*, var. *corporis* ("vagabond's disease"), etiology similar to that of PCa, though eggs laid in seams of clothing, can survive 30 days without host.

Epidemiology

S: Worldwide, 300 million cases. Spread by close bodily contact.

PCa: Annually, 6–12 million US cases. Less common in black Americans; prevalent in African blacks. Spread by head-to-head contact, sharing of combs, hats, etc. Children more susceptible, especially girls, presumably due to longer hair.

PP: Spread generally by sexual contact.

PCo: Predominantly in places of close body contact, eg, homeless shelters, refugee camps. Confined to people who do not change clothes daily. More prevalent in warm humid climates

Ira A. Pion

Treatment

Diet and lifestyle

Launder clothes, towels, linens in hot water, or dry clean. Isolate, in "off limits" closet for 2 weeks, items not readily laundered. Vacuum floors. **PCa**: Avoid sharing combs, brushes, hats, etc. Combs, brushes: boil or soak in pediculocide, 20 minutes. Discard clothes (preferred) or treat with 1% malathion or 10% DDT powder.

Pharmacological treatment

Topical

Apply agents to dry hair; lice shut down respiration, up to 30 minutes, when immersed. Re-treat in 7–10 days to destroy any hatchlings from surviving eggs.

Permethrin: S, PCa, PP. 1% cream rinse applied for 10 minutes, then shampooed (PCa, PP) or 5% cream, applied overnight from neck down (S, PP) or to head with shower cap (PCa). Note: "NIX" most effective over-the-counter (OTC) agent; only one with residual activity in hair (up to 14 days), but patient must not use conditioner; tolerance reported, but may be overcome with 5% cream formulation. Contraindications: Age < 2 months, nursing, pregnancy category B. Main side effects: toxicity low as 2% absorbed; pruritus or mild transient burning possible. **Natural pyrethrins** (most OTC products) (PCa, PP): Shampoo applied for 10 minutes. **Malathion 0.5%** lotion (PCa, PP): Apply every 8–12 hours, then shampoo; avoid occlusion. Contraindications: Infancy; nursing, pregnancy category B. Little documented resistance. Highly flammable. Main side effects: Skin irritation, worsening of dandruff, conjunctivitis with eye contact. **Lindane** 1% (γ benzene hexachloride): Lotion overnight, every 8–12 hours (S); shampoo 4 minutes, add water to lather, rinse (PCa, PP). Contraindications: Age < 2 years, nursing, pregnancy category B. Organochloride (same class as DDT); significant resistance documented. Main side effects: Accumulates in white matter of brain, causing central nervous system toxicity; nausea, vomiting, headaches, seizures reported, mainly with overuse. **Crotamiton** 10% cream, lotion (S): Two to five times daily, wash 24 hours after last application. Less effective, but antipruritic. Irritating to denuded skin; pregnancy category C. **Benzyl benzoate**, 20% to 25% emulsion (S): Three times nightly, wash 24 hours after last application. Less effective than other treatments. High incidence of skin irritation. **Precipitated sulfur** 6% to 10%, in petrolatum (S, PCa, PP): Three times nightly, wash well 24 hrs after last application. Treatment of choice in pregnant women, young children. Malodorous and messy. **Essential oils** (PCa, PP): Peppermint,, tea tree, others. Reports of mild pediculocidal effect. **Ivermectin**, 0.8% solution. Not yet commercially available.

Systemic

Ivermectin: Oral, subcutaneous; 3- and 6-mg tabs; one dose, 200 mug/kg; usually curative; may need to repeat in 10 days. Contraindications: weight below 15 kg, nursing, pregnancy category C. Approved in United States only for *Strongyloides* infection, onchocerciasis; effective in HIV patients with crusted scabies. No apparent major drug interactions or, at standard dosage, major side effects.

Lice: Trimethoprim-sulfamethoxazole (oral; varied dosing) Lice depend on symbiotic gut bacteria sensitive to it. Requires prolonged course; does not kill eggs. Allergic reactions common.

Nonpharmacological treatment

PCa: Petrolatum, mayonnaise, pomade, etc. Apply heavy coating overnight; wash off in morning. Can be effective; difficult to remove from hair. Nit picking: Use nit comb; pretreat with acetic acid (vinegar), 8% formic acid, or enzymatic gel. Helpful as adjunct; mandatory if patient's school has "no nit" policy.

PP: Occlusion; recommended if eyelash involvement. Shaving involved hair may be curative; at least adjunctive.

Special therapeutic considerations

All: All family members and close contacts should be treated simultaneously. Topical steroids, topical antipruritics, oral antihistamines may help with pruritus. In "scabies incognito," symptoms, signs diminished by use of topical steroids. Topical or oral antibiotics needed if secondary infection is present.

Treatment aims

To rid patient of organism; symptoms then resolve.

Prognosis

Most patients are rapidly and successfully treated. Treatment failures may represent drug resistance, improper use of medication, reinfestation.

Follow up and management

Generally, see patients 1–2 weeks after last treatment. If infection persists, ascertain if medication used properly, environmental precautions observed. If so, more aggressive treatment (eg, combined modalities) may be indicated.

Support organizations

National Pediculosis Association, PO Box 149, Newton, MA 02161; www.headlice.org; telephone: (617) 449-6487.

Diagnosis

Signs

Bullous pemphigoid (BP): Tense vesicles, bullae, millimeters to centimeters; urticarial, eczematous plaques, 1 to 3 weeks before bullae. Blisters, leaving superficial erosions, heal without scarring; in normal or erythematous skin; most common: medial aspect of extremities, abdomen, groin, axilla. Usually grouped. Oral and mucosal lesions in 10%. Rare (prepubescent girls, localized to perineum; women, localized to lower extremities): purulent vegetating plaques in groin, axillae (pemphigoid vegetans) . Some bullae on scattered hyperkeratotic nodules, plaques.

Cicatrical pemphigoid (CP): Most common as desquamative gingivitis with patchy, erythematous, tender, erosions and ulcers. Intact blisters rare. After healing, delicate white pattern of reticulated scarring. Commonest ocular lesions: unilateral or bilateral conjunctivitis progressing insidiously to scarring. Erosions, blisters, ulcers possible on genitalia. In 33%, vesicles and bullae (which rupture easily, become crusted eroded papules) on erythematous or urticarial skin of scalp, head, neck, upper trunk. Brunsting-Perry variant: one or more circumscribed, recurrent patches with subepidermal blisters; scarring, usually on head, neck, predominantly in elderly men without mucosal lesions.

Investigations

BP:Perilesional histology: subepidermal blister, mixed inflammatory infiltrate with eosinophils, histiocytes, neutrophils, lymphocytes in dermis, blister cavity. Possible: polymorphic histology, including cell-poor infiltrate variant.

Immunofluorescence (IF): perilesional skin: linear complement band (C3) in 65% to 95% of cases, typically with IgG deposits at dermal-epidermal junction (DEJ); findings shared by epidermolysis bullosa acquista, bullous systemic lupus erythematosus, herpes gestationis, CP; salt-split skin: presence of IgG on epidermal side. In 70% to 80%, serum contains circulating IgG antibodies; in 25%, IgA or IgM that bind linearly at DEJ of normal human skin. Antibody titer has no correlation with clinical disease activity.

CP: Subepidemal blister, often lichenoid inflammatory infiltrate of lymphocytes, histiocytes, neutrophils, eosinophils. Lamellar fibrosis under epidermis. Direct IF studies show linear IgG (rarely IgA or IgM) and C3 in lesional, perilesional skin in 80%.

Complications

BP: Morbidity, mortality from systemic medications, infection.

CP: Eye involvement in 75%; left untreated, progressive scarring, shortened fornices, symblephara, ankyloblephara, conjunctival scarring with entropion and trichiasis, superficial punctate keratinopathy, corneal ulceration, scarred lacrimal ducts, blindness (20%). Oropharyngeal involvement: esophageal or supraglottic stenosis, stricture formation, leading to dysphagia, odynophagia, weight loss, aspiration.

Differential diagnosis

BP: Epidermolysis bullosa acquista, herpes gestationis, bullous systemic lupus erythematosis, cicatricial pemphigoid, linear IgA disease, dermatitis herpetiformis, and erythema multiforme.

CP: Bullous pemphigoid, pemphigus vulgaris, erythema multiforme, erosive lichen planus, linear IgA dermatosis, epidermolysis bullosa. Ocular lesions alone can resemble viral conjunctivitis, ocular rosacea, ocular pseudopemphigoid secondary to use of topical eye medications.

Etiology

BP: Autoantibodies against BPAG1, BPAG2. BP reported with furosemide. Environmental factors (eg, ultraviolet light, therapeutic radiation) may precipitate BP. BP-like drug eruptions with phenacetin, penicillin, furosemide.

CP: Autoantibodies against BPAG2, laminin-5.

Epidemiology

BP: Usually in patients over 60; no evidence of association with underlying malignancy.

CP: Twice as common in women as men; rare in children; usual onset in fifth or sixth decade. Incidence of HLA-B12, HLA-DR4 increases with ocular involvement.

Jeanie Chung-Leddon and M. Joyce Rico

Treatment

Diet and lifestyle

• If systemic corticosteroids, adjust diet to reduce risk of steroid-induced diabetes, hypertension. Against osteoporosis, early calcium (calcium carbonate, 500 mg, t.i.d.), vitamin D (50 000 IU twice weekly); hormone replacement therapy, as appropriate; exercises; no smoking; avoidance of hard foods, brushing dental gums, sunlight.

Pharmacological treatment

Topical

• Corticosteroid (Class I or II) ointments, creams, gels for mild, localized disease, cutaneous or mouthwash; or occlusive base preparations or class I corticosteroid for oral disease. Intralesional injections with triamcinolone acetonide, 5 to 10 mg/mL for cutaneous lesions; up to 20 mg/mL for oral lesions, every 1 to 3 weeks.

Systemic

• Prednisone, 0.5 to 1 mg/kg/d, single morning dose, for severe or refractory disease; if new blisters, increase dose by 50% to 100 % every 3 to 5 days. May need to divide >60 mg into two equal doses. When blister formation stops and erosion healing starts, gradually taper to lowest dose that controls symptoms. Recurrence/flare not uncommon; class I or II topical corticosteroids or small doses of systemic corticosteroids.
CP: Dapsone for mild CP, 25 to 50 mg daily initially, then increased to 100 to 150 mg daily, as tolerated, may be helpful in BP. Prednisone, 1 mg/kg/d if unresponsive to dapsone or for severe or progressive eye, esophageal, laryngeal involvement; usually with cyclophosphamide, 1-2 mg/kg/d, divided. When controlled, slowly taper to alternate-day regimen. If refractory to corticosteroids, add immunosuppressive agents. Prednisone can be discontinued after tapering at 6 months; cyclophosphamide should be continued at gradually tapered doses of 1-1.5 mg/kg/d, 18-24 months, until WBC depressed to 3000-4000/mm3. Immunoglobulin G: refractory BP. Tetracycline (1-2 g/d) with niacinamide (500 mg q.i.d.).
Adjunctive—erythromycin, 1g/d; colchicine, 0.5-0.6 mg, t.i.d.; azathioprine, 1-2 mg/kg/d; cyclophosphamide (1-2 mg/kg/d); mycophenolate mofetil (1 g, b.i.d. to t.i.d.; methotrexate, 25 mg/wk— with prednisone as steroid-sparing agents.

Nonpharmacological treatment

BP: Plasmapheresis, with steroids, immunosuppressants. Photopheresis.
CP: Surgical intervention to release contractures, scarring; only when controlled.
Both: Anesthetics, antiseptics for localized lesions.

Special considerations

• Cyclophosphamide: closely monitor for side effects, such as bone-marrow toxicity, hemorrhagic cystitis, sterility, alopecia, induction of malignancies. Azathioprine: monitor for bone-marrow suppression, hepatotoxicity, induction of malignancies.

Treatment aims

BP: To prevent blister formation, secondary infection, and suppress symptoms.
CP: To prevent lesions, scarring and complications.

Prognosis

BP: Self-limited, months to years; usually responds promptly to systemic corticosteroids. Without treatment, 25% die; 25% go into spontaneous remission by 15 months, 50 to 75% within 2.5 to 6 years. May continue for 10 years, more. Mortality: 10% to 20 %, systemic steroid treatment. Elderly with compromised health: higher fatality risks.
CP: Progressive; scarring: debilitation, life-threatening consequences. Control difficult; episodic exacerbations, waning of disease activity. Ocular cicatricial pemphigoid-only patients: more benign course possible.

Follow-up and management

BP: Long-term, to monitor disease control, side effects.
CP: Multispecialty care may be needed if multiple organs affected.

Support organizations

National Pemphigus Foundation, Atrium Plaza, Suite 203, 828 San Pablo Avenue, Albany, CA 94706, (510) 527-4070, fax (510) 527-8497, http://www.pemphigus.org.

General references

Glied M, Rico MJ: Treatment of autoimmune blistering diseases. *Curr Ther* 1999, 17:431.

Ahmed A, Kurgis B, Rogers R: Cicatricial pemphigoid. *J Am Acad Dermatol* 1991, 24:987.

Leverkus M, Schmidt E, Lazarova Z, *et al.*: Antiepiligrin cicatricial pemphigoid. *Arch Dermatol* 1999, 135:1091.

Diagnosis

Signs

Pemphigus vulgaris (PV): Flaccid blisters, erosions on skin, mucosal surfaces; positive Nikolsky sign, mostly on face, scalp, trunk. Oral erosions usually begin with multiple, painful, nonhealing erosions on buccal mucosa, but may involve larynx or pharynx, as well as conjunctiva; nasal, anal, cervical, or urethral mucosa can be rarely affected. Erosions can evolve into vegetating lesions with excessive granulation, crusting (pemphigus vegetans).
Pemphigus foliaceous (PF): Superficial blisters usually presenting as crusting or erythema with underlying erosions, usually on face, scalp, upper trunk and, rarely, mouth. In pemphigus erythematosus, a variant of PF, lesions develop on malar area. Erythroderma common in fogo selvagem (endemic variant of PF in South America) and in severe PF.

Symptoms

PV: Erosions painful; pruritus common. Hoarseness from laryngeal involvement, nasal stuffiness from nasal involvement may occur.
PF: Pruritus more common than pain.

Investigations

PV histology: Suprabasal intraepithelial blister with acantholysis of epidermis. Direct and indirect immunofluorescence reveals IgG, IgM, IgA, complement (C3) binding to keratinocyte cell surface. Sera: circulating antiepithelial-cell surface IgG, and titer of antibody correlates with disease activity.
PF histology: Acantholysis through most superficial layer of epidermis. Immunofluorescence studies similar to PV, but antibodies often react only to most superficial layers of epidermis. Pemphigus erythematosus: ANA positive

Complications

PV: Untreated, almost invariably fatal. With systemic steroids, mortality is now approximately 5%. However, high-dose corticosteroids and other immunosuppressive drugs can result in multiple complications, including increased risk of life-threatening infections, osteoporosis, gastrointestinal ulcers and perforations, cataracts, leukopenia, and liver toxicity.
PF: Death from PF is less common than from PV. Complications can result from infection of lesions or from systemic therapy.

Differential diagnosis

PV: Epidermolysis bullosa acquisita, bullous pemphigoid, pemphigus foliaceus, bullous erythema multiforme, toxic epidermal necrolysis, linear IgA dermatitis, bullous lupus erythematosus, dermatitis herpetiformis, and bullous impetigo.
Oral PV: Aphthous stomatitis, Behçet's disease, herpes simplex, erosive lichen planus, lupus erythematosus, cicatricial pemphigoid, candidiasis.
PF: Impetigo, pemphigus vulgaris, staphylococcal scalded skin syndrome, pustular psoriasis, subcorneal pustular dermatitis, erythroderma; when restricted to face: seborrheic dermatitis, systemic lupus erythematosus.

Etiology

PV: Autoantibodies directed against desmoglein III (130-kD protein) complexed to plakoglobin (85 kD).
PF: Autoantibodies directed against desmoglein I (165-kD protein), a component of desmosomes. Drugs (captopril, D-penicillamine, rifampin) can rarely induce PF.

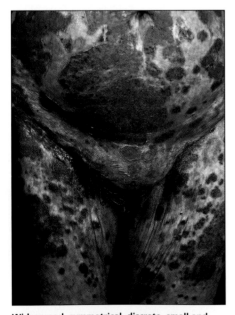

Widespread, symmetrical, discrete, small and large, crusted, erythematous erosions due to ruptured flaccid bullae in a woman with pemphigus foliaceous.

Jeanie Chung-Leddon and Jean-Claude Bystryn

Treatment

Diet and lifestyle

• Patients receiving systemic corticosteroids must adjust their diet to reduce the risk of steroid-induced diabetes and hypertension.

• To prevent osteoporosis, early calcium (calcium carbonate, 500 mg three times daily) and vitamin D (50 000 IU twice weekly) supplementation along with hormone replacement therapy should be provided, when appropriate, in addition to encouragement of weight-bearing exercises and discontinuation of smoking.

• Hard foods, brushing gums, and sunlight should be avoided to prevent further trauma and allow the lesions to heal.

Pharmacological treatment

Topical

• Topical (usually class I) or intralesional corticosteroids (for localized lesions).

Systemic

• Prednisone, 1 mg/kg/d or methylprednisolone (4/5 dose of prednisone), then increasing in 50% increments weekly until activity is controlled. Once most lesions are healed, prednisone can be tapered by 50% every 2 weeks to an alternate-day regimen.

• Immunosuppressives (usually used steroid-sparing agent, but may control disease alone), such as azathioprine (1–3 mg/kg/d), cyclophosphamide (1–2 mg/kg/d), methotrexate (10–25 mg/wk), mycophenolate mofetil (1–3 g/d), oral or intramuscular gold (60% of patients improve, but toxicity in 40%).

• Tetracycline, 2 g/d for 4 weeks, then 1 g/d, has been used as adjuvant with prednisone.

• Intravenous immunoglobulin (for severe, refractory PV unresponsive to conventional therapy), 2 g/kg, i.v., for 4 weeks in addition to prednisone and immunosuppressants.

• Colchicine, 1.5 mg/d for IgA pemphigus of the subcorneal pustular dermatosis type.

• Acitretin, 25 mg for pemphigus vegetans with prednisone.

• Pulse therapy with methylprednisolone, 10–20 mg/kg (250–1000 mg), or dexamethasone, 2–5 mg/kg (50–200 mg), intravenously infused over 1 hour for 1–5 daily or alternate-day doses for severe, recalcitrant disease. Low-dose oral corticosteroids and immunosuppressants are continued after pulse therapy and tapered if possible.

Nonpharmacological treatment

Physical modalities

• Plasmapheresis (with prednisone and azathioprine).

• Extracorporeal photochemotherapy (with prednisone and azathioprine).

Supportive methods

• Gastritis/peptic ulcer disease prophylaxis, preferably with proton-pump inhibitors (omeprazole) or with H_2-blockers (ranitidine).

• Topical antibiotics and compresses (aluminum subacetate) for wound care.

• Analgesics for pain.

Special therapeutic considerations

• Before beginning systemic corticosteroids, a complete history and physical (including blood pressure and eye exam), purified protein derivative, wound cultures, complete blood count, and general chemical profile should be obtained, as well as a 24-hour urine calcium determination and baseline bone densitometry (which should be repeated every 6–12 months).

• In drug-induced cases of PF, therapy with the offending agent must be discontinued.

Treatment aims

To prevent formation of new lesions while allowing old lesions to heal. Ultimate goal is to induce a complete remission with discontinuation of all therapy.

Prognosis

PF: Disease can be chronic and flares can occur.

PV: Mortality with treatment is 5%, but most patients eventually (after years) enter into complete remission and can discontinue therapies. The chronic nature of this disease and flares require patients to receive long-term maintenance systemic therapy.

Follow-up and management

Patients must be monitored carefully by specialists familiar with the use of systemic corticosteroids and other immunosuppressants for life-threatening infections (bacterial and fungal septicemia) and other complications of treatment, including possible development of malignancy.

Support organizations

National Pemphigus Foundation, Atrium Plaza, Suite 203, 828 San Pablo Avenue, Albany, CA 94706; telephone: 510-527-4070; fax: 510- 527-8497; e-mail: pvnews@aol.com.

General references

Bystryn J-C, Steinman NM: The adjuvant therapy of pemphigus. An update. *Arch Dermatol* 1996, **132**:203–212.

Diagnosis

Signs

Perforating folliculitis (PF): Classic lesions are pruritic, pinhead-sized, skin-colored hyperkeratotic papules; most common over extensor surfaces of extremities, also scapular region, buttocks. Lesions can erupt on face, hands, feet during later stages.

Hyperkeratosis follicularis et parafollicularis in cutem penetrans (Kyrle's disease) (KD): Pruritic, flesh-colored or hyperpigmented, folliclar or nonfollicular 2–8 mm papules; central, conical keratinous plugs on extensor surfaces of limbs, dorsa of hands, trunk, face. Lesions may become confluent into verrucous plaques. Postinflammatory changes usually remain after resolution of lesions. A variant, uremic follicular hyperkeratosis, combines features of perforating collagenosis and Kyrle's disease; occurs in patients receiving dialysis.

Elastosis perforans serpiginosa (EPS): usually asymptomatic, eruptive, skin-colored or erythematous, hyperkeratotic, 2–5 mm papules; may be solitary, grouped, or arranged in annular, arched, serpiginous pattern. There is a disseminated form, but involvement is usually localized to one area, usually on neck (70%), face (11%), upper extremities (20%), lower extremities (6%), trunk (3%). May be degree of anatomic symmetry.

Reactive perforating collagenosis (RPC): Haphazardly distributed, small papules; grow to 5–10 mm, become umbilicated with adherent firm plug. Koebnerization common at trauma sites. Typically, lesions involute in 6–10 weeks; residual scaring may remain.

Investigations

Renal function studies (urinalysis, serum creatinine, creatinine clearance) to exclude renal disease.

Serum glucose to exclude diabetes mellitus.

Skin biopsy for histopathologic examination. **PF**: Dilated hair follicle containing keratotic material, basophilic debris. Follicle perforated laterally, creating transfollicular channel topped by central keratotic plug. Degenerated connective tissue extrudes through perforation. At perforation site, focal inflammatory infiltrate invades area of degenerated collagen, elastic fibers. **KD**: Collagen bundles eliminated through invagination in epidermis, forming keratotic, partially parakeratotic plug with cupped epidermal depression. Surrounding epidermis slightly acanthotic. **EPS**: Thickened, swollen eosinophilic-staining elastic fibers in idiopathic and reactive EPS, or thorny fibers (like bramble bushes) in penicillamine-induced cases, extruded through narrow channel, winding through epidermis. In dermis, conglomerates of Orcein-Giemsa–stainable connective tissue impinge on epidermal base. **RPC**: Necrobiotic, deeply basophilic collagen in papillary dermis is eliminated through epidermal perforations that form cupped depressions.

Differential diagnosis

Folliculitis, punctate psoriasis, keratosis pilaris, pityrosporum folliculitis, keratosis follicularis, prurigo nodularis, hypertrophic lichen planus, keratoacanthoma.

Etiology

Transepidermal processes: Cause unknown, but these diseases appear to be variants of a similar process, possibly an abnormal response to trauma (scratching, insect bites, acne/folliculitis). KD may be a more severe form of PF. **Acquired perforating dermatosis**: Usually in association with nephropathies—with, and less often without, diabetes—and in Hodgkin's disease, lymphoma, periampullary carcinoma. **EPS forms**: idiopathic, reactive, drug induced. About 65% of EPS cases are idiopathic. About 25% of cases occur in patients with diseases associated with connective tissue abnormalities, such as Down's syndrome (1% prevalence), Ehlers-Danlos syndrome, Marfan's syndrome, osteogenesis imperfecta, scleroderma, acrogeria, perforating granuloma annulare, pseudoxanthoma elasticum. About 1% of patients treated with penicillamine develop EPS.

Epidemiology

Rare, except for uremic follicular hyperkeratosis, which affects up to 10% of patients treated with maintenance hemodialysis.

Dina Began and Miguel Sanchez

Treatment

Diet and lifestyle
- Renal or diabetic diet, when appropriate.

Pharmacological treatment

Topical
- Tretinoin: 0.05%-0.1% cream twice daily for 1-3 months.
- Salicyclic acid 6% gel.
- High potency corticosteroids: variable (often no) improvement.
- Antipruritic creams, lotions.

Systemic
- Oral retinoids (acitretin 25-50 mg or isotretinoin 80-120 mg per day).
- High-dose vitamin A: 50,000-200,000 U daily, tapered down upon response.
- Antihistamines for pruritus.
- Allopurinol (anecdotally, helps with uremic symptoms)

Nonpharmacological treatment
- UV or narrow band UVB phototherapy.
- Psoralen and UVA photochemotherapy (PUVA).
- PUVA with oral retinoids (Re-PUVA).
- Cryotherapy of each lesion.
- Electrocautery or CO_2 laser ablation of each lesion

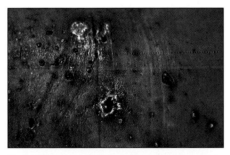

Crop of lesions at various stages of development in a patient with Kyrle's disease. Pinhead-sized scaly papules; excoriated papules with crusted central craters; hard hyperpigmented exophytic nodules surrounded by rims of hyperkeratotic scales; depressed, atrophic hyperpigmented scars.

Treatment aims
To decrease pruritus.

Prognosis
Often recalcitrant to treatment. Lesions self-healing.

Follow-up and management
Monitor for retinoid therapy; if no symptoms, no further treatment.

General references
Morton CA, Henderson IS, Jones MC, *et al.*: Acquired perforating dermatosis in a British dialysis population. *Br J Dermatol* 1996, 135:671–677.

Chang P, Fernandez V: Acquired perforating disease: Report of nine cases. *Int J Dermatol* 1993, 32:874–876.

Patterson JW. The perforating disorders [review]. *J Am Acad Dermatol* 1984, 10:561–581.

Diagnosis

Symptoms

Phototoxic reactions: Burning, pain.

Photoallergic reactions: Pruritus.

Signs

Phototoxic reactions: Erythema, edema; vesicles, or bullae, if severe; blue-gray pigmentation; lichenoid; photoonycholysis.

Photoallergic reactions: Eczematous with erythema, edema, lichenified plaques.

Chronic actinic dermatitis: Eczematous, hyperpigmented, lichenified papules, plaques. Spectrum of disorders includes persistent light reactivity, photosensitive eczema, photosensitivity dermatitis, and actinic reticuloid.

Distribution

Phototoxic reactions: Sites typically affected include the face, forearms, dorsa of the hands, and V-area of the chest with sparing of sun-protected areas.

Photoallergic reactions: Confined to areas of contact with the agent that are subsequently exposed to the sun.

Chronic actinic dermatitis:Sun-exposed areas with some extension to sun-protected areas; may generalize.

Investigations

Laboratory: antinuclear antibody, anti-SSA(Ro) and anti-SSB(La) tests to rule out lupus erythematosus.

Phototests: In chronic actinic dermatitis, the minimal erythema dose for ultraviolet A or B is decreased. Photopatch tests are helpful in identifying photoallergen when either chronic actinic dermatitis or photoallergy is suspected.

Skin biopsy: Phototoxic: Necrotic keratinocytes. Photoallergic: Spongiotic dermatitis. Chronic actinic dermatitis: Spongiosis, acanthosis, and hyperplasia of the epidermis. Perivascular infiltrate with mononuclear cells, occasional neutrophils, plasma cells, eosinophils., and rarely mononuclear cells with hyperconvoluted nuclei resembling those seen in cutaneous T-cell lymphoma.

Complications

Phototoxic reactions: Permanent hyperpigmentation or gray pigmentation.

Photoallergic reactions: Progression to chronic actinic dermatitis.

Chronic actinic dermatitis: Rarely erythroderma.

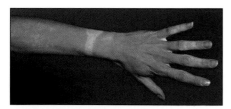

Phototoxic dermatitis, with erythema on the hand and forearm, sparing only the skin shielded by a watch.

Differential diagnosis

Polymorphous light eruption, contact dermatitis from airborne antigens, allergic contact dermatitis, lupus erythematosus, porphyria cutanea tarda.

Etiology

Phototoxic reactions: Result of direct tissue injury (nonimmunologic), mediated by reactive oxygen species and inflammatory mediators. Occur most frequently with systemic agents. Tar and psoralen produce the reaction after topical exposure.
Photoallergic reactions: Have a sensitization phase and occurs on second exposure. Type IV hypersensitivity; a nonallergen is converted by UV to a photoallergen. Require a minimal amount of photoallergen. The allergen is usually topical. Usually mediated by UVA. **Chronic actinic dermatitis**: Endogenous or exogenous antigens persist after the original photosensitizer has been removed.

Epidemiology

Phototoxic reactions: All persons are susceptible. **Photoallergic reactions**: Only in genetically predisposed individuals.
Chronic actinic dermatitis: Uncommon; typically affects older men.

Treatment

Diet and lifestyle

• Patients should minimize sun exposure by using sun-protective clothing and sun-blocks.

Pharmacological treatment

Topical

• Emollients and topical glucocorticoids.

Systemic

• For chronic actinic dermatitis, intermittent courses of the following may be helpful: prednisone, 1 mg/kg per day; azathioprine, 1.0–2.5 mg/kg per day; cyclosporine, 150–300 mg per day; hydroxychloroquine 200–400 mg per day.

Nonpharmacological treatment

• Remove the offending agent. Use broad-spectrum sunscreens with a sun protective factor greater than 15. Phototherapy: PUVA may be used for chronic actinic dermatitis. Should be used with systemic glucocorticoids to avoid a flare.

Special therapeutic considerations

Drugs and substances known to cause phototoxic reactions

NSAIDs, piroxacams, ibuprofen, ketoprofen, naproxen, antimicrobials, chloroquine, quinine, ciprofloxacin, ofloxacin, enoxacin, lomefloxacin, nalidixic acid, norfloxacin, sulfonamides, tetracycline, minocycline, doxycycline, demeclocycline, diuretics, fluorosemide, chlorothiazide, hydrochlorothiazide, hypoglycemics, glyburide, tolazamide, tolbutamide, antianxiety drugs, alprazolam, and chlordiazepoxide.

Miscellaneous drugs and substances that produce other types of reaction

Hypericin (St John's wort), isotretinoin, anticancer drugs, fluorouracil, methotrexate, vinblastine, dacarbazine, antidepressants, desipramine, imipramine, antipsychotic drugs, chlorpromazine, perphenazine, prochlorperazine, thioridizine, trifluoperazine, cardiac medications, amiodarone, quinidine, and fenofibrate.

Treatment aims

Remove underlying cause if known.
Decrease pain or related discomfort.
Educate the patient about the condition.
Control the disease in chronic actinic dermatitis.

Prognosis

Phototoxic reactions: Will cease to progress when the agent is removed. There may be persistent hyperpigmentation or gray pigmentation which may resolve with time.

Photoallergic reactions: Generally resolves on withdrawal of the allergen. May progress to chronic actinic dermatitis.

Chronic actinic dermatitis: Persistent even on withdrawal of agent. May resolve over time with strict sun protection.

General references

Gould JW, Mercurio MG, Elmets CA: Cutaneous photosensitivity diseases induced by exogenous agents. *J Am Acad Dermatol* 1995, **33**:551–573.

Lim HW, Morison WL, Kamide R, *et al.*: Chronic actinic dermatitis: an analysis of 51 patients evaluated in the United States and Japan. *Arch Dermatol* 1994, **130**:1284–1289.

Lim HW, Cohen D, Soter NA: Chronic actinic dermatitis: results of patch and photopatch tests with Compositae, fragrances, and pesticides. *J Am Acad Dermatol* 1998, **38**:108–111.

Fotiades J, Soter NA, Lim HW: Results of evaluation of 203 patients for photosensitivity in a 7.3-year period. J Am Acad Dermatol 1995, 33:597–602.

Samuel Beck and Nicholas A. Soter

Diagnosis

Signs

• Spectrum of recurrent skin lesions, ranging from acute (PLEVA) to chronic (PLC), with an intermediate form in which lesions from both variants are present over a period of weeks to months.

Pityriasis lichenoides et varioliformis acuta (PLEVA), also called Mucha-Habermann disease: Recurrent crops of erythematous, purpuric papules that evolve into hemorrhagic vesicles, bullae, or pustules and papules with scale or crust over several weeks. The skin lesions are concentrated on the trunk, thighs, and arms, especially the flexural areas.

Pityriasis lichenoides chronica (PLC): Recurrent crops of small, asymptomatic red-brown lichenoid papules that flatten over several weeks. Distribution is also mainly on the trunk, arms and thighs.

Symptoms

PLEVA, **PLC** and are usually asymptomatic; rarely, there is itching or burning.

PLEVA is rarely associated with fever, malaise, and headache.

Investigations

• Skin biopsy for diagnosis.

• T cell receptors gene analysis for clonality in unusual or prolonged cases.

Complications

• Impetigo, varioliform scarring (bullous PLEVA).

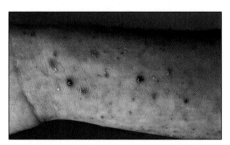

PLEVA on medial aspect of forearm: early, tiny dusky-pink papules; pink papules with central vesiculation; small pustules with erythematous halos; necrotic papules covered with hemorrhagic crust; small erosions; older lichenoid papules with peripheral collarettes of scale.

Differential diagnosis

Dermatitis herpetiformis, drug eruptions, folliculitis, guttate psoriasis, arthropod bites, leukocytoclastic vasculitis, lichen planus, lymphomatoid papulosis, papular eczema, Gianotti-Crosti syndrome, pityriasis rosea, secondary syphilis, small plaque parapsoriasis, and varicella.

Etiology

The etiology remains unclear, although cases have been reported in association with infections, chemotherapeutic agents, estrogen-progesterone therapy, and HIV.

Southern blot or polymerase chain reaction analysis of T cell receptor gene of PLEVA show clonal T cell populations, suggesting a lymphoproliferative response.

Clonal T cell populations have also been found in patients with PLC.

Both PLEVA and PLC are rarely associated with lymphoproliferative disorders and could be reclassified with lymphomatoid papulosis.

Epidemiology

Seen usually in adolescents and young adults, but may be seen rarely in infancy and old age.

No racial or geographic predilection.

Rarely associated with non-Hodgkin's lymphoma and T-cell lymphomas of the skin.

PLC: Male predilection, 70% of reported cases.

PLC: More common than PLEVA.

Special considerations

Rare cases may represent a bridge from benign lymphoproliferative disorders of the skin to non-Hodgkin's lymphoma or T-cell lymphomas of the skin.

Treatment

Diet and lifestyle
- Topical care of lesions to avoid impetigo.
- Loose fitting clothing.

Pharmacological treatment

Topical
- Treatment with topical corticosteroids of low, middle, and high potency twice a day. • •
- Antibiotic creams or ointments (when necessary).

Systemic
- Tetracycline, 500 mg four times daily or doxycycline 100 mg twice daily for 4 weeks in adults.
- Erythromycin, 500 mg four times daily adults or 3-50mg/kg per day in children.
- Antihistamines for itch.
- Methotrexate (for PLEVA), 5-20 mg once weekly, initially, and lowered for maintenance.
- Patients may respond to very low doses.
- Cyclosporine (Neoral), 100 mg twice daily (in selected cases).
- Prednisone, 1 mg/kg/daily (in selected cases).

Nonpharmacological treatment
- UBV light phototherapy.
- Psoralen and UVA chemophototherapy.

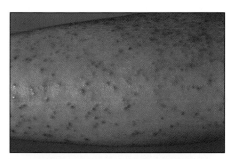

The eruption of PLC is more monomorphous, and consists of crops of asymptomatic, shiny, brownish pink, round, firm lichenoid, planar papules with micaceous scale. The lesions often appear to be forming a retiform pattern.

Prognosis

PLC: Usually involutes within 3–6 weeks with postinflammatory pigmentary changes. Rarely associated with lymphoproliferative disorders.

General references

Patel DG, Kihiczak G, Schwartz RA, *et al*.: Pityriasis lichenoides [review]. *Cutis* 2000, **65**:17–20.

Romani J, Puig L, Fernandez-Figueras MT, *et al*.:Pityriasis lichenoides in children: Clinicopathologic review of 22 patients. *Pediatr Dermatol* 1998, **15**:1–6.

Tsuji T, Kasamatsu M, Yokota M, *et al*.: Mucha-Habermann disease and its febrile ulceronecrotic variant [review]. *Cutis* 1996, **58**:123–131.

Diagnosis

Signs

•Herald patch: Single, oval, slightly raised plaque, 2–10 cm in diameter, with a flesh-colored center surrounded by a pink, elevated border with a fine "collarette" of scale trailing the periphery. A single plaque is seen in 80% of cases. In 5% of cases, multiple herald patches are seen. The herald patch is followed by an eruption 1–2 weeks later.

•Exanthem: Multiple, oval to round, dull pink, 5- to 15-mm papules and plaques with typical marginal collarettes of fine scale, usually symmetrically scattered on trunk and proximal extremities. Characteristically, the long axes of the lesions run parallel to the ribs ("Christmas tree" distribution). An "inverse" distribution pattern affecting the face and distal extremities, as well as localized and unilateral forms, is seen in 20% of cases. Palmoplantar involvement leading to desquamation can develop in severe cases. The lesions may also be vesicular, purpuric, pustular, lichenoid, and erythema multiforme–like. Nail pitting may be present. Mucosal lesions, such as punctate hemorrhages, erosions, or ulcerations, and white or erythematous patches and plaques may affect any mucosal surface, particularly the oral cavity.

Symptoms

•Pruritus: Absent (25% of cases), mild (50%), or severe (25%).

•Constitutional symptoms: Headache, gastrointestinal symptoms, fever, malaise, nausea, weight loss, lymphadenopathy, sore throat, and arthralgias, seen in 5% of cases.

Investigations

•Serologic testing should be performed routinely to rule out syphilis.

•Histopathologic studies may be helpful to support the diagnosis and should be performed if the lesions last for more than 6 weeks. A superficial, perivascular, mononuclear infiltrate is seen in the dermis, often with extravasated erythrocytes in the dermal papillae. The epidermis shows spongiosis and intracellular edema in areas invaded by the infiltrate. Dyskeratotic, eosinophilic keratinocytes are present in some cases.

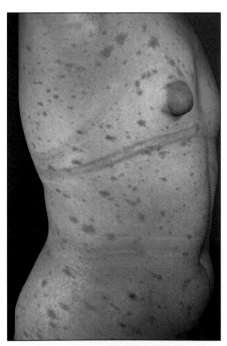

Typical pink, oval macules; patches with central collarettes of scales. long axes of lesions follow lines of cleavage, in inverted "Christmas tree" pattern.

Differential diagnosis

Secondary syphilis, tinea corporis, urticaria, guttate psoriasis, Gianotti-Crosti syndrome, nummular eczema, parapsoriasis, scabies, pityriasis lichenoides, drug-induced pityriasiform eruption (captopril, metronidazole, isotretinoin, D-penicillamine, levamisole, diphtheria toxoid, bismuth, gold, barbiturates, clonidine, arsenic, *beta*-blockers, pyribenzamine, medroxypromazine, omeprazole, griseofulvin, arsphenamine, smallpox immunization), viral exanthems, erythema annulare centrifugum, seborrheic dermatitis, erythema migrans, lichen planus.

Etiology

No clear cause has been found, but many factors have been postulated:

Viral infections (*eg*, echovirus 6, picornavirus), bacterial infection (*eg*, mycoplasma, bacille Calmette-Guéerin vaccines), fungal infection (*eg*, dermatophytes), contact exposure (*eg*, garments), insect bites, autoimmune process, toxins produced by occult infections, psychogenic causes.

Epidemiology

Responsible for 0.35% to 3.0% of dermatologic outpatient visits.

The peak age is 1–35 years, but all ages can be affected.

Slight female predominance; no racial predominance.

More common in the spring and fall and in temperate climates.

Although clustering within close contacts has occasionally been noted, it is not considered contagious.

Atypical and oral pityriasis rosea are more common in children and blacks.

Treatment

Diet and lifestyle
•Because the disease is not contagious, patients should not be isolated or prevented from going to school.

Pharmacological treatment

Topical
•Emollients with menthol and antipruritic agents.

•Corticosteroids, especially in pruritic cases and patients at risk for pigmentation.

Systemic
•Antihistamines for pruritus.

•Dapsone, 50–100 mg/d.

•Prednisone, 0.5–1 mg/kg per day, tapered rapidly, for severe cases.

Nonpharmacological treatment
•Ultraviolet B phototherapy is highly effective.

•Natural sunlight.

Special therapeutic considerations
•Ampicillin should be avoided because it can exacerbate the eruption. Drug-induced pityriasiform eruptions are difficult to manage.

Herald patch: 1 to 3 cm, oval or round; or thin plaque with central, slightly scaly, salmon-pink center, darker peripheral zone. Precedes eruption by up to 10 days.

Treatment aims

Reassure patients of the benign and self-limited nature of their disease, prevent postinflammatory pigmentary changes, and alleviate symptoms.

Prognosis

Herald patch proceeds the exanthematous phase by 1–2 weeks. The exanthem generally develops over 2 weeks, persists for 2 weeks, and resolves over 2 weeks.

Postinflammatory hyperpigmentation and hypopigmentation may remain.

Condition recurs in 2% of cases.

General references

Allen RA, Janniger CK, Schwartz RA: Pityriasis rosea. *Cutis* 1995, **56**:198–202.

Parsons JM: Pityriasis rosea update: 1986. *J Am Acad Dermatol* 1986, **15**:159–167.

Horio T: Skin disorders that improve by exposure to sunlight. *Clin Dermatol* 1998, **16**:59–65.

Mary Ellen Brademas

Diagnosis

Signs

•Pityriasis rubra pilaris (PRP) has been classified into five types, on the basis of clinical characteristics.

All types: Nail changes include distal yellow-brown discoloration, subungual keratosis, nail plate thickening, and splinter hemorrhages. Oral mucous membrane changes occur rarely, and include diffuse hyperkeratosis or macular erythema with white streaks that resemble oral lichen planus.

Classic adult (type I) and **classic juvenile** (type III): Keratotic follicular papules on the dorsal aspects of the proximal phalanges, elbows, and wrists; perifollicular erythema and scaly orange-red plaques, with characteristic islands of normal skin within them, on the trunk and extremities. These plaques may expand and coalesce to cover the entire body **(erythrodermic PRP)**. There is often palmoplantar hyperkeratosis, with fissuring and an intense yellow-red hue.

Adult atypical (type II): Alopecia, ichthyosiform scaling, and eczematous areas.

Circumscribed juvenile (type IV): Stable, focal areas of erythema and hyperkeratosis, characteristically.

Atypical juvenile (type V): Predominantly hyperkeratosis, infrequently erythema, and scleroderma-like changes on the palms and soles.

Symptoms

•Pruritus or burning in approximately 20% of "classic" adult cases.

Investigations

•Diagnosis is generally made clinically. Skin biopsy shows irregular acanthosis, hyperkeratotic stratum corneum with perifollicular parakeratosis, follicular plugging, and a chronic inflammatory infiltrate.

Complications

•Frequently progresses to exfoliative erythroderma.

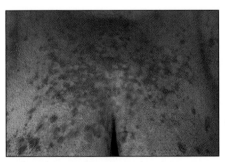

Scaly, orange-red papules that become confluent into large plaques on the chest of a woman with pityriasis rubra pilaris.

Differential diagnosis

Psoriasis (main disease to be differentiated), cutaneous T-cell lymphoma, erythrokeratoderma variabilis, follicular eczema, follicular ichthyosis, lichen planopilaris, seborrheic dermatitis, subacute cutaneous lupus erythematosus.

Etiology

Vitamin A deficiency, abnormal vitamin A metabolism or defective vitamin A receptors have been proposed as the cause; however, patients with PRP frequently have normal vitamin A levels and attempts to produce keratotic lesions by vitamin A deprivation have been unsuccessful.

An additional acidic-keratin (K17), not found in control skin, was found in one kindred with the familial form of the disease.

Epidemiology

This rare disease is estimated to be the presenting problem in 1 of 35,000 to 1 of 50,000 patients with a dermatologic condition. It occurs equally in men and women. Juvenile forms typically present before the age of 2, whereas adult cases most commonly present acutely in the fifth decade. Most cases are acquired, but a familial form (autosomal dominant inheritance with variable expressivity) exists. The familial type generally starts early in childhood, whereas the acquired form may occur at any age.

About 55% of all patients present with type I, 25% with type IV, 10% with type III, 5% with type II, and 5% with type V.

Treatment

Pharmacological treatment

Topical
•Keratolytics containing propylene glycol and salicylic acid or lactic acid under an occlusive plastic dressing for 2–4 hours followed by a potent corticosteroid ointment for 4–8 hours under an occlusive dressing is an effective topical regimen for hyperkeratotic areas such as the palms and soles.

•Tar and calcipotriol may also be effective.

Systemic
•Synthetic retinoids (isotretinoin, usually at 1.0 mg/kg per day, or acitretin, 25–50 mg/d) have replaced vitamin A therapy (toxic doses of 1 million U/d for up to 2 weeks followed by reduced dosages have given the best results) as the treatment of choice. Hyperlipidemia, hepatic dysfunction, and teratogenicity may result from treatment with synthetic retinoids. The use of gemfibrozil is successful in managing retinoid-induced hyperlipidemia.

•Methotrexate, in dosages of 10–25 mg/week, given as a single dose or three divided doses at 12-hour intervals, is an alternative agent for refractory disease. Patients must be followed closely for hepatotoxicity, myelosuppression, teratogenicity, and defective spermatogenesis.

•Combination therapy with oral retinoids and methotrexate has been reported to be effective in cases of severe or resistant PRP, with acitretin, 25–50 mg/d, and a weekly methotrexate dose of 5–30 mg for 16 weeks. Combination therapy should be used with caution given the risk of toxic hepatitis. Frequent clinical and laboratory evaluation, including weekly liver function test monitoring for the first 6–8 weeks, is advised.

•Azathioprine, in dosages of 50–200 mg/d, has been effective in a small number of cases.

•Cyclosporine has had minimal to no effect on PRP, although isolated cases of efficacy have been reported.

Nonpharmacological treatment

•Unlike psoriasis, PRP generally does not respond well to conventional and narrow-band ultraviolet B phototherapy or psoralen plus ultraviolet A light. Extracorporeal photochemotherapy has been used in resistant cases.

Special therapeutic considerations

•Several cases of PRP have been reported in association with HIV infection, and these cases are generally more recalcitrant to therapy than are cases involving HIV-negative patients.

•Topical agents are particularly useful in juvenile disease, because of its overall good prognosis and frequently limited involvement.

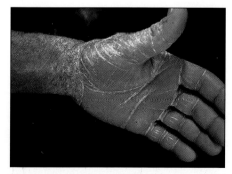

Yellow-orange palm with diffuse hyperkeratosis due to pityriasis rubra pilaris.

Treatment aims
•Treatment is directed toward achieving and maintaining remission of the disease.

Prognosis
Acquired forms of PRP exhibit variable courses of relapse and remission. Clinical improvement and resolution of PRP have been reported within 3 years, in 81% of patients with type I. Type V persists throughout life. Other types typically follow a chronic course of relapse and remission. The percentage of patients who clear in 3 years is 20% for type II, 16% for type III, and 32% for type IV.

Follow-up and management
Follow-up is dictated by severity and treatment. Patients receiving systemic retinoids or methotrexate require frequent clinical and laboratory examination.

Support groups
National Organization for Rare Disorders, Inc. (NORD), PO Box 8923, New Fairfield, CT 06812; telephone, 800-999-6673, Internet, http://www.nord-rdb.com.

General references

Albert MR, Mackool BT: Pityriasis rubra pilaris. *Int J Dermatol* 1999, **38**:1–11.

Cohen PR, Prystowsky JH: Pityriasis rubra pilaris: a review of diagnosis and treatment. *J Am Acad Dermatol* 1989, **20**:801–807.

Dicken CH: Isotretinoin treatment of pityriasis rubra pilaris. *J Am Acad Dermatol* 1987, **16**:297–301.

Goldsmith LA, Baden HP: Pityriasis rubra pilaris. In: *Dermatology in General Medicine*, edn 5. Edited by Freedberg IM, *et al.* New York: McGraw-Hill; 1998:538–541.

Diagnosis

Signs

Polymorphous light eruption (PMLE): Usually erythematous papules, occasionally plaques, uncommonly papulovesicles; morphology same in each patient, with each recurrence; polymorphous from patient to patient.

Actinic prurigo (AP): Erythematous papules or nodules; often excoriated, crusted, or scabbed. Often with associated eczematous skin and lichenification. Face heals to form small linear or pitted scars. Cheilitis and conjunctivitis also occur in an indistinguishable condition seen in Native Americans called hereditary PMLE.

Hydroa vacciniforme (HV): Begins as erythematous macules, progresses to papules, vesicles, or bullae that may become hemorrhagic. Next, umbilication followed by crusting occurs and pock mark scars are left after healing.

Symptoms

PMLE: Follows exposure to sunlight; onset in spring, early summer; improves by fall as skin "hardens" to effects of the sun. Sun exposure necessary to induce eruption varies from 15 minutes to several hours; usually develops several hours after exposure; pruritic; lesions resolve over 2–10 days, without scarring; rarely fever, chills, body aches.

AP: Follows exposure to sunlight; worse in summer, may not clear in winter; pruritic.

HV: Occurs hours following exposure to sunlight. Itching, burning; sometimes fever, malaise, headache; occurs in summer.

Distribution

PMLE: Sun-exposed areas; V of neck, forearms commonest; eruption usually on sun-exposed areas covered in winter. Same symmetrical distribution each recurrence.

AP: Face, distal extremities. Covered skin may be involved (rare in PMLE).

HV: Symmetrical; on some or all sun-exposed skin.

Diagnostic procedures

Polymorphous light eruption

Phototesting: Determine minimal effective dose (MED) for ultraviolet light (UV) A and B (normal values in PMLE) Repetitive exposures or a large single dose of UVA or UVB to elicit eruption. When possible, use skin site typically involved. If lesions elicited, obtain a biopsy. A patient may clearly have PMLE but not respond to phototesting. **Histology**: Characteristic but not diagnostic; perivascular infiltrate in the upper, middle dermis; mainly lymphocytes, occasional neutrophils, eosinophils; papillary dermal edema; liquefactive basal cell degeneration of lupus is absent; variable epidermal changes such as exocytosis, spongiosis. **Laboratory**: Serum antinuclear antibodies (ANA), anti-ssA, anti-ssB to rule out lupus erythematosus. Urine, stool, plasma, and erythrocyte porphyrins to rule out porphyrias.

Actinic purigo

Phototesting: Repetitive testing may produce a PMLE-like eruption. **Histology**: Helpful, acanthosis, spongiosis, mononuclear perivascular infiltrate, edema. **Laboratory**: As in PMLE, to rule out lupus and porphyrias.

Hydroa vacciniforme

Phototesting: This may induce the eruption. **Histology**: Diagnostic; reveals spongiosis, intraepidermal vesiculation, reticular keratinocyte degeneration, epidermal and upper dermal necrosis, sometimes ulceration. Early mononuclear cell infiltrate later includes neutrophils. **Laboratory**: As in PMLE, to rule out lupus and the porphyrias.

Complications

PMLE: No scarring. **AP**: Small linear or pitted scars on the face. **HV**: Poxlike scars.

Differential diagnosis

PMLE: Lupus erythematosus, porphyria, rosacea, chronic actinic dermatitis, phototoxic or photoallergic reactions.

AP: Insect bites, prurigo nodularis, atopic eczema, scabies, erythropoietic protoporphyria.

HV: Erythropoietic protoporphyria

Etiology

PMLE: May be manifestation of type IV hypersensitivity.

AP: May be variant of PMLE. Possibly delayed type hypersensitivity.

Increased frequency of human leukocyte antigen (HLA)-DR4, and HLA-DRB1*0407 may indicate genetic predisposition and autoimmune etiology.

HV: Idiopathic, may be scarring variant of PMLE.

Epidemiology

PMLE: Between 10% and 20% of population report symptoms; 3:1 female predilection. All skin types affected; fair skin most. Typical patient is a young, fair-skinned woman in her 20s. Incidence is higher in temperate and colder climates.

AP: Rare. Affects children and resolves in adolescence. Indistinguishable condition (hereditary PMLE) in Native Americans and persists into adulthood.

HV: Very rare. Affects children and resolves in adolescence.

Treatment

Diet and lifestyle

• Patients should apply broad-spectrum sunblock frequently and wear photoprotective clothing.

Pharmacological treatment

Topical

PMLE: Sunscreen; high sun-protection factor broad spectrum sunscreens; Topical steroids reduce lesions. In more severe cases, 10–15 treatments of UVB or psoralen and UVA (PUVA) phototherapy may prevent outbreaks by "hardening" skin. UVA may be as effective as PUVA.

Systemic

PMLE: Oral glucocorticosteroids used in short courses to treat severe cases; as prophylaxis for patients traveling to tropics in the winter months. Hydroxychloroquine, 200 mg daily is useful in severe cases and may be started 4-6 weeks prior to summer outbreak. Eye examination, G6PD level necessary prior to thearapy with this drug. β-carotene and thalidomide used with variable success, not studied in controlled trials.

AP: Hydroxychloroquine 200 mg daily may be helpful. Thalidomide 100 mg daily reduced to 50 mg daily when disease controlled.

HV: UVB, PUVA, antimalarials may be helpful.

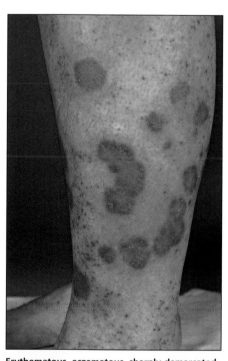

Erythematous, eczematous, sharply-demarcated, round and polygonal plaques with fine scale and darker, prominent borders on the leg of a patient with polymorphous light eruption. Numerous small excoriations are present.

Treatment aims

To prevent eruption of lesions and treat symptoms.

Prognosis

PMLE: Chronic; recurs each spring; may improve or resolve with age.

AP: Resolves by adolescence, except in Native Americans.

HV: Resolves by adolescence or early adulthood. Poxlike scars.

General references

Gonzalez E, Gonzalez S: Drug photosensitivity, idiopathic photodermatoses, and sunscreens. *J Am Acad Dermatol* 1996, **35**:871–885.

Man I, Dawe RS, Ferguson J: Artificial hardening for polymorphic light eruption: practical points from ten years' experience. *Photodermatol Photoimmunol Photomed* 1999, **15**:96–99.

Lim HW, Epstein J: Photosensitivity diseases. *J Am Acad Dermatol* 1997 **36**:84–90.

Lane PR, Hogan DJ, Martel MJ, et al.: Actinic prurigo: clinical features and prognosis. *J Am Acad Dermatol* 1992, **26**:683–692.

Goldgeier MH, Nordland JT, Lucky AW, et al.: Hydroa Vacciniforme: Diagnosis and therapy. *Arch Dermatol* 1982, **118**:588–591.

Diagnosis

Signs

Classic porokeratosis of Mibelli (PKM): Small, red-brown keratotic papules; slowly form annular/serpiginous plaques; atrophic, hairless, anhidrotic, hyperpigmented or hypopigmented centers; raised margins. Mature lesions: a few millimeters to several centimeters in diameter. Raised border may measure 1–10 mm in height; characteristic furrow at apex. Few lesions, usually localized, unilateral; bilateral or symmetric lesions reported. Koebner phenomenon noted, commonly on acral regions of extremities. Possible on palms, soles, face, genitals, oral mucosa.

Disseminated superficial/actinic porokeratosis (DSP/DSAP): Small, red-brown keratotic crateriform papules, gradually form 0.5- to 1-cm circinate lesions with slightly atrophic anhidrotic centers and superficial peripheral ridge. Peripheral border <1 mm high; slight furrow in apex. Few to several hundred lesions; typically bilateral, symmetric. Palms, soles, mucosal surfaces not involved. DSP develops regardless of sun exposure; generalized. DSAP only on sun-exposed areas, especially extensor surface of limbs, shoulders, and back; spares face.

Porokeratosis palmaris et plantaris disseminata (PPPD): Keratotic red-brown papules initially on palms, soles; form 0.5- to 1-cm circinate lesions; fine peripheral rim, superficial peripheral border, < 1 mm high. Border may be keratotic on palms, soles; pronounced furrow. In months to years, lesions disseminate to extremities, anterior and posterior trunk, regardless of sun exposure. Mucous membranes may be involved; multiple, small, asymptomatic, opalescent ring-like lesions.

Linear porokeratosis (LPK; minimal to >1 mm high): Small keratotic papules; evolve over years into discrete or confluent, variably sized, hypopigmented or hyperpigmented plaques with atrophic center, peripheral furrowed ridge. Few to many lesions, strictly unilateral. Primarily on distal extremities; less often, trunk. Linear or elongated arcuate patterns. Palms, soles may be involved; mucous membranes spared.

Punctate porokeratosis (PPK): Discrete, minute punctate keratotic spine-like papules; fine raised border. Linear or coalesce into plaques that do not enlarge centrifugally. Many lesions confined to palms, soles. Usually associated with LK, PKM.

Symptoms

PKM: Usually asymptomatic. **DSP/DSAP**: Pruritus/stinging common in DSAP; in 50% of cases, DSAP exacerbated during the summer from heat, sun or after exposure to ultraviolet light. Pruritus less common in DSP. **PPPD**: Disseminated lesions may be pruritic; in 25% of cases, exacerbation in summer; palm, sole lesions often painful. **LPK**: Occasionally pruritic. **PPK** may be moderately tender to pressure.

Investigations

• Skin biopsy: cornoid lamella (parakeratotic column at lesion periphery angles away from center, extends through surrounding orthokeratotic stratum corneum). Granular layer absent beneath parakeratotic column; dyskeratotic and vacuolated keratinocytes present at base. Cornoid lamella most prominent in PKM and LPK; less pronounced in DSP, DSAP, and PPPD.

Complications

• Malignant degeneration (squamous-cell carcinoma, basal-cell carcinoma). Incidence of malignancies about 7.5%. One third of patients develop multiple tumors. Malignancy most common in LP; rare in DSAP. Factors increasing malignancy risk: large coalescing lesions, older patient age, long-standing disease (average latency, 36 years), history of ionizing radiation exposure. Malignant lesions more common on extremities. Fatal metastatic disease reported. Role of UV irradiation unclear; most reported malignancies in nonexposed skin; DSAP malignancies rare.

Differential diagnosis

PKM: Atrophic lichen planus, verrucae, actinic keratosis, basal-cell carcinoma, squamous-cell carcinoma, elastosis perforans serpiginosa. **DSP/DSAP**: Actinic or seborrheic keratosis, annular lichen planus, granuloma annulare. **PPK**: Basal-cell nevus syndrome, Darier's disease, pitted keratolysis, punctate keratoderma. **LPK**: Epidermal nevus, lichen striatus, verrucae, linear lichen planus, psoriasis, or Darier's disease.

Etiology

Most widely accepted theory: develops from peripheral expansion of mutant clone of epidermal keratinocytes at base of cornoid lamella; concept supported by presence in affected keratinocytes of abnormal DNA content, overexpression of *p53* tumor suppression protein, immunophenotypic changes similar to those seen in malignant transformation. Dermal influence also suggested in pathogenesis. Dermal infiltrate of Langerhans and T-helper cells located beneath cornoid lamella may participate in establishment. Defects in immune surveillance by these cells may promote development, proliferation of mutant clone of keratinocytes. Porokeratotic lesions recur after epidermal destruction but not after dermal destruction.

Expansion of epidermal clone and induction of porokeratosis promoted by trauma, natural or artificial UV light exposure (particularly in DSAP), immunosuppression associated with organ transplantation, liver disease, hematologic malignancies, HIV infection, immunosuppressive therapy, possibly, electron-beam radiation.

Epidemiology

Inheritance: PKM, PPPD, DSAP/DSP—autosomal dominant; LPK—unknown, but familial cases have been identified. **Incidence:** DSAP/DSP—most common clinical type; PKM, PPPD, LPK—rare. **Age at onset:** PKM—usually childhood; may occur at any age; DSP/DSAP—third to fourth decade; PPPD—childhood to early twenties; LPK—birth to adulthood.

Treatment

Diet and lifestyle
• Sun screen use, avoidance of excessive UV exposure particularly in DSAP.

Pharmacological treatment

Topical
• General: lubrication, keratolytics (salicylic acid, urea, lactic acid) may relieve symptoms.
• Topical or intralesional corticosteroids and topical tretinoin; results variable.
• Calcipotriene reported to clear lesions of DSAP after once-daily use for 6–12 weeks.
• 5-Fluorouracil 5% cream effective in PKM, LPK, DSAP, DSP. Treatment end point: development of a marked inflammatory response.

Systemic
• Acitretin, 25–50 mg/d, isotretinoin, 0.5–1.5 mg/kg/d: good response in DSAP, widespread PKM, PPPD, LPK. High recurrence rate after cessation of therapy; significant potential toxicity. Exacerbations noted during therapy.

Surgical
• Isolated circumscribed lesions: excision and grafting, cryosurgery, electrodesiccation, dermabrasion, carbon dioxide laser, 585-nm pulsed-dye laser.

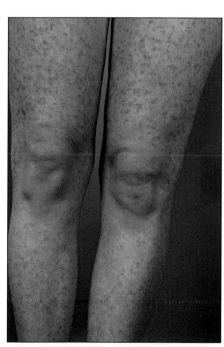

Disseminated superficial actinic porokeratosis of the lower extremities; close inspection shows that crops of papules may form circinate patterns.

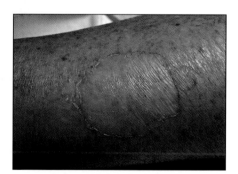

Lesion of porokeratosis of Mibelli on leg: sharply-demarcated, atrophic, shiny, annular patch bordered by white pink, hyperkeratotic, thin, raised rim; threadlike groove.

Treatment aims
To clear cutaneous lesions, relieve symptoms, decrease risk of malignant degeneration. Treatment usually palliative, not curative.

Special therapeutic considerations
Must avoid all therapies that may increase the risk of malignant transformation: x-rays, immunosuppression, excessive UV light exposure.

Prognosis
PK usually progresses slowly; lesions increasing in size/number over years. Exposure to natural or artificial UV irradiation may exacerbate DSAP. PK may be associated with immunosuppression (usually PKM/DSAP/DSP): may parallel level of immunosuppression. Complete regression may occur when immune function normalizes. Facial porokeratosis with extensive destructive changes reported. Rarely, spontaneous regression after marked inflammatory response. If sudden rapid exacerbation of DSAP/DSP, evaluate for underlying cause of immunosuppression.

Follow-up and management
Malignant potential warrants, at minimum, careful observation.

General references
Kanitakis J, et al.: Porokeratosis and immunosuppression. *Eur J Dermatol* 1998, 8:459–465.

Schamroth JM, et al.: Porokeratosis of Mibelli. *Acta Derm Venereol* 1997, 77:207–213.

Sehgal VN, et al.: Porokeratosis. *J Dermatol* 1996, 23:517–525.

Diagnosis

Definition

Porphyrias are *erythropoietic* (erythropoietic protoporphyria, **EPP**; erythropoietic porphyria, **EP**) or *hepatic* (porphyria cutanea tarda, **PCT**; variegate porphyria, **VP**; acute intermittent porphyria, **AIP**; hepatoerythropoietic porphyria, **HEP**; hereditary coprporphyria, **HCP**), depending on where the enzyme deficiency is predominately expressed.

Signs

PCT: Skin overexposed to sun, especially dorsa of hands, face: skin fragility, bullae, erosions; lanugo hypertrichosis; hyperpigmentation; milia; sclerodermoid changes; scarring alopecia; calcifications. Photoonycholysis. In VP, skin lesions can be indistinguishable from PCT. Some 20% to 30 % of patients with HCP have a delayed-type photosensitivity similar to PCT.
AIP: Not associated with cutaneous findings.
EPP: Early: Erythema, edema, subsequent purpura shortly after exposure to ultraviolet. Late: Thickened, waxy scarring on sun-exposed areas, perioral furrows; vesicles, bullae rare. In EP (Gunther's disease), vesicles, bullae; may result in mutilating deformities. Erythrodontia. Face, nose, dorsa of hands most affected.

Symptoms

VP, AIP, HCP: Neurovisceral symptom complex (episodic abdominal pain; may mimic acute abdomen), or neurologic, psychiatric findings (neuropathy, seizures, delirium, mood disorders).
EPP: Burning, stinging, pruritus on sun exposure.

Investigations

All: Screen all patients with suspected porphyria for total porphyrin levels in plasma. Characteristic porphyrin patterns in plasma, erythrocytes, urine, feces. Normal porphyrin profiles suggest alternate diagnosis. If elevated: Wood's light examination of urine reveals coral pink fluorescence; urine has elevated uroporphyrin, coproporphyrin; stool has elevated isocoproporphyrin. Assess baseline hemoglobin, hematocrit, iron studies, liver function tests, hepatitis C antibody, HIV status, fasting blood glucose.
VP, AIP, HCP: Increased urine and delta-aminolevulinic acid and porphobilinogen during attacks. VP: Elevated coprporphyrin, uroporphyrin in urine; protoporphyrin, coproporphyrin in stool. In AIP, levels also elevated between attacks. HCP characterized by increased urinary and fecal coproporphyrin. **EPP**: Elevated protoporphyrin in erythrocytes, plasma, feces. Urine levels normal. Monitor liver function tests. **EP**: Elevated uroporphyrin I, coproporphyrin I in erythrocytes, plasma, urine; elevated coproporphyrin in feces.

Complications

PCT: Increased iron stores in liver; increased serum iron. Abnormal glucose tolerance in 25%. Hepatocellular carcinoma is rare complication.
AIP, other "acute attack" porphyrias: Misdiagnosis may lead to inappropriate interventions.
EPP: Early gallstone formation. Liver disease, including hepatic failure in 5%.
EP: Hemolytic anemia; splenomegaly; ectropion.

Differential diagnosis

PCT: VP, pseudoporphyria secondary to drugs or hemodialysis, epidermolysis bullosa acquisita, or HCP. Pseudoporphyria induced by medications resembles PCT but urine porphyrin levels normal. Drugs associated with pseudoporphyria: nonsteroidal anti-inflammatory drugs, diuretics, chemotherapeutic agents, immunosuppressants, vitamin A derivatives, *et al*. **VP**: AIP, HCP, PCT. **EPP**: Solar urticaria, polymorphous light eruption, hydroa vacciniforme, systemic lupus erythematosus. **EP**: Other porphyrias, epidermolysis bullosa, xeroderma pigmentosum, bullous pemphigoid.

Etiology

Caused by specific enzyme deficiencies in biosynthesis of heme. Reduced enzyme activity leads to toxic accumulation of porphyrin precursors, porphyrins (photoactive molecules that absorb light radiation maximally at 400–410 nm; Soret band). Cutaneous manifestations result from generation of reactive oxygen species, effects of porphyrins on cells, soluble mediators. **PCT**: Deficient enzyme: uroporphyrinogen decarboxylase. Acquired form frequently associated with exposure to alcohol, estrogens, iron, chlorinated hydrocarbons. PCT associated with hepatitis C virus, HIV infection. **VP**: Deficient enzyme: protoporphyrinogen oxidase. **AIP**: Deficient enzyme: porphobilinogen deaminase. Acute attacks may be precipitated by medications (barbiturates, estrogens, hydantoins, sulfonamides, griseofulvin), infection, pregnancy, decreased caloric intake. **HCP**: Deficient enzyme: coproporphyrinogen oxidase. **EPP**: Deficient enzyme: ferrochelatase, which catalyzes insertion of iron into protoporphyrin. **EP**: Deficient enzyme: uroporphyrinogen III synthase.

Epidemiology

PCT: Most common porphyria; onset in third, fourth decade; familial form may be earlier. VP: Onset typically at puberty, young adulthood; men, women equally affected; most common in South Africans of Dutch ancestry. AIP, HCP: Rare, onset in early adulthood. EPP: Most common erythropoietic porphyria; onset in early childhood; men, women equally affected. EP: Very rare: onset in infancy, childhood.

Katherine L. White and Nicholas A. Soter

Treatment

Diet and lifestyle

All: Sun avoidance by sensitive persons. **PCT, HCP, VP, EP, EPP**: Sun protection. Physical sunblock agents.

Pharmacological treatment

Topical

PCT, HCP, VP, EP, EPP: Topical antibiotic ointments for skin erosions.

Systemic

PCT: Phlebotomy to achieve hemoglobin count of 10–11 g/dL is treatment of choice. Alternatively, low dose antimalarials (*eg*, chloroquine 125, mg twice weekly, or hydroxychloroquine, 200 mg, twice weekly.

VP, AIP, HCP: During acute attacks, i.v. glucose or i.v. heme analogues to suppress heme biosynthesis.

EPP: Antioxidant therapy with beta-carotene to achieve plasma level of 600 µg/dL (60–180 mg/day, adults; 30–90 mg/day, children); result in carotenoderma. Maximum effect at 1 to 2 months after therapy starts. In liver failure, cholestyramine, iron, vitamin E, heme analogues, charcoal used with limited success. End-stage disease: liver transplantation.

EP: Hypertransfusion protocols, splenectomy, oral beta-carotene; variable success.

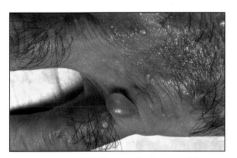

Erythema, bullae and milia over the dorsum of the hand of a man with porphyria cutanea tarda.

Katherine L. White and Nicholas A. Soter

Treatment aims

Identification, and withdrawal of exacerbating factors and drugs; prevention of acute attacks; patient education and support.

Prognosis

PCT: In absence of HIV disease or complications of hepatitis C, normal life expectancy, with appropriate therapy.

VP, AIP, HCP: Acute attacks potentially life-threatening, may have lasting neurologic consequences.

EPP: Life expectancy normal, absent liver disease.

EP: Reportedly normal life expectancy, but quality of life adversely affected.

Follow-up and management

Regular dermatologic follow-up; referral to appropriate medical specialists; team approach to care.

Support organizations

American Porphyria Foundation. P.O. Box 22712, Houston, TX 77227; phone (713) 266-9617.

Diagnosis

Signs

Pressure ulcer (PU): Agency for Healthcare Research and Quality pressure-ulcer classifications: **Grade 1**: Nonblanchable skin erythema; On dark skin, changes are subtle. **Grade 2**: Epidermis, dermis ulcerated; no extension into subcutaneous fat; Clinical appearance: blister, superficial crater. **Grade 3**: Full-thickness skin loss, subcutaneous involvement, no muscle involvement; clinically, a deep crater. **Grade 4**: Full-thickness skin loss, tissue necrosis or damage to deep fascia, muscle, bone, or supporting structures.

Neuropathic ulcer (mal perforans; MP): Skin in ulcer area usually dry (due to sensory neuropathy). Ulcers round, deep, covered with brown eschar, rim of thick callus. Induration, edema possible.

Distribution

PU (in order of frequency): sacral bone and coccyx, heels, greater trochanter, ischial tuberosity, malleolus, elbows, knees, scapula, shoulder, occiput. In spinal cord injury, sacrum, ischium most common sites.

MP: Commonly on great toe, soles of feet, metatarsals.

Symptoms

PU: Pain common; worsened by superinfection.

MP: Usually asymptomatic.

Investigations

• Culture: Bacteria may play a perpetuating role in PU and MP.

• Biopsy: May be used to rule out other causes, especially malignancy.

• Laboratory evaluation: Albumin and, preferably, prealbumin, to follow nutritional status; hemoglobin, hematocrit to exclude anemia.

• Semmes Weinstein test: Monofilament test is one of the most cost-effective, cost-efficient ways to assess loss of sense in a diabetic foot; can help prevent MP.

• Radiography and magnetic resonance imaging: To exclude osteomyelitis.

Complications

• Infection: If increased pain, search for infection. Septicemia, osteomyelitis, pyoarthrosis most common. Enlarging ulcers:higher rate of infection with *Pseudomonas aeruginosa*, *Providenica* species, anaerobic organisms.

• Squamous-cell carcinoma: Rarely may develop in long-standing pressure ulcers.

• Amputation: 5% to 15 % of diabetic patients, eventually.

• Other: Dehydration, anemia, electrolyte imbalance.

Differential diagnosis

Pyoderma gangrenosum, deep fungal infection, necrotic malignancy, radiation injury, vascular ulcers, vasculitic skin condition.

Etiology

PU: Pressure impedes diffusion of oxygen to tissue, stopping nutrient blood blow and causing tissue ischemia. Reperfusion injury by oxygen free radicals can significant perpetuate PUs.

MP: Sensorimotor neuropathy results in decreased sensation; repetitive trauma to foot eventually damages soft tissues.

Epidemiology

PU:70% occur in patients 70 years or older. 7% to 8% of inpatients have pressure sores. Risk factors: spinal cord lesions, neurologic disease, inability to ambulate and change weight.

MP: 5% of US population is diabetic; of these 12–13 million, 15% will develop a diabetic foot or ankle ulcer.

Leonard Kim and Miriam Pomeranz

Treatment

Diet and lifestyle

Both: Adequate diet vital; ascorbic acid plays key role in collagen synthesis, and may aid healing.

PU: Constant attention to relief of pressure.

MP: Constant foot inspection, care.

Pharmacological treatment

• For Grade 1 and 2 PU and for superficial MP, simple topical antibiotic ointment (*eg*, bacitracin, silver sulfadiazene) to enhance reepithelialization.

Nonpharmacological treatment

All Grades PU: Preventive methods are primary treatment. Turn patient every 2 hours. Keep patient in 30-degree oblique position, relieving pressure on sacrum, greater trochanters, ischial tuberosities, lateral malleoli, heels. Avoid elevating bed greater than 30 degrees, because shearing forces increase at this angle. Clean area of urine, feces; keep area dry.Air mattress to help reduce pressure, friction.

Grade 2 and 3 PU: Gentle undermining to determine full extent of defect. Wound debridement: sharp, autolytic (hydrocolloid dressings), chemical (collagenase, fibrinolysin, streptokinase). If wound is exudative, absorb excess with foam, alginate, or hydrocolloid dressing. Surgery if necrotic debris is extensive.

Grade 4 PU: Wound debridement. If osteomyelitis is suspected, confirm with bone culture and treat immediately. Flap procedures may be best option to fill large defects. Anemia, nutrition must be corrected. Currently favored: sharp debridement, excise bursal sac, contoure bony prominences, then myocutaneous flaps.

MP: Edema control vital; if arterial blood-flow allows, use Unna boots, compression stockings, compression bandage. Debridment of callus around MP may help healing. Treat superficial MP like Grade 1 and 2 PU. Pressure control and off-loading with appropriate footwear are paramount. If nonsurgical methods fail, elective surgical procedures to correct deformities; amputation is last resort.

Supportive methods

MP: Educate patient to inspect foot daily, look into shoes for objects before wearing, avoid avoiding walking barefoot, wear comfortable shoes. If patient has no deformity, regular athletic shoes should be adequate; if deformity, extra-depth/ custom-made shoes, podiatrist visits necessary.

Special therapeutic considerations

• Becaplermin (once daily; two-thirds of an inch of gel from a 15-g tube, spread evenly over entire ulcer) or recombinant platelet-derived growth factor to accelerate healing in chronic diabetic foot ulcers.

• Autologous split-thickness and pinch grafts.

• Bioengineered grafts if ulcer resistant to standard therapy.

• Hyperbaric oxygen chamber may enhance epithelialization, reduce bacterial growth.

Treatment aims

PU: Heal ulcers, relieve pressure, restore tissue perfusion, prevent additional ulcers. Also, treat underlying diseases, assess nutritional status, prevent and treating infection, provide good local wound care, maintain moist wound environment.

MP: Prevention is key. Also, control of diabetes, patient education, daily personal foot inspection, comfortable footwear, meticulous foot care.

Prognosis

PU: 80% heal without surgery. More than 60% of PU remain > 6 months. Mortality rate in patients with PU more than five times that in patients without PU.

MP: Prognosis poor. At 20 weeks, ulcer healing occurs in only 31%. Reulceration rate is 70% at 5 years. Amputation: 50% mortality rate at 3–5 years.

Follow-up and management

Constant attention to PU and MP essential. Patient and caretaker education and continual follow-up enhance epithelialization and reduce recurrences.

General references

Orlando PL: Pressure ulcer management in the geriatric patient. *AnnPharmacother* 1998, **32**:1221–1227.

Goode PS: Pressure ulcers. Local wound care. *Clin Geriatr Med* 1997, **13**:543–552.

Jacobs AM: Foot ulcer prevention in the elderly diabetic patient. *Clin Geriatr Med* 1999, **15**:351–369.

Thomas DR: The role of nutrition in prevention and healing of pressure ulcers. *Clin Geriatr Med* 1997, **13**:497–511.

Diagnosis

Signs

Primary varicella (PV): Small red macules progress over 12-14 hours to papules, umbilicated vesicles, pustules, eventually crusts; on face, trunk, then proximal upper extremities; distal, lower extremities mainly spared. Characteristic: "dewdrop on a rose petal." Subsequent crops: lesions in all stages simultaneously present.

Herpes zoster (HZ): Erythematous macules, papules progress to vesicles (12-24 hours), pustules (3-4 days), crusted erosions (7-10 days). Arise in unilateral, linear, dermatomal (zosteriform) distribution, often at sites most severely affected by PV; usually on facial, midthoracic to upper lumbar dermatomes; any may be affected. Lesions on bridge of nose: Involvement of nasociliary branch of ophthalmic nerve. Regional lymphadenopathy usually present.

Symptoms

PV: Pruritus. Occasional headache, myalgias, nausea, anorexia, vomiting; more common in older children, adults).

HZ: Intense pain in involved dermatome, usually 1-3 days before rash. Rarely, fever, malaise, headache (usually children). Occasionally, dermatomal pain without cutaneous lesions (zoster sine herpete).

Diagnostic procedures

Clinical diagnosis: characteristic lesion structure, distribution; confirmation: multinucleated giant cells and epithelial cells containing acidophilic intranuclear inclusions from scraping of vesicle floor, on Tzanck smear; skin biopsy specimen.

Serologic tests for varicella zoster virus (VZV) infection; be aware of herpes simplex virus (HSV) cross-reaction.

Culture more specific, but VZV cultured much less readily than HSV.

Direct immunofluorescence of cellular material from skin biopsy specimens for VZV infection.

Complications

PV: Most common: bacterial superinfection (rarely, streptococcal toxic shock syndrome). Scarring due to infection or excoriations. Extracutaneous complications: varicella pneumonia (16% to 33% of adults), central nervous system (CNS) complications, disseminated intravascular coagulation; rarely, myocarditis, glomerulonephritis, appendicitis, pancreatitis, hepatitis, Henoch-Schönlein vasculitis, orchitis, arthritis, optic neuritis, keratitis, iritis. In pregnancy (especially first trimester), maternal varicella can cause congenital defects. Immunocompromised patients: high morbidity, mortality; persistent viremia, prolonged fevers, extensive rash (hemorrhagic or purpuric lesions), increased incidence of lung, liver, CNS involvement.

HZ: Secondary bacterial infection, scarring. Postherpetic neuralgia common, can be debilitating. Also, ophthalmic zoster, Ramsay-Hunt syndrome, meningoencephalitis, myelitis, motor paralysis, granulomatous cerebral angiitis, asymptomatic cerebrospinal fluid abnormalities. Immunocompromised patients: high risk for dissemination (up to 40% with lymphoma); visceral involvement follows cutaneous dissemination (> 20 vesicles outside primary and immediately adjacent dermatomes) in 10%.

Differential diagnosis

PV: Other viral exanthems, rickettsialpox, insect bites, scabies, papular urticaria, drug eruptions, dermatitis herpetiformis, other vesicular dermatoses.

HZ: Zosteriform herpes simplex, contact dermatitis, burns, arthropod reactions, localized folliculitis, bullous impetigo. Intense preceding dermatomal pain may be mistaken for herniated disc, acute myocardial infarction, pleuritis, cholecystitis, appendicitis, duodenal ulcer.

Etiology

VZV, a herpesvirus (subfamily α Herpesviridae).

Epidemiology

PV: Most (90%) cases in children < 10 years. Immunocompromised persons may be more susceptible to recurrent varicella.

HZ: Any age, but most patients are > 50 years or immunocompromised. About 20% with varicella history develop HZ. Immunosuppressed patients: incidence increased 20–100 times; recurrences also increased.

Infectivity/incubation period

PV: Acquired by inhalation of respiratory secretions or contact with skin lesions. Invades epidermis around day 14–16. Patients contagious approximately 48 hours before onset of skin eruption, during period of vesicle formation (generally 4–5 days), and until all vesicles are crusted.

HZ: VZV spreads from mucocutaneous lesions into sensory nerve endings during PV, remains latent in dorsal root ganglion. During reactivation, which may be triggered by decline in VZV-specific cell-mediated immunity, replication within affected sensory ganglion produces active ganglionitis, causes severe neuralgia, which intensifies as virus travels down sensory nerve to skin.

Elizabeth K. Hale and Philip Orbuch

Treatment

Pharmacological treatment

Topical

PV: Emollient "shake" lotions, creams with calamine, pramoxine, 0.25% to 0.5% menthol, 0.25% to 0.5% camphor.

HZ: Acyclovir, penciclovir ointment not beneficial. Possible benefit: lidocaine cream, wet-to-dry compresses, shake lotions; topical idoxuridine (40%) in dimethylsulfoxide base for rash, acute pain, postherpetic neuralgia prevention.

Systemic

PV: Oral acyclovir (20 mg/kg, 4 times daily, 5 days) decreases severity, duration; high cost, possible development of resistant strains preclude routine use. Oral antihistamines help alleviate pruritus. Immunocompromised patients: acyclovir, 500 mg/m$_2$, i.v., every 8 hours, 7–10 days.

HZ: Acyclovir, 800 mg, 5 times daily, 7 days; valacyclovir, 1g, three times daily, 7 days (limits pain duration better than acyclovir); famciclovir, 500 mg, three times daily, 7 days.

Nonpharmacological treatment

• Tepid baths with colloidal oatmeal, cool compresses. Acetaminophen or ibuprofen for children with PV. Cornstarch or baking soda to hasten drying of vesicles.

Special therapeutic considerations

• Immunocompromised patients with significant exposure to varicella: varicella-zoster immune globulin (VZIG), 125 U/10 kg.

• OKA varicella vaccine US approved, recommended for universal childhood use.

• Acyclovir suppressive doses may prevent zoster in immunocompromised; long-term use in HIV-infected may promote acyclovir-resistant strains, cause neutropenia.

• Disseminated, complicated infection: acyclovir, 10 mg/kg (ideal body weight) every 8 hours (i.v., given over 1 hour), 7 days, if normal renal function. If acyclovir resistance: foscarnet, 60 mg/kg every 8 hours, infused slowly over at least 1 hour, or ganciclovir 5 mg/kg every 12 hours, infused over 1 hour, 7 days. Oral ganciclovir, 1000 mg, three times daily, with food. Sorivudine, 40 mg/d, 7–10 days, may be alternative in moderately ill, resistant cases.

Treatment aims

PV: To decrease duration, severity of symptoms. Antiviral therapy not recommended in otherwise healthy children; considered in certain situations (*eg*, to relieve parental stresses).

HZ: To expedite cutaneous healing, resolve acute pain, prevent complications.

Prognosis

PV: In otherwise healthy children, usually benign, low rate of complications. Primary infection results in lifelong immunity, eliminates varicella risk in immunocompetent adult. Mortality 25 times greater in adults than in children.

HZ: Immunocompetent children, young adults: typically resolves rapidly. Elderly, immunocompromised: more pain, delayed healing, scarring, increased risks for dissemination, severe neuralgia in up to 20% of untreated patients; persists months, years.

Follow-up and management

HZ: Ophthalmologic consultation for all ophthalmic zoster. HZ transmission by direct contact with lesions, aerosol.

General references

Grose C: Variation on a theme by Fenner: the pathogenesis of chickenpox. *Pediatrics* 1981, **68**:735–737.

Juel-Hensen BE, MacCallum FO, Mackenzie AM, *et al.*: Treatment of zoster with idoxuridine dimethyl sulfoxide: results of two double-blind control trials. *Br Med J* 1970, **4**:776–780.

McCrary ML, Severson J, Tyring SK: Varicella zoster virus. *J Am Acad Dermatol* 1999, **41**:1–14.

Whitney RJ: Varicella-zoster infections. In *Antiviral Agents and Viral Diseases of Man*. Edited by Galasso GJ, Whitley RJ, Merigan TC. New York: Raven Press; 1990:235.

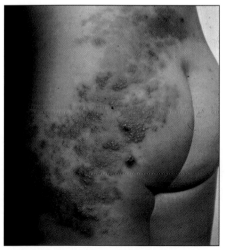

Dermatomal band of erythema, with superimposed grouped and scattered vesicles due to herpes zoster infection.

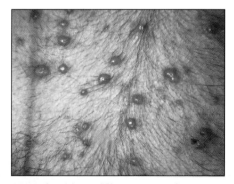

Crops of vesicles at different stages of development in a circumscribed area in a child with varicella. Some vesicles have become cloudy and umbilicated; others are clear and surrounded by an erythematous halo ("dewdrop on a rose petal").

Diagnosis

Signs and symptoms

• Itchy or unpleasant sensation limited to the anus and immediate surrounding area.

• Excoriations and lichenification may be present.

Investigations

• A cause can usually be found. Diagnosis requires a detailed history, careful skin inspection, digital rectal examination, and proctoscopy or sigmoidoscopy.

• Patch testing is indicated in cases in which allergic contact dermatitis is suspected.

• When specific secondary lesions are present, biopsy and cultures can help determine the cause.

Complications

• Itching may be intractable.

• Secondary bacterial infection, usually with *Staphylococcus aureus*, may occur.

• Group A *Streptococcus* infection can cause Fournier's gangrene, a fulminant, destructive infection requiring rapid and aggressive intervention.

Differential diagnosis

Many diseases can involve the anal/perianal area. These include diaper dermatitis; lichen sclerosis et atrophicus; cicatricial pemphigoid; hidradenitis suppurativa; and acanthosis nigricans. Perianal erythema is often seen in Kawasaki's disease.

Etiology

Causes

Pruritus ani may be primary or secondary to a number of diseases.

Secondary causes include eczema, especially allergic contact and irritant dermatitis; psoriasis; dermatophytosis (candidiasis or tinea); herpes simplex; syphilis; human papillomavirus infection (subclinical or clinical); parasites, especially pinworm; perianal cellulitis; squamous cell carcinoma; extramammary Paget's disease; hemorrhoids; anal fissures; proctalgia fugax; and levator ani syndrome

Contributing factors

Fecal incontinence; suboptimal hygiene; spicy foods; diarrhea; constipation; sweating; tight, occlusive clothing; anal manipulation; anxiety.

Once itching develops, an itch-scratch-itch cycle ensues.

Epidemiology

Primary pruritus ani may occur at any age, but elderly men are most commonly affected.

Casey Gallagher and Miguel Sanchez

Treatment

Diet and lifestyle

• Gentle cleaning, with only water, of anal/perianal area after defecation, followed by tap drying with towel, is preferable to the use of tissue paper, which can be abrasive and exacerbate the itch-scratch cycle. Overvigorous cleansing should be discontinued.

• If allergies have been excluded, patients may use glycerin-impregnated pads; Balnetar (2.5% coal tar in an emollient lotion); gentle cleansers (Cetaphil, Aveeno); or a mild soap.

• Eliminate, spices, peppers, citrus fruits from the diet.

Pharmacological treatment

Topical

• Low potency corticosteroids: Patients must be educated about the potential for atrophy and striae.

• Iodoquinol: 1% hydrocortisone 1% (Vytone) cream

• Pramoxine: 1%, in lotion (Prax) may provide relief without high risk of sensitization. Coal tar: 2%–3%, is compounded into a lotion by some dermatologists.

• Azole antifungal creams, only if dermatophytosis is proven or suspected.

• Zinc oxide paste or triple cream protects skin from irritants.

• Methylene blue (methylthionine chloride) 0.5% injected intracutaneously on the anodermal and perianal skin (incidences of long-term cure after a single treatment have been reported).

Systemic

• Antihistamines should be administered, as needed, to control itching.

Special therapeutic considerations

• Allergic patch testing can be helpful in recalcitrant cases in which allergic contact dermatitis is suspected. Common sensitizers include preservatives, antiseptics, corticosteroids, anesthetics, and fragrances (eg, in tissue paper or lotion).

• Sitz baths, with or without colloidal oatmeal or tar emulsion. Avoid ointments.

• Hypnosis has been reported to be helpful in some cases.

• Test to rule out effect of drugs (gemcitabine, antibiotics, drugs causing diarrhea).

• Psychogenic anal pruritus is not common, and should be considered when all other possibilities have been excluded.

General references

Dasan S, Neill SM, Donaldson DR, et al.: Treatment of persistent pruritus ani in a combined colorectal and dermatological clinic. Br J Surg 1999, 86:1337*1340.

Daniel GL, Longo WE, Vernava AM 3rd: Pruritus ani. Causes and concerns. Dis Colon Rectum 1994, 37:670–674.

Eusebio EB, Graham J, Mody N: Treatment of intractable pruritus ani. Dis Colon Rectum 1990, 33:770–772.

Hanno R. Murphy P: Pruritus ani. Classification and management [review]. Dermatol Clin 1987, 5:811–816.

Casey Gallagher and Miguel Sanchez

Diagnosis

Signs

Primary pruritus (PP): No primary lesions; linear excoriations, erosions, ulcerations; generalized or localized.

Secondary pruritus (SP): Same as for PP, plus signs related to underlying internal or cutaneous disease or exogenous causes.

Lichen simplex chronicus (neurodermatitis circumscripta; LSC): Well-circumscribed, erythematous, hyperpigmented plaques; accentuated skin markings. Localized to areas of severe pruritus; usually on nape, extensor forearms, wrists, upper thighs, calves, ankles anogenital region.

Prurigo nodularis (PN): Papules, nodules; often scale, erosions, crusts, pigmentary change. More common on extremities; lesions may be superimposed on plaque of LSC.

Symptoms

Pruritus: Unpleasant sensation provoking desire to scratch, rub. In lichen simplex chronicus and prurigo nodularis, may be paroxysmal.

Investigations

PP: Examine for dermographism, skin biopsy; diagnostic work-up for pruritus of unknown cause, to rule out systemic diseases.

SP: Work-up for pruritus of unknown cause. Detailed history; review of systems; medication history. Full physical examination. Laboratory testing: complete blood count with differential, liver function tests, renal function tests, thyroid function tests, stool examination for ova and parasites (three samples), stool examination for occult blood, with or without erythrocyte sedimentation rate. Chest radiography. Examination for dermographism. Skin biopsy to rule out primary or secondary dermatosis. Further diagnostic testing, as indicated by history and physical examination.

LSC: Potassium hydroxide (KOH) preparation to rule out dermatophytosis.

LSC, PN: Skin biopsy to exclude underlying cutaneous disease.

Complications

• Secondary infection (impetiginization), postinflammatory pigmentary alteration, scarring.

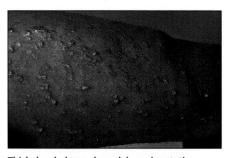

Thick, hard, dome-shaped, hyperkeratotic exophytic nodules with central hypopigmentation and peripheral hyperpigmentation on extensor surface of thighs, secondary to chronic picking. Some lesions are grouped or linear. There are numerous excoriations.

Differential diagnosis

SP: Autoimmune disease, endocrine/metabolic disease, cholestatic liver disease, neurologic disease, pregnancy disorders, psychiatric disorders, chronic uremia (affects 80% of patients undergoing dialysis), HIV infection, parasitic diseases, cutaneous diseases.

LSC: Psoriasis, atopic dermatitis, contact dermatitis, seborrheic dermatitis, lichen planus, lichen amyloidosus, dermatophytosis, parapsoriasis, cutaneous T-cell lymphoma.

PN: Hypertrophic lichen planus, persistent arthropod bite reactions, nodular scabies, epidermal neoplasms, perforating disorders, verrucae.

Etiology

Skin itch can be precipitated locally by histamine, endopeptidases (trypsin, papain), biogenic amines and kinins (serotonin, kallikrein), tachykinins (substance P), opiates. Prostaglandins may also augment itch stimulus. Chronic rubbing of pruritic skin results in "itch-scratch" cycle, which progresses to LSC or PN, and which may complicate underlying dermatosis. Pathophysiology of LSC includes epidermal hyperplasia secondary to cutaneous trauma and proliferation of nerves in epidermis, causing increased cutaneous sensitivity and hyperexcitability to touch.

Epidemiology

LSC: Peak incidence: ages 30 to 50; women affected more then men.

PN: Peak incidence: ages 20 to 60; no sex predilection. In 20%, lesions begin after arthropod assault.

Joshua P. Fogelman and David E. Cohen

Treatment

Diet and lifestyle

• Instruct sensitized patients to avoid allergenic foods and additives.

Pharmacological treatment

Topical

All: Emollients, shake lotions, and aqueous creams with menthol, camphor, and phenol, to cool the skin; capsaicin; doxepin cream, t.i.d. to q.i.d., up to 10% of body surface area.

• Anesthetic agents (*eg*, lidocaine, prilocaine .075% cream, t.i.d. to q.i.d.). Avoid ester anesthetic agents because of risk for contact sensitization. In the absence of acute or chronic inflammation of the skin, topical corticosteroids may not be useful. Avoid topical diphenhydramine because of risk of contact sensitization.

LSC and **PN**: Potent topical corticosteroid ointments (may be enhanced by occlusive dressings); corticosteroid impregnated adhesive tape; intralesional corticosteroids (triamcinolone, 5–105 mg/mL, up to 20 mg, every month); coal tar preparations.

Systemic

All: Antihistamines may reduce itching and inflammation. Soporific antihistamines, such as hydroxyzine HCl, chlorpheniramine, and promethazine, may provide greater relief of pruritus. Caution should be exercised in elderly patients because of anticholinergic side effects (*eg.*, urinary retention) and in patients operating vehicles or potentially dangerous equipment. Nonsedating antihistamines, such as fexofenadine, loratadine, and cetirizine, may have limited efficacy. Doxepin, 10–25 mg/hr, may be added to antihistamines.

• Systemic corticosteroids (*eg*, prednisone, 0.5–0.7 mg/kg/d, tapering off over a 3-week period) may help intractable pruritus. Cyclosporine in severe, recalcitrant cases (malignancy must be ruled out before therapy begins).

Pruritus due to cholestasis: Cholestyramine, phenobarbital, rifampicin, plasmapheresis, plasma superperfusion over charcoal-coated glass beads; ursodeoxycholic acid, ondansetron.

Pruritus due to renal disease: Dialysis, ultraviolet B (UVB) phototherapy, psoralen plus ultraviolet A (PUVA) photochemotherapy.

Pruritus due to polycythemia rubra vera and aquagenic pruritus: UVB phototherapy, PUVA photochemotherapy, aspirin.

PN: Thalidomide, 50–200 mg, at night.

Nonpharmacological treatment

Psychogenic pruritus: See chapter on **Psychocutaneous disorders**.

• Light clothing and bedding, air-conditioning, humidification of the ambient environment, and avoidance of central heating; proper dry skin care (*ie*, infrequent [daily or less frequent], short, tepid showers; avoidance of long, hot showers and baths; use of oatmeal baths; avoidance of harsh soaps), cool shower before retiring to facilitate sleep.

LSC and **PN**: Protect affected areas from scratching and rubbing. Unna boot provides occlusion for up to 1 week.

• For localized pruritus, acupuncture and transepidermal electrical nerve stimulation, which may be administered through a pain-management service; may help, but are of unproven efficacy.

PN: Cryotherapy

Special therapeutic considerations

• Any pruritic condition can lead to LSC; thus, scratching and rubbing must be avoided. Systemic antihistamines, antidepressants, and topical doxepin may cause sedation. Certain systemic medications should be avoided, or doses should be adjusted, in patients with hepatic or renal disease. Monitor renal function, blood pressure, and electrolytes in patients taking cyclosporine.

Treatment aims

All: To identify and treat underlying systemic or cutaneous disease, exogenous cause. To relieve symptoms.

LSC and **PN**: To decrease pruritus and prevent scratching and rubbing of skin to stop the "itch-scratch" cycle.

Prognosis

Depends on cause of pruritus. **LSC** and **PN** are chronic conditions that are difficult to treat; PN is more resistant to therapy than is LSC.

Follow-up and management

Patients may need psychiatric referral if severe pruritus interferes with activities of daily living or causes secondary psychiatric disease.

General references

Teofoli P, Procacci P, Maresca M, *et al*.: Itch and pain. *Int J Dermatol* 1996, **35**:159–166.

Greaves MW, Wall PD: Pathophysiology of itching. *Lancet* 1996, **348**:938–940.

Fleischer AB Jr: Pruritus in the elderly. *Adv Dermatol* 1995, **10**:41–59.

Kantor GR, Bernhard JD: Investigation of the pruritic patient in daily practice. *Semin Dermatol* 1995, **14**:290–296.

Diagnosis

Signs

Plaque psoriasis (Pl): Well-demarcated, erythematous plaques; characteristic mica-like scale on extensor surfaces, scalp, intergluteal cleft, areas of trauma.

Guttate psoriasis (G): Multiple erythematous, small, round, rain-drop–like plaques, mainly on trunk. **Pustular psoriasis (Pu)**: Sheets of superficial sterile pustules, erythematous background; fever, arthralgia, malaise. Localized variant, "palmoplantar pustulosis:" erythematous plaques studded with pustules, limited to palms, soles.

Impetigo herpetiformis (IH): Grouped erythematous plaques rimmed with small sterile pustules, typically in flexural areas; expanding peripherally, in pregnancy.

Inverse psoriasis (IP): Erythematous patches, plaques, characteristically without scale; intertriginous sites.

Subcorneal pustular dermatosis : Sneddon-Wilkinson disease: rare, chronic, recurrent, pustular eruption; nail changes: pitting, subungual hyperkeratosis, onycholysis, yellow-brown discoloration.

Symptoms

• Pruritus in 10% to 20% of patients.

Investigations

Diagnosis: Lesions structure, distribution.
Biopsy may aid in differentiation.
Auspitz sign: Bleeding with mechanical removal of scale.

Complications

Exfoliative erythroderma.
Psoriatic arthritis (PA): Asymmetrical oligoarticular arthritis; periarticular swelling of small joints of fingers, toes.

Differential diagnosis

Pl: Pityriasis rubra pilaris, lichen planus, eczema, cutaneous T-cell carcinoma.
G: Secondary syphilis, pityriasis rosea.
Pu: Subcorneal pustular dermatitis.
IP: Candidiasis, erythrasma.

Etiology

Genetic predisposition: positive family history in 30%, strong association with histocompatibility antigens. Central pathophysiologic event may be skin infiltration by activated T lymphocytes responding to unknown antigenic stimulus. Precipitating factors: streptococcal infections (especially in G); drugs, including lithium, β-blockers, antimalarials; steroid withdrawal (Pu); possibly smoking, alcohol use.

Epidemiology

Relatively common in Scandinavians, Ashkenazi Jews; uncommon in Asians, Native Americans, West African and North American blacks. No sexual predilection. Any age, but usually develops between second and fifth decades.

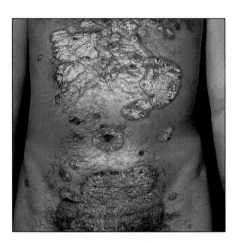

Sharply demarcated, erythematous plaques with silvery-white, micaceous scales on lower chest, abdomen and pubic area, characterisitic of psoriasis.

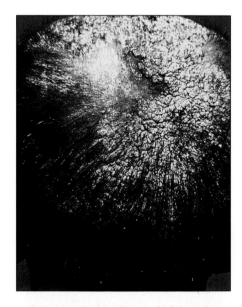

Scalp is covered with adherent thick, hyperkeratotic scaling due to psoriasis. Small bleeding points on skin where scales were scraped off: Auspitz sign.

Jonathan Dosik and Jerome Shupack

Treatment

Diet and lifestyle

- Stress reduction, cessation of smoking, alcohol use may benefit some.

Pharmacological treatment

Topical

Corticosteroids: Effective, relatively cosmetically elegant; efficacy may be limited by steroid side effects, tachyphylaxis. Intralesional triamcinolone acetonide (2.5–10 mg/mL) particularly effective for treating localized areas resistant to standard topical therapy. **Calcipotriene and tazarotene**: Effective steroid-sparing agents; associated irritation usually dictates, at least initially, concomitant topical-steroid use. Tar, anthralin preparations less cosmetically appealing alternatives.

Scalp psoriasis: Tar or salicylic-acid shampoos in conjunction with corticosteroid solutions, foam, gels; calcipotriene solution; tazarotene gel. Fluocinolone (0.025%) in peanut oil, under occlusion overnight. May be particularly resistant to topical therapy, and require intralesional triamcinolone injections or systemic therapy.

Systemic

Methotrexate: Test dose of 2.5 mg, gradually increased to 7.5–30 mg, weekly; single three divided doses administered every 12 hours; for widespread Pl, acute Pu, PA. **Acitretin**: 25–50 mg, once daily, for acral psoriasis or acute pustular psoriasis as monotherapy; for widespread Pl, in combination with phototherapy. Short-term isotretinoin therapy may be useful in patients of childbearing age, especially for acute Pu. **Cyclosporine**: 2.5–4.0 mg/kg, daily, for severe refractory psoriasis. **Mycophenolate mofetil**: 1–8 g, daily or **Thioguanine**: 2–3 mg/kg, daily, for severe refractory Pl. **Hydroxyurea**: 100 mg, b.i.d.; may be increased to t.i.d., if recalcitrant.

Nonpharmacological treatment

Psoralen with ultraviolet light A (PUVA) photochemotherapy: For widespread psoriasis; long-term: substantial increase in nonmelanoma skin cancer; statistically significant increase in malignant melanoma, premature skin "aging." **Ultraviolet B (UVB) phototherapy**: Less efficacious than PUVA, but possibly far less skin-cancer risk; especially useful in G. **Narrow-band (311 nm) UVB phototherapy**: May be more effective than UVB; less skin-cancer risk than PUVA.

Special therapeutic considerations

Avoid prednisone because of risk for rebound Pu on discontinuation; but may be required for IH. **Methotrexate** contraindicated in hepatic disease, alcohol abuse, malignancy, pregnancy. **Avoid alcohol use** concomitant with trimethoprim-sulfamethoxazole (solution form is lower-cost alternative to tablets) or nonsteroidal anti-inflammatory drugs (NSAIDs); renal insufficiency increases levels. **Acitretin**: Contraindicated in hepatic and renal damage, during pregnancy; Recipients must avoid becoming pregnant for 3 years after discontinuation. Reduces minimal erythemogenic dose of phototherapy. **Cyclosporine** contraindicated in renal disease, uncontrolled hypertension, cancer. **NSAIDs** may increase nephrotoxicity; liver cytochrome p450 inhibitors increase NSAID levels; liver cytochrome p450 inducers may reduce NSAID levels.

Risk of chronic toxicity from systemic therapy fosters combination and rotational therapies. **Systemic sequential therapy** phases: clearing (cyclosporine); transitional (cyclosporine and acitretin); maintenance (acitretin, alone or in combination with phototherapy). **Analogous topical sequential therapy** may involve initial concomitant calcipotriene, corticosteroids; then weekday calcipotriene, weekend corticosteroids; then daily calcipotriene.

Main adverse effects

Methotrexate: Hepatic fibrosis (liver biopsy should be done after every 1.5-g cumulative dose), acute bone-marrow suppression (test dose required), stomatitis, dyspepsia. **Acitretin**: Hyperlipidemia, elevated liver enzyme levels, alopecia. **Cyclosporine**: Dose-related hypertension, nephrotoxicity. **Mycophenolate mofetil**: Leukopenia, diarrhea. **Thioguanine**: Acute bone-marrow suppression (any time during treatment), gastrointestinal symptoms.

Treatment aims

To control extent, severity. Limited, localized disease: usually topical regimens; widespread disease may require phototherapy, systemic therapy. Tailor therapeutic regimen to quality of life, by case.

Prognosis

Chronic: relapses, remissions. G may exhibit longer remissions than Pl. IH usually remits after delivery; may recur in subsequent pregnancies.

Follow-up and management

Generally dictated by severity. In systemic therapy, usually more intensive clinical, laboratory evaluation. Phototherapy: regular total-body screening for skin cancer.

Support organizations

National Psoriasis Foundation, important educational resource for physicians, patients: http://www.psoriasis.org.

General references

Koo J: Systemic sequential therapy of psoriasis: a new paradigm for improved therapeutic results. *J Am Acad Dermatol* 1999, **41**:S25–S28.

Jonathan Dosik and Jerome Shupack

Diagnosis

Signs

Neurotic excoriations (NE): Symmetrical excoriations, healed dyschromic scars.
Trichotillomania (TM): Typically, relatively well-circumscribed patch of incomplete alopecia, hairs of varying lengths (usually on scalp). Hairs usually plucked, twisted.
Delusions of parasitosis (DOP): Excoriations, erosions, gouges.
Dermatitis artefacta (DA): Unilateral lesions (due to picking, chemical or thermal burns, injection of foreign materials) at various stages of healing; bizarre, often angulated or geometric outlines; normal skin at inaccessible sites.

Symptoms

NE, TM: Shame, embarrassment, denial. **DOP:** Complaints of formication; production of "evidence." Anxiety, obsession. Also delusions of bromosis, dysmorphosis. **Dermatitis artefacta (DA):** Typical denial of responsibility for self-infliction.

Investigations

• Clinical picture, personality behavioral traits often diagnostic, with absent findings, thus ruling out other causes. Features of obsessive-compulsive personality (OCP) in NE, TM, DOP; of borderline personality in DA.

NE: Biopsy nonspecific.
TM: On skin biopsy, empty follicles, retained fractured hair shafts, corkscrew configurations. Hair growth under occlusive dressing.
DOP: Exclude drug allergy, neurologic disease, vitamin deficiency. Biopsy only if dermatologic disease suspected. Microscopic examination of "specimens." Evaluation by entomologist experienced in DOP.
DA: Appearance of lesions, patient history (typically "hollow" or vague), affect, personality. Birefringent crystals under polarized light suggest foreign bodies. Healing if lesion protected (*eg*, with cast).

Complications

• Vary widely, depending on underlying psychopathology, manifestations of disease. Permanent alopecia can result from TM.

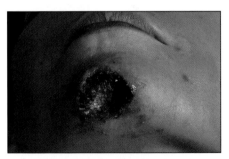

Disfiguring ulceration on the chin of a patient who picks and digs in the area.

Differential diagnosis

NE: Secondary causes of pruritus, scabies incognita, notalgia paresthetica, and other skin disorders associated with excoriations.
TM: Tinea capitis, alopecia areata, inflammatory diseases of scalp (may coexist TM).
DOP: Arthropod infestation; abuse of alcohol, amphetamines, cocaine; organic brain syndromes; formication without delusional belief.
DA: Infection, arthropod bite, vasculitis, collagen vascular disease, coagulopathy (may mimic nearly any dermatosis).

Epidemiology

NE: Most severe cases start at age 30–50. Female predilection. Associated with OCP. Depression common.
TM: Peak onset in childhood, as early as 18 months. Female predilection (5:1) until 2 years of age, then male predilection. Associated with OCP.
DOP: Highest incidence, ages 50–80). Female predilection over age 50. Anxiety; paranoid, schizoid, obsessional personality traits common. Actual pruritus or paresthesia may set stage for subsequent delusion. Suggestible contact adapts delusion ("folie a duex").
DA: Most common in adolescents, young adults. Female predilection. Associated with borderline personality disorder, psychosis. Produced consciously or unconsciously; possibly on another.

Edwin Joe and Miguel Sanchez

Treatment

Pharmacological treatment

NE: Selective serotonin-reuptake inhibitor antidepressants (SSRIs): Paroxetine, 10mg up to 50 mg, daily; fluoxetine, 20 mg up to 80 mg, daily; nafazodone, 100mg up to 200 mg, twice daily; fluvoxamine, 25 up to 150 mg, twice daily; sertraline, 50 mg up to 200 mg, twice daily; citalopram, 8 mg up to 40 mg, daily; mirtazapine, 20 mg up to 60 mg, daily. Intolerance, no response: bupropion, 75 mg up to 200 mg, twice daily; doxepin, 25 up to 150 mg, qhs.

TM: SSRIs as described, including fluvoxamine (approved for obsessive-compulsive disease).

DOP: Pimozide; start at 0.5 mg, daily, increase by 1 mg every 1–2 weeks until marked improvement, usually by 4 mg. Complete resolution may not be possible; higher doses increase risk of extrapyramidal effects. Maximum dose: 12 mg daily. Follow electrocardiograms (pretreatment, at 4 mg daily, and then after every 2 mg increase) for QT prolongation and arrhythmia. Maintain dose at least 1 month, then decrease dose 1 mg every 1–2 weeks. Re-start regimen for relapse. Observe for dyskinesia, extrapyramidal symptoms, orthostasis, withdrawal dyskinesia after discontinuation of drug. If intolerant of or unresponsive to pimozide: olanzapine, 5 mg up to 20 mg, daily, or risperidone,1 mg, twice daily, increased by 1 mg every 2 days. up to 3 mg. twice daily).

DA: Psychopharmacotherapy best managed by one experienced with these agents.

Nonpharmacological treatment

Psychotherapy: All psychocutaneous disorders, if patient is willing to see a mental health professional.

Behavioral therapy: Brief, cost effective, but does not address underlying psychopathology, making recurrence more likely.

Insight-oriented psychoanalysis, psychotherapy address underlying psychopathology; best long-term prognosis.

Special considerations

Dermatologic care: Conventional wound care. Protective dressing may prevent further self-injury.

SSRIs: Inhibit hepatic cytochrome P450 isoenzyme inhibition, can cause drug interactions. Dosage can be increased every 4–7 days, if no significant adverse effects, until desired response is achieved; decrease dosage for elderly patients to about half the usual dose. Sertraline, citalopram: best safety:efficacy ratio.

DOP: Pay attention to skin; perform complete skin examination; however, do not reinforce delusions by agreeing with patient. Depressed, elderly: antidepressants may be used with pimozide. Dermatographia can keep patients from improving.

Treatment aims

To address underlying condition; appropriate wound care

Prognosis

General: Supportive, empathic approach helps. Often periods of remission, exacerbation. Insight-oriented psychoanalysis, psychotherapy: best prognosis.

NE, TM: Prognosis variable. **DOP**: Untreated, tends to become chronic; 60% to 80% improve with pimozide; most require maintenance therapy. **DA**: Usually, factitious disease does not occur as a single event, but over a longer period of time. Recovery often seems to depend on changes in life circumstances.

General references

Garewal HS, Schantz S: Emerging role of beta-carotene and antioxidant nutrients in prevention of oral cancer. *Arch Otolaryngol Head Neck Surg* 1995, **121**:141–144.

Popovsky JL, Camisa C: New and emerging therapies for diseases of the oral cavity [review]. *Dermatol Clin* 2000, **18**:113–125.

Porter SR, Scully C, Pedersen A: Recurrent aphthous stomatitis [review]. *Crit Rev Oral Biol Med* 1998, **9**:306–321.

Dent CD, Svirsky JA, Kenny KF: Large mucous retention phenomenon (mucocele) of the upper lip. Case report and review of the literature. *Va Dent J* 1997, **74**:8–9.

Purpura

Diagnosis

Signs

Morphology

Ecchymoses: Any collection of blood in the skin.

Petechiae: Circumscribed collection of blood ≤ 0.5 cm in diameter.

Purpura: Circumscribed collection of blood ≥ 0.5 cm.

Palpable purpura: Typically, lesions of leukocytoclastic vasculitis.

Contusions/hematomas: Deep or subcutaneous collection of blood.

Progressive pigmented purpura: Most commonly, orange-brown patches dotted with numerous cayenne pepper–colored pinpoint-sized macules, usually on lower extremities, occasionally trunk. Lesions usually asymptomatic, but variants may be very pruritic. Variants: annular, lichenoid, golden lichenoid, eczematous, extensively lichenified.

Itching purpura.

Distribution

Any area: Trauma.

Legs, dependent areas: Cutaneous necrotizing venulitis, progressive pigmented purpura.

Segmental: Systemic vasculitis, emboli.

Acral: Erythema migrans, cryoglobulinemia.

Head, distal extremities: Acute hemorrhagic edema of childhood.

Symptoms

Pain (trauma), pruritus, burning (especially with vasculitis).

Investigations

Diascopy: Purpura does not blanch.

Complete blood count, including platelet count.

Hess test (sphygmomanometry testing of vascular fragility).

Bleeding time.

Coagulation screen.

Skin biopsy.

Complications

• Dependant upon primary disease; Progressive pigmented purpura: None.

Differential diagnosis

Nonpalpable petechiae: Thrombocytopenia, platelet dysfunction, pigmented purpura, valsalva maneuver, benign hypergammaglobulinemic purpura, drug effect.

Nonpalpable ecchymoses: Coagulation defect, vascular fragility, psychogenic purpura, drug effect.

Discrete palpable purpura: Cutaneous necrotizing vasculitis (CNV), systemic vasculitis, erythema migrans, pityriasis lichenoides et varioliformis acuta, pigmented purpura, benign hypergammaglobulinemic purpura.

Retiform palpable purpura: Livedoid vasculitis, pernio, systemic vasculitis, warfarin necrosis, thrombotic thrombocytopenic purpura (TTP), myeloproliferative disorders, cryoglobulinemia, intravascular infection, disseminated intravascular coagulation, coagulation defects, emboli (septic, cholesterol, other), calciphylaxis, sickle cell anemia, drug effect.

Etiology

Nonpalpable purpura is caused by hemorrhage due to abnormal hemostasis, vascular fragility, Valsalva maneuver, or trauma.

Discrete palpable purpura is caused by inflammatory hemorrhage due to CNV, systemic vasculitis, nonleukocytoclastic vessel inflammation.

Inflammatory retiform palpable purpura is caused by systemic vasculitis, livedoid vasculitis, and septic vasculitis.

Noninflammatory retiform palpable purpura is caused by occlusion due to platelet aggregation, cryoglobulins, cold agglutinins, infectious microorganisms, coagulation defects, emboli, crystal deposition, or red cell sickling.

Drug purpura may be due to direct capillary damage or hypersensitivity reactions.

Pigmented purpura consists of a heterogeneous group of disorders that bear in common red cell extravasation, hemosiderin deposition in macrophage, capillary endothelial damage, inflammation, and exacerbation with gravity and increased venous pressure.

Epidemiology

Depends on cause.

Macrene Alexiades-Armenakas and Andrew Franks, Jr.

Treatment

Diet and lifestyle
• Low-fat diet for hypercholesterolemia. Rest and hydration for sickle cell disease. Avoid grapefruit juice when taking warfarin. Vitamin C (vascular fragility).

Pharmacological treatment

Topical
Corticosteroids: Class I–III, for pigmented purpura.

Vitamin K cream: Anecdotally for senile purpura.

Systemic
• H_1 antihistamines, nonsteroidal anti-inflammatory drugs, colchicine, hydroxychloroquine, dapsone, corticosteroids, azathioprine, cyclosporine, cyclophosphamide, methotrexate, and plasmapheresis may be beneficial for cutaneous necrotizing (leukocytoclastic) vasculitis (palpable purpura).

• Anticoagulation and antiplatelet agents: Aspirin, dipyridamole, pentoxifylline, heparin.

• Lipid-lowering agents for cardiac and atherosclerotic (cholesterol) emboli.

• Intravenous γglobulin for idiopathic thrombocytopenic purpura.

• Antibiotics for purpura fulminans.

• Platelet transfusion for thrombocytopenia.

Nonpharmacological treatment
• Plasma exchange for TTP.

• Compression stockings for venous insufficiency in pigmented purpura. Not to be used in arterial insufficiency.

• Emollients

• Leg elevation in venous insufficiency

• Avoidance of trauma in bleeding diatheses.

Surgery
• Vascular surgery and angioplasty, as appropriate.

• Amputation of extremities and skin grafting, as necessary.

Special therapeutic considerations
• Change suspected agent in purpuric drug reactions or warfarin necrosis.

Treatment aims
To treat underlying disease.

Prognosis
Varies depending on cause. Of special note, the mortality rate associated with purpura fulminans is very high.

Follow-up and management
Follow coagulation profile and platelet counts when appropriate. Pigmented purpuric dermatoses are often recalcitrant to therapy and vary in their course.

General references
Kottke-Marchant K: Laboratory diagnosis of hemorrhagic and thrombotic disorders. *Hematol Oncol Clin North Am* 1994, **8**:809.

Piette WW: Hematologic diseases. In *Dermatology in General Medicine*, edn 5. Edited by Freedberg IM, *et al*... New York: McGraw-Hill; 1999:2044–2053.

Sams W Jr: Macular purpuras. In *Principles and Practice of Dermatology*, edn 2. Edited by Sams W Jr, Lynch P. New York: Churchill Livingstone; 1996:559–564.

Sham R, Francis C: Evaluation of mild bleeding disorders and easy bruising. *Blood Rev* 1994, **8**:98.

Soter NA: Cutaneous necrotizing venulitis. In: *Dermatology in General Medicine*, edn 5. Edited by Freedberg IM, *et al*... New York: McGraw-Hill; 1999:2044–2053.

Diagnosis

Signs

• Irregular ulcer with necrotic, boggy base, often with raised, tender, undermined borders. Lesion can start as painful, deep nodule or pustule that breaks down, ulcerates.

• Purulent or hemorrhagic exudate may occur with elevated, tender, undermined borders. Base is irregular, granulating, often with small abscesses. Usually on lower extremities, buttocks, abdomen; also, face, neck, scalp, genitalia. Mucous membranes usually spared.

Clinical variants

• Ulcerative: Ulcerations with undermined borders, surrounding erythema, rapidly enlarging purulent base.

• Pustular: Discrete painful pustules with inflammatory border.

• Bullous: Painful; bullae progress to erosions, then ulcerations with erythematous halos.

• Vegetative: Ulcers without undermining borders; slowly progressive; may be exophytic, vegetative.

Symptoms

• Pain from pustule; fever, general toxicity may occur early.

Investigations

• Diagnose by clinical features; no pathognomonic serologic or hematologic markers. History: Ingestion of iodides, bromides, recent spider bite, viral symptoms, syphilis risk factors, current medications, systemic symptoms (gastrointestinal, rheumatologic).

• Blood tests: Complete blood count with differential and erythrocyte sedimentation rate, chemistry profile, rapid plasma reagin test, antiphospholipid antibodies.

• Histologic stains, cultures of skin biopsy specimens for bacteria, deep fungi, atypical mycobacteria, mycobacteria.

• Biopsy: Neutrophilic infiltrate, often involving follicular structures.

• Vascular damage: None to fibrinoid necrosis.

Complications

• Scarring, disfigurement may occur. Ulcerative variant: Malignant pyoderma of head, neck; can rapidly progress, be fatal.

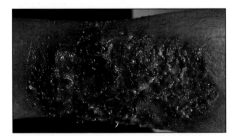

Irregular, painful ulcer; raised inflammatory, crenulated, dusky-red borders, undermined edges, surrounding halo of erythema; boggy, soggy base with exuberant tissue that weeps purulent, hemorrhagic exudate.

Differential diagnosis

Deep mycoses, insect bite(s), neoplasms, halogenodermas, factitial ulcers, mycobacteria infection, gummatous syphilis, drug reactions, synergistic gangrene, antiphospholipid syndrome, systemic vasculitis.

Etiology

Autoimmunity believed to play role. New lesions often follow trauma, suggesting uncontrolled inflammatory process.

Epidemiology

No sex predilection. Usually occurs between 25 and 54 years; rare in childred.

Special considerations

Associated with ulcerative colitis in 30% to 60% and Crohn's disease in approximately 1% of patients. Other associations: monoclonal gammopathies, specifically IgA/IgG paraproteinemias, polyarthritis, myeloid leukemias.

Leonard Kim and Michael Whitlow

Treatment

Diet and lifestyle
• Keeping wound clean, avoiding trauma to affected area are absolute musts.

Pharmacological treatment

Topical
Intralesional triamcinolone, 30-40 mg/mL, is often ineffective alone, but can be useful as adjunctive agent in systemic therapy. Cyclosporine (100 mg/mL, t.i.d.), disodium cromoglycate (2% solution, t.i.d.), as adjunctive agents.

Systemic
• Prednisone: Most effective. Initial dosage: 100-200 mg/d. Response usually very rapid; systemic toxicity may resolve in 24 hours. Taper slowly (10 mg or less per week), only after complete resolution.

• Methylprednisolone: Pulse therapy, 1 g/d for 3-5 days, very effective. In-hospital cardiac monitoring needed due to rare cardiac fatalities from this therapy.

• Cyclosporine: Effective in severe or refractory disease, at dosage of 6-10 mg/kg/d; alone or in combination with systemic corticosteroid treatment. Often, significant improvement by 1-3 weeks; complete healing by 1-7 months.

• Sulfonamides: Response is best when combined with prednisone. Sulfasalazine (reportedly most effective): initial, 1-4 g/d; maintenance, 0.5-1 g. Sulfapyridine: 4-8 g/d, usually concomitant with prednisone. Dapsone: 100-200 mg/d when G6PD levels are normal.

• Clofazamine: Anti-inflammatory; enhances neutrophil phagocytosis. At 200-300 mg/d, can induce healing in 1-2 weeks; not all patients respond.

• Azathioprine, mercaptopurine: Azathioprine dosage is 100-150 mg/d. May take 6-8 weeks to show any effect; often useful as steroid-sparing agent. Most serious side effects: bone marrow toxicity, hepatotoxicity. Mercaptopurine, active metabolite of azathioprine, used with varying success. Standard dosage is 75 mg/d.

• Alkylating agents: Cyclophosphamide, 100-150 mg/d, in combination with prednisone; monitor myelosuppression, hemorrhagic cystitis (2%-40% of patients), hepatotoxicity. Chlorambucil, 4 mg/d, in combination with steroids; less toxic, slower acting than cyclophosphamide.

• Minocycline, 200-300 mg/d; longer-term maintenance therapy often needed; anti-inflammatory effects may be main reason for effectiveness.

Nonpharmacological treatment

Hyperbaric oxygen chamber: Increased oxygen tension in ulcers may diminish pain, enhance healing. **Plasma exchange**: Acecdotal: in 7 of 10 patients, progression halted in 24 hours; healing in several weeks. **Intravenous immune globulin**: Anecdotal: 0.4 mg/kg for 5 days healed pyoderma gangrenosum refractory to prednisone, dapsone, cyclophosphamide. **Tacrolimus**, at 0.15 mg/kg, b.i.d.: complete response in most treated patients. **Remicade**: anti-tumor necrosis factor, **Micophenolate mofetil**, combined with cyclosporine.

Combination therapy for severe cases; especially prednisone and cyclosporine. Multiple immunosuppressive agents increases risk of opportunistic infections.

Vacuum-assisted closure dressing (placing open-cell foam dressing into wound cavity and applying controlled subatmospheric pressure) efficacious for therapy-resistant wounds.

Wet compresses: Saline or Burrow's solution, for gentle debridement; hydrophilic occlusive dressings for clean, moist wound environment good for epithelialization. Topical antimicrobials may prevent secondary infection.

Treatment aims
To eliminate both ulcer and any underlying systemic disorder; prevent scarring, disfigurement, possible loss of limb; reduce risk of fatality.

Prognosis
Prognosis is usually good with aggressive, early treatment. Spontaneous healing can occur, but new lesions can always develop. Scarring, disfigurement risks.

Follow-up and management
Follow closely for development of new lesions and appropriate response to treatment. If condition progresses with one medication, others may be added.

Special therapeutic considerations
Absolutely avoid surgical debridement. Aggressive treatment of underlying ulcerative colitis or malignancy often keeps pyoderma gangrenosum under control.
Immunosuppressive regimens increase risk for bacterial infection of the ulcer. Periodic wound cultures, especially if increased pain, wound drainage, sudden halt in improvement despite no change in therapy.

General references
Chow RK: Treatment of pyoderma gangrenosum. *J Am Acad Dermatol* 1996, **34**:1047–1060.

Powell FC: Pyoderma gangrenosum: classification and management. *J Am Acad Dermatol* 1996, **34**:395–409.

Callen JP: Pyoderma gangrenosum [review]. *Lancet* 1998, **351**:581–585.

Huang W: Neutrophilic tissue reactions. *Adv Dermatol* 1997, **12**:33–64.

Argenta LC: Vacuum-assisted closure: a new method for wound control and treatment: clinical experience. *Ann Plast Surg* 19997, **38**:563–576.

Diagnosis

Signs

Rosacea (R): Flares of granulomatous papules, nodules, papulopustules associated with episodic blushing, erythema, permanent teleangiectases, edema of central face Most commonly affected areas are cheeks, nose, glabella, forehead, chin. Progressive deforming enlargement of nose, due to increased numbers and size of sebaceous glands, may develop. May affect eyelids, conjunctivae. Rosacea conglobata: predominantly nodules. Fulminant rosacea (pyoderma faciale) in persons who flush after emotional stress: draining erythematous nodules, associated with fever and leukocytosis. **Perioral dermatitis (PD)**: Recurrent erythema with numerous erythematous papules and occasionally papulovesicles and papulopustules periorally; zone of sparing adjacent to vermilion border. Nasolabial folds, glabella, periocular areas sometimes involved. **Both**: Comedones, cysts notably absent.

Symptoms

R: Recurrent flushing, blushing. **PD**: Occasional stinging, pruritus.

Complications

R: Eye involvement in 58% (initial manifestation in 20%), such as blepharitis (scaling, erythema, itching of eyelids), conjunctivitis, recurrent chalazia, eyelid margin telangiectases, corneal vascularization, and corneal scarring.

Investigations

Skin biopsy: Dilated capillaries, perivascular lymphocytic infiltrate, perifollicular infiltrate with neutrophils, granulomatous infiltrate with or without *Demodex* mites, severe elastosis, disruption of collagen fibrils, hyperplastic sebaceous glands. **PD**: Scraping of pustules to examine for overgrowth of *Demodex* mites.

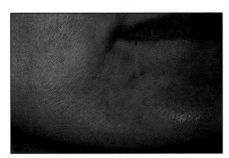

Perioral dermatitis with pinhead-sized erythematous papules and papulopustules predominantly on erythematous skin with fine scaling.

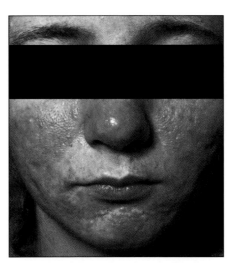

This young woman with rosacea, exhibits vivid erythema and telangiectasias over the nose, cheeks and chin, as well as granulomatous papules and papulopustules, but no comedones.

Differential diagnosis

R: Acne vulgaris, *Demodex* folliculitis, pityrosporum folliculitis, seborrheic dermatitis, malar eruption of systemic lupus erythematosus, carcinoid syndrome, tinea barba, drug eruptions. **PD**: Rosacea, acne vulgaris, seborrheic dermatitis, contact dermatitis, necrolytic migratory erythema, acrodermatitis enterohepatica.

Etiology

R: *Helicobacter pylori* gastrointestinal infection causes increased gastric hormone, leading to flushing, but eradicating organism has not shown conclusive benefit. *Demodex* mites in approximately 50% of rosacea patients; role controversial: may occlude follicles, induce inflammatory reaction. Vascular activity, induced either endogenously or exogenously, may precipitate papular and pustular activity. **PD**: Use of topical corticosteroids, fluorinated toothpaste associated with onset, aggravation of eruption. Attempts to isolate bacterial, fungal, demodicidal agents unsuccessful. Hormonal influences substantiated. Irritant or allergic effects of topical products may aggravate, but not causative.

Epidemiology

R: Affects 13 million Americans; onset usually between ages 30 and 60. Prevalence in women slightly greater than in men. More common in persons with fair skin. **PD**: Most common in women ages 20 to 30 (range, 16–45) with fair complexion. Number of reported cases in children has been increasing.

Linda K. Franks

Treatment

Diet and lifestyle

• Patients must identify and avoid personal trigger factors that cause flushing and worsen rosacea, such as alcohol (especially red wine), spicy foods, foods high in histamine (tomatoes, spinach, eggplant, citrus, cheese, chocolate) or niacin (liver, some yeast products), vinegar, vanilla, soy sauce, citrus fruits, hot liquids, caffeine withdrawal, sun exposure, extremes of weather, saunas, emotional stress, medications (vasodilators, angiotensin-converting enzyme inhibitors, cholesterol-lowering agents), topical irritants (scrubs, exfoliating agents, soap cleansers), alcohol or acetone solutions (toners, astringents, perfumes, sunscreens, and medications), ingredients (menthol, peppermint, eucalyptus oil, clove oil). Patients must avoid emotional stress, anxiety, embarrassment, rage, straining, chronic cough, vigorous exercise, and vasodilators. Menopause may need to be treated hormonally.

Pharmacological treatment

Topical

• Avoid corticosteroids and nonfluorinated, low-potency steroids (such as 2.5% hydrocortisone cream), except for brief periods. If patients are receiving fluorinated corticosteroids, dose should be progressively tapered, using lower potencies.

• **Metronidazole**, 0.75% cream or lotion once to twice daily (clinical results may take 8-12 weeks): treatment of choice for R and PD. **Sodium sulfacetamide**, 10% lotion. **Sulfacetamide sodium**, (10%) and sulfur (5%). **Retinoic acid**, 0.025%-0.1%, for 6 months, decreases erythema, telangiectasias. **Azeleic acid**, 20%. **Permethrin, lindane, or crotamiton**, twice to three times daily, for recalcitrant cases. **Sulfacetamide eye ointment** for ocular rosacea. **Tacrolimus**, especially for rosacea in patients with atopic reactions. **Intralesional corticosteroids**, 3 mg/mL for nodules or cysts.

Systemic

• Systemic antibiotic therapy initially, to reduce inflammation quickly and control eye disease. Initial doses are listed below. Tapering may begin after 4-6 weeks and should proceed slowly. **Tetracycline**, 500 mg twice daily. **Doxycyline**, 50-100 mg twice daily. **Minocycline**, 50-100 mg twice daily. **Erythromycin**, 500 mg twice daily. **Clarithromycin**, 250 mg twice daily. **Isotretinoin** for granulomatous, nodular variants; begin at 10-20 mg/d, may increase up to 1 mg/kg/d; may aggravate blepharitis, conjunctivitis. **Prednisone** (with antibiotics or isotretinoin), 40 mg/d, to control rosacea fulminans.

Surgery

• **Laser surgery** for telangiectasias, erythema. **Rhinophyma** can be treated with ablation using pulsed CO_2, erbium, or Nd:YAG lasers or with dermabrasion, electrosurgery, cryotherapy, scalpel ablation, and trichloroacetic acid.

Supportive methods

• Cosmetics and green concealers to camouflage telangiectasias, erythema.

Treatment aims

R: To control flushing, clear lesions, prevent progression to hyperplasia/rhinophyma, decrease ophthalmologic complications. **PD**: To eradicate eruption, usually over 4–8 weeks.

Special therapeutic considerations

A combination of agents may be needed to treat either disease.

Testing and eradication of *H. pylori* in patients with a history of gastritis or ulcer disease: lansoprazole, 30 mg (or omeprazole, 20 mg) twice daily, plus clarithromycin, 500 mg twice daily, plus amoxicillin, 1 g twice daily, for 10–14 days (≥90% efficacy); or omeprazole, 40 mg/d, plus clarithromycin, 500 mg three times daily, for 2 weeks, followed by omeprazole, 20 mg/d, for additional 2 weeks; or Pepto-Bismol, 525 mg four times daily, plus metronidazole, 250 mg four times daily, plus doxycycline, 100 mg twice daily, plus H_2-receptor antagonist therapy for 2 weeks, followed by H_2-receptor antagonist therapy for an additional 2 weeks (less effective).

Prognosis

R: Successful management with combination systemic/topical therapy. Prognosis excellent with early intervention, good patient compliance. **PD**: Resolution, low incidence of recurrence expected with proper treatment; if untreated, chronic activity over 2–3 years is usual.

Follow-up and management

Monthly follow-up during weaning from systemic therapy; then follow every 3–6 months to monitor activity and emphasize adherence to therapy. Ophthalmologic follow-up necessary for any patient with eye symptoms.

Support organizations

National Rosacea Society, 800 South Northwest Highway, Suite 200, Barrington, IL 60010; Phone: 847-382-8971; e-mail: rosaceas@aol.com; Internet: www.rosacea.org.

Diagnosis

Signs

Papular sarcoid: Yellow-brown to violaceous, waxy, translucent, 3- to 6-mm papules; face, neck, trunk, extremities. Common in blacks; lesions pigmented.

Maculopapular sarcoid: 0.5–1.0 cm, erythematous, widespread eruption lasting approximately 1 month; trunk, face, extremities.

Plaque sarcoid: Firm, brownish, violaceous infiltrated plaques; new or result of confluence of papules; trunk, extremities, buttocks, face. Plaques annular, serpiginous, polycyclic. If dark skin, flat, hypopigmented and hyperpigmented lesions.

Lupus pernio: Violaceous, symmetrical, infiltrated, doughy nodules; nose, cheeks, earlobes, hands, fingers, toes. If perinasal sarcoid, increased risk for upper respiratory tract involvement, pulmonary fibrosis.

Angiolupoid sarcoid: Infiltrated purple plaques or nodules; telangiectasia on or around nose. Frequent, persistent, progressive pulmonary manifestations.

Subcutaneous/nodular sarcoid (Darier-Roussy): Skin-colored or violaceous, asymptomatic, round or oval deep nodules; trunk, legs.

Scar sarcoidosis: Purple, translucent nodules in scars. Occurs in patients with active sarcoidosis elsewhere.

Symptoms

•Lesions asymptomatic unless they ulcerate. Systemic symptoms: include dyspnea, cough, chest pain/tightness, fever, night sweats, chills, fatigue, weight loss.

Investigations

•Clinical, radiologic, laboratory findings, demonstration of noncaseating granulomas in tissue.

Diascopy: Yellow-brown color during blanching of skin lesions with glass slide. **Chest radiography**: Hilar adenopathy, pulmonary fibrosis. **Pulmonary function tests**: Restrictive impairment. **Broncheoalveolar lavage**: Increased number of T lymphocytes. **Laboratory investigations**: Complete blood count (5%: anemia; leukopenia frequent; 24%, eosinophilia), erythrocyte sedimentation rate (elevated in 66%), calcium level (elevated secondary to increased intestinal absorption); angiotensin-converting enzyme (increased in 60%, especially with hilar adenopathy, pulmonary infiltrates; false negative results, 40%; false-positive, 10%), delayed-type hypersensitivity reactions, γ-globulin (high), Kveim intradermal skin test no longer used. **Biopsy**: Granulomas composed of epithelioid cells with occasional giant cells and little or no caseation necrosis (special stains must all be negative for infectious organisms and foreign bodies).

Complications

•Skin lesions can be highly disfiguring; may ulcerate, scar. Other: blindness, debilitating fatigue and dyspnea, increased risk for malignancy. Mortality: 3% to 6%, secondary to cardiac disease, progressive pulmonary disease, neurosarcoidosis.

•Erythema nodosum: Sarcoid causes 25% of cases. Löfgren's syndrome: Erythema nodosum with uveitis, arthritis, fever. Heerfordt's syndrome: Parotid enlargement, facial nerve palsy, uveitis, fever. Erythema multiforme. Exfoliative erythroderma. Scarring alopecia.

Differential diagnosis

Granuloma annulare, granuloma faciale, cutaneous lupus erythematosus, deep fungal or mycobacterial infection, foreign-body granulomas, cutaneous T-cell lymphoma, psoriasis, secondary and tertiary syphilis, lupus vulgaris, amyloidosis, lichen planus, flat warts, syringoma, trichoepithelioma, lymphoma, xanthoma.

Etiology

Genetic predisposition. T-cell–mediated response to unknown antigen processed and presented to macrophages. No infectious agent, or toxin found.

Epidemiology

Cutaneous involvement in 25%. Incidence: 11/100 000. More prevalent in blacks, women. Usually ages 20–40; range: 12–70 years.

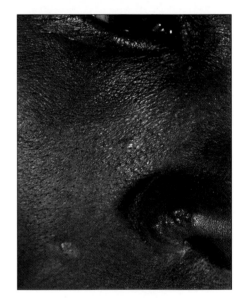

Smooth, violaceous, granulomatous papules that become annular on the nasal alae of a man with lupus pernio.

Rhonda J. Pomerantz

Treatment

Pharmacological treatment

Topical
- Corticosteroid creams (class I–III), two to three times daily.
- Intralesional corticosteroids (triamcinolone, 3–5 mg/mL, every week).

Systemic
- Corticosteroids: Prednisone 20–40 mg/d, gradually tapered to 10 mg/d for 3–6 months, for acute sarcoidosis. Use with caution in patients with uncontrolled hypertension, diabetes, infection, peptic ulcers.
- Methotrexate: 5–25 mg/d weekly, especially in ulcerative sarcoid. Contraindicated in liver dysfunction and preexisting blood dyscrasias.
- Azathioprine: 1 mg/kg/d. Contraindicated in patients with known hypersensitivity and patients previously treated with alkylating agents.
- Chlorambucil: 4–6 mg/d. Contraindicated patients with in hepatic dysfunction.
- Cyclosporine: 3–6 mg/kg/d. Monitor blood pressure, magnesium levels, and renal function.
- Chloroquine (250–500 mg/d) or hydroxychloroquine (200 mg, twice daily): main side effects are retinopathy, blindness (especially chloroquine), corneal opacities, gastrointestinal reactions, electrocardiographic changes; may precipitate severe psoriatic flare, exacerbate porphyria.
- Thalidomide: Initial dosage is 200 mg/d; may be increased to 400 mg/d, then reduced to smallest dose needed for maintenance. Main side effects: teratogenicity, peripheral neuropathy, neutropenia.
- Isotretinoin (40–80 mg/d) or acitretin (25–50 mg/d).
- Colchicine: 0.6 mg three times daily.

Surgery
- Excision of small lesions.
- Skin grafting of extensive sarcoidal ulcers; keloids may form in donor site in blacks.
- Flash-lamp pulsed-dye laser.

Special therapeutic considerations

Löfgren's syndrome is usually self-limited and does not require specific therapy. **Ocular sarcoid** and **progressive pulmonary disease** warrant aggressive treatment (usually systemic corticosteroid therapy). **Corticosteroid dose** may be decreased by addition of antimalarial agents. **Other**: Allopurinol (100 mg three times daily), photophoresis.

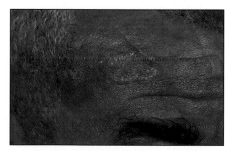

Annular, skin colored plaque on the forehead of a man with sarcoidosis.

Treatment aims

To prevent scarring and disfigurement. Skin lesions are not life-threatening. Treatment is based on severity and progression of the involvement. Antimalarial agents and topical corticosteroids are usually the initial treatments.

Prognosis

Chronic; remissions occur. Spontaneous resolution in up to 50%.

Follow-up and management

Angiotensin-converting enzyme levels can be used to follow disease. Close clinical and laboratory follow-up is required.

Support organizations

National Sarcoidosis Resource Center, PO Box 1593, Piscataway, NJ 08855; telephone: 732-699-0733;
Internet: www.nsrc-global.net.

General references

Carlesimo M, et al.: Treatment of cutaneous and pulmonary sarcoidosis with thalidomide. *J Am Acad Dermatol* 1995, **32**:866–869.

Muthiah MM, MacFarlane JT: Current concepts in the management of sarcoidosis. *Drugs* 1990, **40**:231–237.

Webster GF, Razsi LK, Sanchez M: Weekly low-dose methotrexate therapy for cutaneous sarcoidosis. *J Am Acad Dermatol* 1991, **24**:451–454.

Zic JA, et al.: Treatment of cutaneous sarcoidosis with chloroquine. Review of the literature. *Arch Dermatol* 1991, **127**:1034–1040.

Samtsov AV: Cutaneous sarcoidosis. *Int J Dermatol* 1992, **31**:385–391.

Diagnosis

Signs

- Hypertrophic scars and keloids are broad, thick papules, plaques. and nodules caused by overgrowth of dense fibrous tissue resulting from of injury. Hypertrophic scars remain confined to the area of injury and may regress over time. Keloids extend beyond the confines of the initial wound. Scars are initially pink to purple, but eventually become skin-colored or pigmented. The surface of hypertrophic scars is usually smooth, but the surface of keloids tends to be convoluted, with claw-like extensions. Body areas with high skin tension, such as the presternal area, upper chest, shoulders, upper back, ear lobes, beard area and face, are the sites of predilection.

- Striae are linear atrophic scars, usually on the abdomen, thighs, upper arms and back; they result from breakdown of collagen and elastin, usually due to skin stretching (pregnancy, weight gain, sudden growth, mechanical factors) or hormones (topical corticosteroids). Early scars are pink or violaceous (striae rubra) but over time become white (striae alba).

Symptoms

- Some patients experience hyperesthesia, pain, or pruritus.

Investigations

- Diagnosis is simple if an inciting trauma or inflammatory skin lesion is present.

Complications

- Disfigurement, contractures, and possible restriction of movement depend on the location.
- Alopecia in hair-bearing areas.
- Malignant degeneration of keloids has been reported but is exceedingly rare.

Differential diagnosis

Dermatofibrosarcoma protuberans can resemble keloids. Blastomycosis and lobomycosis should be considered in endemic areas. The Rubinstein-Taybi syndrome is characterized by spontaneous keloids during adolescence, mental retardation, microcephaly, and beaking of nose.

Etiology

These proliferative scars are characterized by increased collagen and glycosamino-glycan content, as well as increase collagen turnover. Trauma (lacerations, burns, tattoos, vaccinations, and inflam-matory lesions) is the most significant factor, although keloids can occur sponta-neously and patients may fail to report injury before their appearance. The inciting event usually occurs within 1 year. Keloids tend to occur after puberty, regress after menopause, and may be stimulated by pregnancy, suggesting hormonal influences.

Epidemiology

Higher incidence in darker-pigmented persons (blacks, Hispanics, and Asians).

Equal incidence in males and females, most commonly between the ages of 10 and 30.

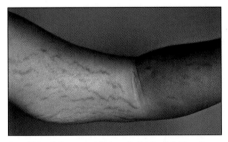

Purplish pink, atrophic bands (striae) following aggressive weight loss.

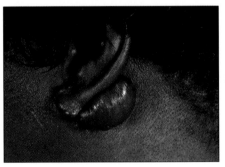

Smooth, hard, skin-colored exophytic keloid on the earlobe.

Erick Mafong and Christopher Nanni

Treatment

Pharmacological treatment

Topical

• Intralesional triamcinolone acetonide (10–40 mg/mL) directly suppresses collagen synthesis and accelerates collagen breakdown. For keloids, higher concentrations (usually 40 mg/mL) are needed. Concentration is reduced as lesions flatten to avoid atrophy. To decrease risk for effects from systemic corticosteroids, total dose should not exceed 20 mg per month. The speed of injection is an important determinant of pain.

• Silicone gel dressings may decrease the size and firmness of the scar or keloid, but requires application for 12 hours daily for at least 2 to 4 months.

• Intralesional 5-fluorouracil (50 mg/mL) mixed with triamcinolone acetonide (1 mg/mL) OW-TIW plus concomitant use of the pulsed-dye laser.

• Recombinant interferon-γ}, 0.01 to 0.1 mg injected intralesionally into keloids three times per week, was shown to reduce the size of the lesions.

• Recombinant human interferon-α2b, 1.5 million U per injection, was shown to decrease keloid size; 0.5 million U per cm^2 of keloid has been reported to decrease the postsurgical recurrence rate. However, injections can be painful.

• Tretinoin 0.5% emollient cream daily and glycolic acid 20% daily improves both striae rubra and striae alba.

Systemic

• No proven systemic therapy available. In patients prone to keloidal acne scars, aggressive acne treatment with antibiotics and retinoids is recommended.

Nonpharmacological treatment

Surgery

• Surgical excision (45%–100% recurrence, depending on area). Recurrence rate is markedly higher for keloids. It is of vital importance to pay attention to lines of tension during closure. Wound closure may require the use of skin grafting. Excision may be combined with intralesional corticosteroids (reduces recurrence rate to > 50%), cryotherapy, or silicone sheeting for added efficacy.

Carbon dioxide, argon, and neodynium:yttrium-aluminum-garnet lasers are initially effective but are associated with high recurrence rates.

• The 585-nm flashlamp pumped pulsed-dye laser may offer the best alternative for the treatment of hypertrophic scars, particularly scars that have an erythematous quality, are located on the face, and are of less than 2 years' duration; it also alleviates symptoms. Keloids tend to be more resistant to laser treatment. This laser, when used with 10 mm spot size using 3.0J/cm^2 fluence, also improves the appearance of striae rubra.

• Excision of scars (e.g., abdominoplasty) for striae.

Physical modalities

• Radiation therapy, usually in conjunction with compression and intralesional corticosteroids, reduces the rate of postsurgical recurrences to less than 10%.

• Compression with bandages or pressure earrings (for earlobe keloids) is essential after surgery.

• Massage of abdomen with emollient cream during pregnancy may decrease risk for developing striae.

Special therapeutic considerations

• Vitamin E, aloe vera, polysiloxane gel, onion (Allium cepa) extract gel, elastomer, or silicone ointment have not been scientifically proven to benefit hypertrophic scars or keloids.

Treatment aims

To prevent further trauma or treatment of associated inflammatory conditions, to ameliorate symptoms, if present, and to improve appearance and functionality of scar. Although improvement of hypertrophic scars is often possible, complete regression of keloids is not a reasonable expectation. Therapeutic studies are difficult to interpret because of lack of differentiation between hypertrophic scars and keloids (which have a worse treatment response) or because data are based on ear keloids. A combined therapeutic approach offers the most promise for preventing keloid recurrence.

Prognosis

Hypertrophic scars tend to flatten over time and remain stable in size after the initial growth period. Keloids demonstrate continued slow growth. In one study, the rate of recurrence was 51.1% after excision without postoperative injections, 58.4% after intralesional TAC injections1, and 18.7% after intralesional interferon-α 2b injections. Postoperative TAC injections did not reduce the number of keloid recurrences.

Follow-up and management

Intralesional injections can be repeated at monthly intervals.

Scars treated with the pulse-dye laser can be evaluated at 4- to 6-week intervals. Occasionally, retreatment may be necessary.

General references

Alster TS: Laser treatment of hypertrophic scars, keloids and striae. Dermatol Clin 1997, 15:419–429.

Urioste SS, Arndt KA, Dover JS: Keloids and hypertrophic scars: review and treatment strategies. Semin Cutan Med Surg 1999, 18:159–171.

Berman B, Bieley HC: Adjunct therapies to surgical management of keloids. Dermatol Surg 1996, 22:126–130.

Berman B, Flores F: Recurrence rates of excised keloids treated with postoperative triamcinolone acetonide injections or interferon α-2b injections. J Am Acad Dermatol 1997, 37:755–757

Erick Mafong and Christopher Nanni

Diagnosis

Signs

Systemic sclerosis: Diffuse skin thickening, early widespread indurated plaques (lilac borders; atrophic, ivory centers), predominantly on upper trunk, abdomen, buttocks, legs. Early findings: Raynaud phenomenon; hand, foot, periorbital edema; sclerodactyly. *Limited sclerosis*: progression to acral sclerosis; masklike face, microstomia, lip thinning, rhagades; flexion contractures, ulcerations; distal digit resorption; cutaneous calcifications; mat-like telangiectasias; scarring alopecia. *Diffuse sclerosis*: rapid progression to generalized hidebound skin; findings as in limited form, plus generalized hyperpigmentation, hypopigmentation; frequently poikilodermatous. Other findings: dysphagia, dyspnea, angina, muscle weakness, nailfold capillary dilatation, tenosynovitis, tendon friction rubs, migratory polyarthritis, digital osteoarthritis.

CREST (**C**alcinosis, **R**aynaud, **E**sophagus, **S**clerodactyly, **T**elangiectasia) **syndrome**: Prominent calcinosis, Raynaud's phenomenon, esophageal dysmotility, sclerodactyly, telangiectases prominent on face, erosive digital osteoarthritis.

Localized sclerosis (morphea): Usually asymptomatic; single or few indurated plaques, absent Raynaud's phenomenon, acrosclerosis, organ involvement. Variants: linear morphea on head, extremities, trunk (coup de sabre: linear, depressed, atrophic plaque in frontal or frontoparietal forehead or scalp). With facial hemiatrophy, extensive furrowing), guttate morphea (multiple small chalk-white plaques on neck, trunk—lichen sclerosus overlap), morphea profunda (deep, bound-down, indurated plaques usually without color change, trunk and upper extremities).

Investigations

• Nailfold capillary microscopy. Deep skin biopsy. Laboratory studies: radiography of digits, gastrointestinal imaging (barium upper gastrointestinal swallow with small bowel follow-through), pulmonary function tests, electrocardiography, echocardiography, blood pressure monitoring, renal chemistries, urinalysis (in systemic sclerosis). Antinucler antibody; anti-topoisomerase antibody (Scl-70); anti-centromere antibody (ACA); anti-SSA (Ro), anti-SSB (La), anti-Smith, anti-nuclear ribonuclearprotein antibodies; serum protein electrophoresis testing.

Linear morphea: Antinuclear antibody–positive in 67% of cases.
Limited sclerosis: Sensitivity of ACA 57%; anti-Scl-70–positive in 17% of cases (specificity, 83%).
Diffuse sclerosis: Sensitivity of anti-Scl-70, 40%; ACA positive in 9% of cases (specificity, 92%).
Other connective-tissue diseases: ACA-positive in 5% and anti-Scl-70–positive in 2% (specificity, >95%).
Disease-free controls: Both antibodies positive in less than 1% (specificities > 99%)

Complications

Morphea: Scarring, contractures, muscle atrophy.
Limited sclerosis: Main cause of death is pulmonary hypertension with cor pulmonale; biliary cirrhosis (especially CREST).
Diffuse sclerosis: Eesophageal dysfunction (90%), myocardial fibrosis (50% to 70%), pulmonary fibrosis (a major cause of death), renal failure (45%), hypertension (renal hypertensive crisis is major cause of death).

Etiology

Autoimmune antibodies directed at cellular and extracellular targets, including centromere proteins and topoisomerase I. Autoantibodies are T-cell–dependent and show strong HLA class II associations. Topoisomerase I binds to specific DNA sequences and relaxes supercoiled DNA, enabling transcription and replication to proceed. Its binding sequences have been found flanking fibrillar collagen genes. Antitopoisomerase antibodies may therefore explain the altered collagen gene expression that is pathogenic of the disease. *Borrelia* species have been implicated in the pathogenesis of morphea in Europe and Japan.

Epidemiology

Localized: Onset between ages 20 and 50.
Linear morphea: Mean age of onset is 5 years.
Systemic sclerosis: Female:male ratio is 4:1; prevalence, 240 cases in 1 million; predominate in blacks; onset peaks between ages 30 and 50.

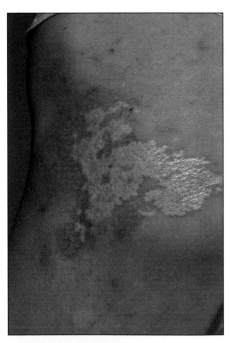

Localized scleroderma presenting as a sharply demarcated atrophic, ivory-colored patch with surrounding hyperpigmentation.

Macrene Alexiades-Armenakas and Andrew Franks, Jr.

Treatment

Diet and lifestyle
• Smoking cessation necessary, especially in Raynaud phenomenon.

Pharmacological treatment

Topical
Morphea: Class I and II corticosteroid preparations, calcipotriene.
Morphea profunda: Triamcinolone acetonide, 5–7.5 mg/mL, intralesionally.
Raynaud: Nitroglycerine (1% glyceryl trinitrate) cream, t.i.d. and p.r.n.

Systemic
Morphea: Antibiotics (doxycycline or penicillin); antimalarials (hydroxychloroquine, 200–400 mg/d; quinacrine, 50–100 mg/d; chloroquine, 250–500 mg/d), D-penicillamine, 2–5 mg/kg/d; corticosteroids, 0.5 mg/kg/d.
Raynaud: Calcium-channel blockers (oral diltiazem [sustained release], 60–120 mg, b.i.d.; oral verapamil [sustained release], 240–480 mg/d); dipyridamole, 25–75 mg, p.o., t.i.d.

Immunosuppressants
For systemic sclerosis: Chlorambucil, < 10 µg/d; methotrexate, 2.5–25 mg/wk; 5-fluorouracil; cyclosporine, 3 mg/kg/d; azathioprine, 25–200 mg/d; thalidomide; stem-cell transplantation.
Early, or for myositis, alveolitis or myocarditis: Corticosteroids, 0.5–2.0 mg/kg/d.
Pulmonary fibrosis: Cyclophosphamide.

Collagen inhibitors
• Colchicine, 0.6 mg, p.o., t.i.d., for morphea and systemic sclerosis. D-penicillamine 250 mg, p.o., q.d., on empty stomach, increased at 2- to 3-month intervals to maximum of 1500 mg/d, for diffuse disease. Monitor for hematologic abnormalities and drug-induced pemphigus, nephrotic syndrome, lupus erythematosus, polymyositis, Goodpasture syndrome, myasthenia gravis. Diethylsulfoxide. Interferon-gamma, 50 µg, SC, three times weekly.

Nonpharmacological treatment

Supportive treatments
• Angiotensin-converting enzyme inhibitors for renal disease; omeprazole and other proton-pump inhibitors for reflux; octreotide, 30–100 µg/d, for small bowel dysfunction.

Physical modalities
• Physical therapy to prevent contractures; phototherapy (ultraviolet A I); plasmapheresis, photopheresis for systemic sclerosis.

Macrene Alexiades-Armenakas and Andrew Franks, Jr.

Treatment aims
To prevent scarring, flexion contractures, ulcerations, and digital resorption and to reverse sclerosis. In systemic sclerosis, also to prevent organ-related sequelae and prolong survival. There is no current proven effective treatment for systemic sclerosis. Patients should be treated specifically for organ system involvement.

Prognosis
Systemic sclerosis: 60% of cases are limited (older women with 10- to 15-year history of Raynaud, early onset of telangiectasias, delayed systemic involvement). Many die of other causes. 40% of cases are diffuse; (usually abrupt onset and rapid progression to internal organ involvement). Few cases do not develop severe organ involvement ("chronic diffuse systemic sclerosis") and have 75% survival at 7 years. Progonsis poor for older patients, men, black women with diffuse disease.

Ten-year survival: With sclerodactyly alone, 71%; with skin stiffness proximal to metacarpophalangeal joint and sparing trunk, 58%; with diffuse skin stiffness, 21%. Survival rates at 1, 6, 12 years: Limited disease, 98%, 80%, 50%, respectively; diffuse disease, 80%, 30%, 15%, respectively.

Follow-up and management
Monitor closely for progression to systemic disease, particularly pulmonary and renal involvement, which respond to prompt therapy.

Support organizations
Scleroderma Info Exchange, Inc., 150 Hines Farm Road, Cranston, RI 02921; Phone: 401-943-3909.
Scleroderma Research Foundation, Pueblo Medical Commons, 2320 Bath Street, Suite 307, Santa Barbara, CA 93105; Phone: 800-441-CURE; Web site: http://www.srfcure.org.

General references
Franks AG Jr: Topical glyceryl trinitrate as adjunctive treatment in Raynaud's disease. *Lancet* 1982, **1**:76–77.

Seibold JR, Furst DE, Clements PJ: Treatment of systemic sclerosis by disease modifying agents. In *Systemic Sclerosis*. Edited by Clements PJ and Furst DE. Baltimore: Williams & Wilkins; 1996.

Spencer-Green G, Alter D, Welch HG: Test performance in systemic sclerosis: anti-centromere and anti-Scl-70 antibodies. *Am J Med* 1997, **103**:242–248.

Diagnosis

Signs

Adult form: Erythematous patches with oily-looking scales and crusts in areas rich in sebaceous follicles, usually the scalp, eyebrows, glabella, nasolabial folds, retroauricular folds, external ears, beard area, axillae, groin, and V-shaped areas of the chest. Blepharitis, with honey-colored crusts, along the rim of the eyelid and keratinaceous casts around the eyelashes.

Infantile form: Cradle cap (greasy-looking, thick, fissured crusts on the frontal and parietal scalp) is most characteristic. Intertriginous dermatitis with greasy scale is common, particularly in the folds of the neck, axillae, and diaper area.

Symptoms

•Occasionally, mild pruritus.

Investigations

•Skin biopsy shows a superficial perivascular lymphohistiocytic infiltrate with acanthosis, variable elongation of rete ridges, slight to moderate spongiosis, and focal areas of parakeratosis in the stratum corneum.

Complications

•Rarely, progression to exfoliative erythroderma.

•Red face syndrome is usually due to long-term topical corticosteroid use.

•Patients with Leiner's disease (seborrheic erythroderma in infants) become severely ill, with anemia, diarrhea, vomiting, and secondary bacterial infections; the disease occurs in both familial (associated with functional deficiency of C5) and nonfamilial forms.

Differential diagnosis

Psoriasis, atopic dermatitis, contact dermatitis, nummular eczema, impetigo, rosacea, tinea versicolor, pityriasis rosea, scabies (in infants), Langerhans-cell histiocytosis (in infants).

Etiology

The cause may be multifactorial. Pityrosporum ovale counts in lesional skin are high in about half of patients; in the other half, counts are similar to or even lower than those of uninvolved skin. Not all patients respond to antifungal therapy. Increased sebum production cannot always be detected in patients with seborrheic dermatitis. Risk factors include stress; immunodeficiency, especially AIDS; acne; obesity; neurologic disease, especially Parkinson's disease; drugs (neuroleptic agents, cimetidine, methyldopa, gold); low temperature and low humidity.

Epidemiology

Affects 2% to 5% of the population. There are two age peaks, one in the first 3 months of life and the second around the fourth to the seventh decades of life. Males are more often affected than females in all age groups. In HIV infection and neuropsychiatric disease, the disorder is exceedingly common (60%) and often severe.

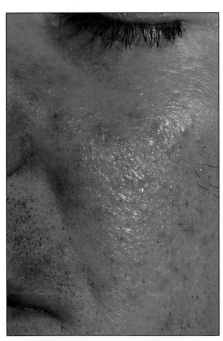

Prominent follicular openings; follicular erythema; pink papules, patches with fine scale; on oily skin over nasolabial region, cheeks. Perinasal erythema evident.

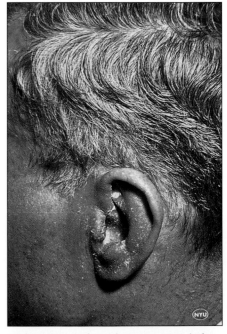

Erythematous, scaly patches cover preauricular area, pinna; scaling on scalp.

Jonathan Dosik and Paul Possick

Treatment

Diet and lifestyle

- Help patients decrease stress.
- Supplementary zinc therapy is not beneficial.
- The use of a humidifier may be helpful in dry climates or rooms.

Pharmacological treatment

Topical

- Scalp shampoos containing selenium sulfide (1% to 2.5%), ketoconazole (1% in over-the-counter form, 2% by prescription), zinc pyrithione, salicylic acid, or coal tar may be used daily or three times weekly.
- Corticosteroids in aqueous solution (halcinonide), alcohol-base (betamethasone dipropionate, clobetasol), propylene glycol-base (fluocinolone), gels (flucinonide, clobetasol), oil-in-water emulsion (hydrocortisone butyrate), foam-base (betamethasone valerate), or peanut oil (fluocinolone) used daily or up to two times daily.
- Salicylic acid in olive oil (3% to 5%) or 60% alcohol used for up to 1 hour to reduce scale.
- Phenol, glycerin, and mineral oil (eg, P&S Liquid) used overnight under shower-cap occlusion to remove scale.
- Corticosteroid creams, low-potency (hydrocortisone acetate, alclometasone) for the face and mid-potency (fluticasone, desonide) for the body; use can be tapered upon improvement.
- Lotions containing hydrocortisone, 1% to 2.5%, lactic acid 5%, and an antifungal agent.
- Antifungal creams may be used on a longer-term basis to reduce yeast colonization. Ketoconazole 2% cream, used twice daily, has been shown to be 75% to 95% effective in double-blind studies.
- Other treatments include topical metronidazole, sodium sulfacetamide 10% lotion, ammoniated mercury 5% and salicylic acid 2.5%, and glycolic acid and coal tar lotion.

Systemic

- Oral antifungal agents (fluconazole, itraconazole) for widespread disease.
- Prednisone, tapered over 5–10 days, for severe (erythrodermic) disease.
- Isotretinoin, in daily doses as low as 0.1 mg/kg, for 4 weeks. Relapse may not occur for months, years. High-dose isotretinoin may initially exacerbate disease.

Special therapeutic considerations

Infants: Low-potency corticosteroids (hydrocortisone 0.05%–1%) on body; rub scalp with oil, wash with baby shampoo or ketoconazole shampoo.

Intertriginous areas: High risk for striae from topical corticosteroids; use low-potency creams (with or without 3% cliquinol). Drying lotions (0.5% clioquinol in zinc oxide lotion), imidazole creams (ketoconazole 2%) may be effective.

Blepharitis: Hot compresses, gentle debridement with a cotton-tipped applicator, baby shampoo; severe cases: ophthalmic ointment containing low-potency corticosteroids (dexamethasone) or antibiotics (sodium sulfacetamide), alone or in combination.

In HIV-positive patients, seborrheic dermatitis may be more difficult to treat.

Treatment aims

Treatment is aimed toward removal of scales and crusts, reduction of erythema and itching, and inhibition of yeast colonization. Patients must understand that the disease is chronic and that therapy controls but does not cure it.

Prognosis

Adult disease generally lasts for years to decades, with remissions in warmer seasons and relapses during colder months. Infantile disease usually persists for weeks to months. Infants with seborrheic dermatitis have no higher risk for developing adult disease.

Follow-up and management

Depends on severity.

General references

Faergemann J, et al.: Pityrosporum ovale (Malassezia furfur) as the causative agent of seborrheic dermatitis: new treatment options. Br J Dermatol 1996, **134(Suppl 46)**:12–15.

Hay RJ, Graham-Brown RAC: Dandruff and seborrhoeic dermatitis: causes and management. Clin Exp Dermatol 1996, **22**:3–6.

Peter RU, Richarz-Barthauer U: Successful treatment and prophylaxis of scalp seborrheic dermatitis and dandruff with 2% ketoconazole shampoo: results of a multicentre, double-blind, placebo controlled trial. Br J Dermatol 1995, **132**:441–445.

Plewig G, Jansen T: Seborrheic dermatitis. In Dermatology in General Medicine, edn 5. Edited by Freedberg IM, et al. New York: McGraw-Hill; 1998:1482–1489.

Diagnosis

Signs

Gonorrhea (G): Men: most commonly, urethritis with purulent, yellow, clear or white mucosal urethral discharge often with accompanying dysuria. Women: urethral and vaginal discharge, purulent or mucopurulent endocervical exudate possible. **Chlamydia (Chl)**: Asymptomatic in about 75% of infected women; 30% of infected men. Most common: clear or white mucous urethral discharge (men), vaginal discharge (women). Dysuria, testicular tenderness, edema, lower abdominal pain, urinary frequency or hesitancy, painful ejaculation, dyspareunia, vaginal itching. **Chancroid (Cha)**: Soft, erythematous papules; ulcerated within 2 days to form tender, friable, malodorous ulcer with ragged, undermined borders, red base, grayish exudate. In men, prepuce often edematous. In women, vulva most commonly involved. Tender inguinal lymphadenopathy. Rarely, urethritis. **Granuloma inguinale (GI)**: Erythematous papules ulcerate, become painless, progressive, irregular highly vascular ulcers with rolled borders, beefy red, friable base. Subcutaneous granulomas (pseudobuboes) in inguinal region. **Lymphogranuloma venereum (LV)**: Initially, fleeting, nontender, small ulcers at inoculation site. Tender inguinal or femoral lymphadenopathy, usually unilateral. Women, homosexually active men might have procto-colitis or inflammatory involvement of perirectal or perianal lymphatic tissues.

Investigations

G: Gram stain: gram-negative diplococci in cells in discharge. Cultures from urethra, anus, throat. **Chl**: Fluorescent antibody (FA) examination of direct smear; enzyme immunoassay (EIA) and polymerase chain reaction (PCR) on genital swab or urine specimen. Cultures expensive, not routine.

Complications

G: Pelvic inflammatory disease, proctitis, epididymitis, prostatitis, periurethral abscess, urethral stricture, prostatitis, seminal vesiculitis, cowperitis, conjunctivitis. **Disseminated gonococcemia (DG)**: perihepatitis; rarely, endocarditis or meningitis. Minimal genital inflammation. **Chl**:Women: Up to 40% develop pelvic inflammatory disease (PID); of those, 20% become infertile; 18% experience debilitating, chronic pelvic pain; 9% have one or more ectopic pregnancies. Higher risk of premature labor, delivery. Newborns of infected mothers delivered vaginally have more than 1 in 3 risk of conjunctivitis, 15% chance of pneumonia, higher risk of death. Men: Epididymitis, orchitis, prostatitis, sterility. Other (either gender): proctitis, parahepatitis, Reiter's syndrome.

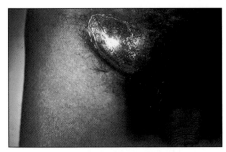

A man with lymphogranuloma venereum showing massive, discrete, fixed, fluctuant, tender, suppurative adenopathy with overlying warm and erythematous skin. The groove sign due to swelling above and below the Poupart ligament is not present in this case.

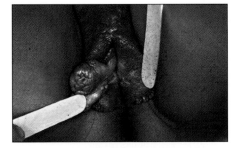

A young woman with granuloma inguinale presenting as vulvar edema, irregular ulcerations with granulomatous borders arising at the periphery of a granulomatous plaque on the labia minora, and a subcutaneous nodule with a vegetating surface.

Treatment

Pharmacological treatment

G: Single dose of: cefixime, 400 mg, p.o.; ciprofloxacin, 500 mg, p.o; ofloxacin, 400 mg, p.o.; ceftriaxone, 125 mg, i.m., (pregnant women, conjunctivitis). Alternatives: spectinomycin, 2 g, i.m., single dose; azithromycin, 2 g, p.o. (gastrointestinal distress); enoxacin, 400 mg, p.o.; lomefloxacin, 400 mg, p.o.; norfloxacin, 800 mg, p.o.

DG: Ceftriaxone, 1 g, i.m. or i.v., q. 24h. Alternatively, cefotaxime, 1 g, i.v., q. 8h; ceftizoxime, 1 g, i.v., q. 8h; (if allergic to beta-lactam drugs); ciprofloxacin, 500 mg, i.v., q. 12h; ofloxacin, 400 mg, i.v., q. 12h; spectinomycin, 2 g, i.m., q. 12h. All regimens: continue for 24–48 hours after improvement begins, then may switch to cefixime, 400 mg, p.o., b.i.d., or ciprofloxacin, 500 mg, p.o., b.i.d., or ofloxacin, 400 mg, p.o., b.i.d., 1 week of antimicrobial therapy. Hospitalization recommended for initial therapy.

Chl: Azithromycin, 1 g, p.o., single dose, or doxycycline, 100 mg, p.o., b.i.d., 7 days. Alternatives: erythromycin base, 500 mg, p.o., q.i.d., 7 days; erythromycin ethylsuccinate, 800 mg, p.o., q.i.d., 7 days; ofloxacin, 300 mg, p.o., b.i.d., 7 days. Pregnant women: eythromycin base, 500 mg, p.o., q.i.d., 7 days; amoxicillin, 500 mg, p.o., t.i.d., 7 days. If allergy or adverse effect, erythromycin base, 250 mg, p.o., q.i.d., 14 days; erythromycin ethylsuccinate, 400 mg, p.o., q.i.d., 14 days; azithromycin, 1 g, p.o., single dose.

Cha: Azithromycin, 1 g, p.o., single dose; Ceftriaxone, 250 mg, i.m., single dose; ciprofloxacin, 500 mg, p.o., b.i.d., 3 days; erythromycin base, 500 mg, p.o., q.i.d., 7 days. Ulcers: improvement within 7 days of treatment; healing within 2 weeks. Treat sexual partners within 10 days of ulcer's onset. Avoid ciprofloxacin and, if possible, azithromycin in pregnant women. No adverse effects on pregnancy or fetus reported in pregnant women with chancroid. HIV-infected patients and uncircumcised patients may require longer treatment. Incision and drainage of buboes preferred to needle aspiration.

GI: Trimethoprim-sulfamethoxazole, one double-strength tablet, b.i.d.; doxycycline, 100 mg, p.o., b.i.d. Treat at least 3 weeks, until all lesions healed completely. Alternatives: ciprofloxacin, 750 mg, p.o., b.i.d.; erythromycin base, 500 mg, p.o., q.i.d. Consider addition of aminoglycoside (gentamicin, 1 mg/kg, i.v., q. 8h) if no response within a few days therapy and if HIV infected. Prolonged therapy often required to enable granulation, reepithelialization. Relapse can occur 6–18 months later despite effective initial therapy. Observe until resolution. Examine, treat sex partner if sexual contact with patient in 60 days preceding onset of patient's symptoms and if signs, symptoms.

Recurrent/persistent urethritis (with negative cultures and after adequate treatment of G and Chl): Metronidazole, 2 g, p.o., single dose, plus erythromycin base, 500 mg, p.o., q.i.d., 7 days, or erythromycin ethylsuccinate, 800 mg, p.o., q.i.d., 7 days.

LV: Doxycycline, 100 mg, p.o., b.i.d., 21 days; erythromycin base, 500 mg, p.o., q.i.d., 21 days (choice if pregnant). Azithromycin, 250 mg, daily, over 2–3 weeks appears effective. Prolonged treatment may be needed in HIV-infection. Buboes may require aspiration through intact skin or incision and drainage to prevent formation of inguinal/femoral ulcerations. Examine, test for urethral or cervical Chl infection, and treat sex partners from the 30 days preceding onset of symptoms in patient.

Treatment aims

To cure infection of patient and sexual partners, to prevent complications and to prevent sexual transmission.

Follow-up and management

G: If no complication and compliance with recommended regimen, no retest needed. Encourage reculture if Asian transmission, due to high rate of quinolone resistance. Infection after recommended treatment usually reinfection, not treatment failure; need for improved patient education, referral of sex partner(s). Persistent urethritis, cervicitis, proctitis may be caused by *C. trachomatis*, other. **Chl**: Follow-up in 1 week if diagnosis not clearly established or compliance uncertain. **Cha**: Follow-up 3–7 days after treatment. If no improvement by 1 week, consider another etiology. **LV**: Observe until resolved.

Special considerations

All patients with STDs should be encouraged to undergo HIV testing, especially those with genitoulcerative disease. Even after complete diagnostic evaluation, at least 25% of patients who have genital ulcers have no laboratory-confirmed diagnosis.

General references

U.S. Centers for Disease Control and Prevention: 1998 Guidelines for treatment of sexually transmitted diseases. *MMWR Morb Mortal Wkly Rep* 1998, 47 (No. RR-1): 18–26, 28–41.

Rosen T, Brown TJ: Genital ulcerations: Evaluation and treatment. *Dermatol Clin North Am* 1998, 16: 673.

Diagnosis

Signs

Seborrheic dermatitis (SD): Erythematous patches, oily-looking scales, crusting; scalp, eyebrows, nasolabial folds, retroauricular folds, external ears, beard area; also axillae, groin, chest.

Psoriasis (P): Plaques, guttate papules, pustules simultaneously; intertriginous areas, genitals, nails, palms, soles involved; plaques flat, large, irregular, finer scale.

Pruritus (Pr): Widespread excoriations.

HIV-associated papular eruption: Pink urticarial papules.

Eosinophilic pustular folliculitis (EPF): Intensely itchy, folliculocentric, erythematous urticarial papulopustules, papules; pinpoint vesicles, pustules; face, neck, upper chest, back, proximal arms; few intact lesions but many excoriations.

Squamous cell carcinoma (SCC), basal cell carcinoma (BCC), melanoma (M): Risk factors: fair skin, actinic damage, immunosuppression. SCC on scalp; BCC, trunk. Oncogenic human papilloma virus–induced SCC in situ: cervix, anorectal area, genitals, perineum: may become invasive.

Major aphthous ulcers (AU): Oral, genital mucosa.

Chronic actinic dermatitis (CAD): Pruritic, hyperpigmented, lichenified eczematous plaques on face, neck, hands, chest.

Porphyria cutanea tarda: Blisters, erosions, milia, scars, hyperpigmentation, hypertrichosis of exposed body areas; HIV/hepatitis C or B coinfection, alcohol-induced liver disease.

Emaciation and wasting syndrome (EWS): Progressive or rapid weight reduction, loss of muscle tissue, decreased subcutaneous fat; progeric countenance; 10% or more unintentional weight loss, fever or diarrhea more than 30 days.

Lipodystrophy (L): Subcutaneous fat deposits; cervical, upper thoracic, waist, abdomen, preauricular area; after treatment with protease inhibitors; loss of fat, muscle; prominent visualization of veins.

Drug eruptions: Usually maculopapular or exanthematous; bullous eruptions, fixed drug reaction, erythema multiforme, toxic epidermal necrolysis. Intravenous foscavir: Irritation of distal urethral membrane; may ulcerate. Zidovudine (ZDV): Pseudomelonychia striata. Hivid: Oral ulcers. Protease inhibitors: Ichthyotic-appearing skin, cheilitis, persistent paronychia, increased eczema. Nevirapine: Maculopapular, sometimes pruritic eruptions; mainly upper body, upper arms; decreasing intensity on face, neck; low incidence of Stevens-Johnson syndrome, erythema multiforme, TEN. Nevirapine and efavirenz: Rarely, Stevens-Johnson. Abacavir: Hypersensitivity reaction, fever, chills, lethargy, aches, malaise, truncal morbilliform eruption; in 3% to 4%, cardiopulmonary collapse on rechallenge. Antiretroviral cocktails: Acute generalized exanthematous pustulosis, high fever, nonfollicular sterile pustules, edematous erythema, purpura. Protease inhibitors: Lipodystrophy; hypertriglyceridemia in 78.5%.

Etiology

SD: Inability to contain *Pityrosporum ovale,* in these areas is presumed.

EPF: *Demodex folliculorum* mite implicated; induces eosinophilic response, production of specific Ig-E antibodies, which bind to mast cells and Langerhans' cells.

Pruritic papular eruptions (PPE): Immune restoration syndrome with inefficiently targeted T cells, during antiretroviral therapy, proposed.

EWS: Malabsorption, anorexia, drug-induced adverse effects, or cryptosporidiosis contributory; increased metabolism coupled with the effect of cytokines accelerate EWS.

L: Unclear if natural progression of HIV infection; an adverse effect of protease inhibitors or other antiretrovirals suspected.

Epidemiology

HIV infection: Worldwide, 33 million HIV infected; US, 650,000 to 900,000; 44,000 (half under age 25) new cases annually. Leading cause of death of men 25–44; fourth leading among same-age women.

SD: At some point in 50% to 60% of HIV-infected; more common if CD4 count below 200 cells/mm3.

P: Incidence is similar to general population; severity increases as immunosuppression worsens.

Investigations

SD: Skin biopsy: superficial perivascular lymphohistiocytic infiltrate with acanthosis, variable elongation of rete ridges, slight-to-moderate spongiosis, focal areas of parakeratosis in stratum corneum. Often, leukoexocytosis, dyskeratotic keratinocytes in epidermis, plasma cells, neutrophils more common in dermal infiltrate.

EPF: Peripheral eosinophilia in up to one third; flares more common if CD4 counts 50–100 cells/L. Gram stain of scraped pustules: predominance of eosinophils. Skin biopsy of an intact lesion is test of choice.

Histopathologic studies: To confirm diagnosis of other diseases.

Miguel Sanchez and Patrick Hennessey

Treatment

Diet and lifestyle

EWS: High calorie and protein diet, appetite stimulants (megestrol acetate, cannabis derivative such as Marinol).

Pharmacological treatment

Topical

CAD: Sunscreens. Medium-to high-potency topical corticosteroids. **SD**: Scalp disease: shampoos containing selenium sulfide, 1% to 2% ketoconazole, zinc pyrithione, salicylic acid, or coal tar; intermittent topical corticosteroids. Solutions, gels, oils, foams are better-accepted media. Corticosteroid creams, lotions (low-potency on face, intertriginous areas; midpotency), with or without antifungal creams, such as ketoconazole 2% cream twice daily.

Pr: Antipruritic lotions

PPE: If mild, medium-to-high potency topical corticosteroids; daily permethrin for efficacious in eosinophilic folliculitis.

Systemic

CAD: Antiretroviral therapy. Oral antihistamines. Thalidomide, 100–200 mg daily, if recalcitrant prurigo.

P: High-dose ZDV; other antiretrovirals; acitretin. Methotrexate, cyclosporine if unresponsive; essential to avoid interactions with antiretroviral agents and to monitor liver functions carefully, to avoid drug induced– and chronic hepatitis–associated hepatotoxicity.

Pr: Antihistamines.

PPE: If mild, antihistamines, with or without topical antibacterial solutions. Systemic corticosteroids. Isotretinoin (20–40 mg daily), itraconazole (200–400 mg daily), metronidazole (250 mg three times daily for 3 weeks) for eosinophilic folliculitis.

EWS: Anabolic steroids, glucocorticosteroid replacement, Thalidomide.

L: Anabolic androgens and growth hormone.

Nonpharmacological treatment

P: Narrow band or conventional UVB phototherapy, PUVA.

Pr: UVB phototherapy.

L: Liposuction of fatty deposits to improve appearance.

Special therapeutic considerations

•Highly active antiretroviral therapy (HAART), initially the combination of one protease inhibitors and two reverse transcriptase inhibitors, currently denotes any highly effective combination of antiretrovirals that rapidly reduces HIV-viral loads and boosts helper T-cell counts. HAART is the treatment of choice for such HIV-associated skin diseases as mucosal candidiasis, oral hairy leukoplakia, disseminated molluscum contagiosum, aggressive seborrheic dermatitis and Kaposi's sarcoma, which have long been known to be common initial manifestations of HIV infection.

PPE: Chronic cases of pruritic papular eruptions may progress to prurigo nodularis, which requires aggressive treatment with a combination of antihistamines, intralesional corticosteroid injections, phototherapy, and, if needed, thalidomide, 100–200 mg daily.

SCC: At-risk patients, such as those with history of anogenital warts, should be observed particularly closely with cervical and anal cytology as well as colposcopic-guided biopsies.

AU: Painful; may continue to expand unless treated with intralesional or topical corticosteroids, colchicine and, in resistant cases, thalidomide.

Treatment aims

To reduce symptoms and, when possible, cure the skin disease.

General references

Majors MJ, Berger TG, Blauvelt A, *et al.*: HIV-related eosinophilic folliculitis: a panel discussion. *Sem Cut Med Surg* 1997, **16**:219–223.

Berger T: Cutaneous manifestations in patients infected with the human immunodeficiency virus. *West J Med* 1996, **164**:516–517.

Meola T, Sanchez M, Lim HW, *et al.*: Chronic actinic dermatitis associated with human immunodeficiency virus infection. *Br J Dermatol* 1997, **137**:431–436.

Smith KJ, Skelton HG, Yeager J, *et al.*: Cutaneous findings in HIV-1-positive patients: a 42-month prospective study. *J Am Acad Dermatol* 1994, **31**:746–754.

Miguel Sanchez and Patrick Hennessey

Diagnosis

Signs

Squamous cell carcinoma (SCC): A persistent erythematous, scaly patch or plaque; a shallow ulcer surrounded by wide, elevated, indurated border; or a flesh-colored to erythematous firm nodule with verrucous, papillomatous, or hyperkeratotic surface, often on background of actinically damaged skin (head, neck, and upper extremities, especially in fair-skinned persons).

Bowen's disease (SCC in situ): Usually an erythematous patch/plaque with adherent scale, sharp irregular outline and minimal infiltration; or a cutaneous horn. Bowen's disease of glans penis (erythroplasia of Queyrat) is a pink to red, smooth, macerated or ulcerated patch. Verrucous carcinoma typically develops on the plantar aspect of the foot as a cauliflower-like mass (epithelioma cuniculatum). When on the genitalia, it is called Buschke-Löwenstein tumor. Bowenoid papulosis are multifocal, flesh-colored, hypopigmented or hyperpigmented, slightly raised papules on the anogenital area

Actinic keratosis (AK): Small (<1 cm), barely raised pink papules with slightly scaly and rough surfaces typically located on the dorsal aspect of the hands and on the forearms, face, and bald scalp of men. Actinic cheilitis is an AK on the lip and presents with hyperkeratosis, fissures or erosions, and loss of vermilion border.

Symptoms

• Pain in SCC should raise suspicion of perineural invasion (present in 41% of metastasizing SCCs). Facial or trigeminal neuropathy may signal recurrence. Some AKs may be tender.

Investigations

• Skin biopsy shows irregular masses containing atypical squamous cells that proliferate downward into dermis. In Bowen's disease, the border between the epidermis and dermis is always sharp and the tumor is limited to the epidermis. In AK, the atypia is partial. In grade 4 SCC, the cells become spindle-shaped.

• Hypercalcemia without metastases or parathyroid gland abnormalities (very rare).

Complications

• Metastases and death. Disfigurement secondary to tumor growth and ulceration, neural invasion or tumor eradication. Ulcerated lesions may become infected.

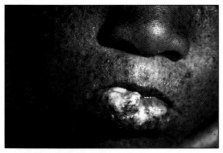

Erythematous leukoplakic plaque with eroded malignant nodule (invasive SCC) in a child with xeroderma pigmentosum.

Kenneth A. Mark and Deborah S. Sarnoff

Treatment

Diet and lifestyle

• Sunscreen and sun avoidance can prevent AK and subsequently SCC via decreased induction of *p53* mutations. Low-fat diet (> 20% of caloric intake) decreased development of AK in one study. Smoking and ethanol cessation, particularly for oral SCC; avoidance of arsenic.

Pharmacological treatment

Topical

• 5-fluorouracil 1%–5% twice daily, with or without topical steroids (for widespread AK); severe irritation, including ulceration and infection, may limit therapy.

• 5-fluorouracil/epinephrine gel intralesionally weekly for up to 6 weeks (96% success rate, but no long-term follow-up data are available).

Systemic

• Isotretinoin reported to cause regression or chemoprevention of SCC.

• Results are enhanced when combined with interferon-α2a.

Surgery

• Curettage and electrodesiccation: 90% cure for nonaggressive superficial SCC, but, like, cryosurgery and radiation, lack "true" margin control.

• Carbon dioxide laser ablation: Excellent for digit, periungal, penile, vulvar SCC in situ and actinic cheilitis.

• Excision: Over 90% cure with up to 6- to 9-mm margins, but not as successful as Mohs surgery.

• Mohs micrographic surgery: Cure rate approaches 98% and offers 100% margin control. Treatment of choice for recurrent tumors, locations in which tissue conservation is paramount, aggressive subtypes, and larger, poorly circumscribed lesions.

• Lymph node histologic sampling and/or fine-needle aspiration (if clinically indicated).

Nonpharmacological treatment

Physical modalities

• Cryosurgery very efficient for AK. Other treatments for AK include curettage, dermabrasion, microdermabrasion, laser resurfacing, tretinoin, trichloroacetic acid (TCA), and peels (glycolic acid, TCA, or salicylic acid).

• Cryosurgery (for SCC).

• Photodynamic therapy (for SCC).

• Radiation therapy: Conserves anatomy; good for nose, lip, eyelid, and canthus, but requires fractionation of dose and prolonged treatment course with more than 10 visits over several weeks. Radiation therapy has also been advocated after surgery for SCC in patients with high risk for metastasis or recurrence.

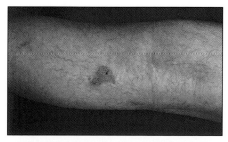

Red, irregular plaque on an extremity; proven, on biopsy, to be squamous cell carcinoma

Treatment aims

To eradicate neoplasm and prevent recurrence and additional lesions.
Lymph node involvement must be excluded. Choice of treatment depends on convenience to patient; overall health of patient; cosmetic result; function of affected site; and aggressiveness, size, and subtype of tumor.

Prognosis

Malignant conversion rate of untreated AK ranges from 1% to 20%, but lifetime risk is 10%. About 5% of cases of Bowen's disease, and 10% of cases of erythroplasia of Queyrat become invasive. Most grow slowly, but rapid invasion may occur.
Metastatic rate for SCC: 0.5% of those on sun-damaged skin, 2%–3% overall, 16% of lip, 18% of burn scars, 20% of radiation-induced.
5-year survival rate: 50% for scar SCC, 80% for lip SCC, 22% for head or neck SCC metastatic to lymph node.
HIV: Aggressive, rapidly growing tumors, recurrences, and metastases uncommon.
Transplant recipients: Aggressive, recurrent, and metastatic disease not uncommon.

Follow-up and management

Total skin and lymph node examinations at regular intervals for recurrences and new lesions. Consider oral retinoids for immuno-suppressed patients.
Toluidine blue rinse to rule out oral SCC.

General references

Goldman GD: Squamous cell cancer: a practical approach. *Semin Cut Med Surg* 1998, **17**:80–95.
Allison RR, Mang TS, Wilson BD: Photodynamic therapy for the treatment of nonmelanomatous cutaneous malignancies. *Semin Cut Med Surg* 1998, **17**:153–163.
Kuflik EG: Cryosurgery for cutaneous malignancy. An update. *Dermatol Surg* 1997, **23**:1081–1087.
Geohas J, Roholt NS, Robinson JK: Adjuvant radiotherapy after excision of cutaneous squamous cell carcinoma. *J Am Acad Dermatol* 1994, **30**:633–636.

Kenneth A. Mark and Deborah S. Sarnoff

Diagnosis

Signs

Dermatophytosis: Tinea capitis, patchy or diffuse scaling, erythema, with or without alopecia on scalp; tinea favosa: yellow adherent thick crusts; tinea barbae: kerion-like, folliculitis-like, or erythematous pustules in advancing border, on beard area; tinea corporis: erythema and scale the advancing border, often annular pattern, pale center, on body; bullous tinea: bullae, erythema; tinea faciale: erythematous scaly patches on face; tinea imbricata: concentric rings of erythema; tinea cruris: erythematous annular scaly patches in groin; tinea pedis: mocassin distribution of scale, interdigital web space maceration, erythema and scaling on feet; Majocchi's granuloma: Erythematous nodules on hair bearing surfaces; kerion: pustules, erythematous nodules. **Tinea nigra**: Scaly brown/green/black patches or macules on volar surfaces. **Black piedra**: Hard brown/black nodules on hair shafts on scalp. **White piedra**: Soft white/light brown concretions on hair shafts on scalp. **Candidiasis**: Cutaneous candidiasis—red pustules, macules, or papules on skin, often in intertriginous areas; oral thrush—yellow/white patches on tongue and palate; paronychia—red swollen periungual area. **Tinea versicolor**: Hypopigmented or hyperpigmented or pink scaly oval/round macules and patches on the trunk and body.

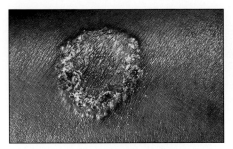

Typical ringworm lesion of tinea corporis consisting of a gradually expanding erythematous annular plaque with raised, scaly indurated border, tiny pustules, and central hyperpigmentation.

Symptoms

Dermatophytosis: Pruritus, discomfort, burning possible. **Tinea nigra**, **Piedra**: Asymptomatic. **Candidiasis**: Pruritus, burning, itching, discomfort. **Tinea versicolor**: Pruritus possible.

Investigations

Potassium hydroxide examination for branching hyphae. Wood's light in tinea capitis. **Skin biopsy**: Superficial perivascular lymphohistiocytic infiltrate, often with neutrophils in stratum corneum; obvious dermatophyte organisms in stratum corneum or hair shaft on periodic acid–Schiff stain.

Tinea nigra: Potassium hydroxide—brownish/olive hyphae and budding yeast; culture—brownish-black growth; skin biopsy—hyperkeratosis, hyphae brown/black in stratum corneum. **Candidiasis**: Potassium hydroxide— branching pseudohyphae and budding yeast forms; culture—can be positive; skin biopsy—superficial perivascular infiltrate of lymphocytes and histiocytes, yeast forms, and pseudohyphae in stratum corneum in subcorneal pustules, also with papillomatosis and hyperkeratosis. **Tinea versicolor**: Potassium hydroxide—yeast and hyphal forms; culture—with olive oil, positive culture is possible; Wood's light—yellow fluorescence; skin biopsy—superficial perivascular infiltrate of lymphocytes and histiocytes with yeast and hyphal forms in stratum corneum.

Complications

Dermatophytosis: Scarring alopecia in tinea capitis, bacterial superinfection if excoriated, id reaction, especially for tinea pedis. **Candidiasis**: Bacterial superinfection, odynophagia, systemic infection if immunocompromise. **Tinea versicolor**: Postinflammatory hypopigmentation.

Differential diagnosis

Dermatophytosis: Atopic dermatitis, psoriasis, seborrheic dermatitis, lupus, bacterial folliculitis, candidiasis, erythrasma.

Tinea nigra: Nevi, melanoma, syphilis.

Piedra: Nits, hair casts, trichomycosis axillaris.

Cutaneous candidiasis: Tinea, eczema, seborrheic dermatitis, inverse psoriasis, erythrasma, intertrigo, Hailey and Hailey disease; paronychiae—bacterial paronychiae; thrush—mucositis, herpes, erythema multiforme, lichen planus, pemphigus.

Tinea versicolor: Vitiligo, pityriasis alba, confluent and reticulated papillomatosis of Gougerot and Carteaud, secondary syphilis.

Etiology

Responsible organism varies, by condition

Epidemiology

Dermatophytosis: Adults and children; zoophilic, anthropophilic, geophilic.

Tinea nigra: Tropical, subtropical; rare in North America.

Black piedra: South America, Far East, Pacific Islands.

White piedra: South America, Europe, Asia, Japan, southern United States.

Candidiasis: Contributing factors: diabetes, pregnancy, immunocompromise, antibiotic therapy, extremes of age; trauma or occlusion.

Tinea versicolor: Hot weather.

Rebecca Baxt and Janet Moy

Treatment

Pharmacological treatment

Topical

Dermatophytosis: Tinea capitis: Selenium sulfide or ketoconazole shampoo 3 times a week. Tinea corporis, tinea faciale, tinea imbricata, tinea cruris, tinea pedis: Topical antifungal cream, 2 to 4 weeks. **Tinea nigra**: Topical antifungal cream for 2-3 weeks and adjuvant therapy with topical keratolytic agent. **Candidiasis**: Topical mycostatin or azole cream twice daily for 2-3 weeks. **Tinea versicolor**: Topical antifungals twice daily if limited, or selenium sulfide 2.5% lotion for 30 minutes every day for 10-14 days or for 2 hours every other day for 5 days. Once-monthly application prevents recurrences.

Systemic

Dermatophytosis: Tinea capitis: Griseofulvin, ultramicronized, 10-15mg/kg/d, with fatty foods, 6-8 weeks; itraconazole, 3-5mg/kg/d, 4-6 weeks; terbenafine, 3-6mg/kg/d, 4-8 weeks; fluconazole, 3-6 mg/kg/d, 6 weeks. Tinea favosa: Griseofulvin, ultramicronized, 10-15mg/kg/d, with fatty foods, 6-8 weeks. Tinea barbae: Griseofulvin 1g/d, for 2-3 weeks after clinical resolution. Tinea corporis: Griseofulvin 1g/day; fluconazole, 150 mg/wk, 2-4 weeks; itraconazole, 100-200 mg/d, 1-2 weeks; terbenifine, 250 mg/d, 1-2 weeks. Bullous tinea: Oral antifungal agent and topical steroid and antibacterial soaks, continue for 2-3 weeks after clinical resolution. Tinea pedis: Fluconazole, 150 mg/week, 3-4 weeks; itraconazole, 400 mg/d, 1 week; terbenafine, 250 mg/d, 2 weeks. Majocchi's granuloma: Oral antifungal for 2-3 weeks after clinical resolution. Kerion: Oral antifungal for 2-3 weeks after clinical resolution; prednisone, 1mg/kg/d, 10 days to 2 weeks. **Cutaneous candidiasis**: Fluconazole, 200 mg/d, 7-10 days. **Oral thrush**: Nystatin, 200,000 U, as lozenge, four times daily, or 500,000 U, as solution, swish and swallow four times daily, 14 days; clotrimazole troches, 10 mg 5 times a day for 14 days; fluconazole, 200-mg single dose or 100 mg/d for 5-14 days; itraconazole oral solution, 200 mg (20 mL), daily, without food, 7 days. **Tinea versicolor**: Fluconazole, 400 mg single dose; or itraconazole, 200 mg/d, 5-7 days.

Nonpharmacological treatment

Piedra: Shaving infected hair, with or without oral or topical antifungal agents.

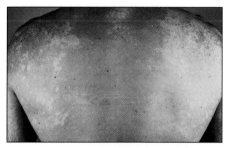

Hypopigmented, finely scaly, macules becoming confluent into irregular, geometric patches on the back of a man with tinea versicolor. The lesions may also be hyperpigmented or pink.

General references
Lesher JL: Oral therapy of common superficial fungal infections of the skin. J Am Acad Dermatol 1999, **40**:31–34.
Hay RJ: The management of superficial candidiasis. J Am Acad Dermatol 1999, **40**:S35–42.
Elewski BE: Treatment of tinea capitis: beyond griseofulvin. J Am Acad Dermatol 1999, **40**:S27–30.
Drake LA, Dinehart SM, Farmer ER, et al.: Guidelines of care for superficial mycotic infections of the skin: Pityriasis (tinea) versicolor. Guidelines/Outcomes Committee. American Academy of Dermatology. J Am Acad Dermatol 1996, **34**:287–289.

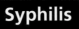

Syphilis

Diagnosis

Signs

Primary syphilis (PS): Round or oval ulcer approximately 1–2 cm; sharply defined, raised, indurated borders; ham-colored, smooth base. "Hunterian" chancre is firm, rubbery, painless unless traumatized, secondarily infected; on squeezing, thin serous exudate teeming with spirochetes. Untreated, chancre persists 1–6 weeks; treated, resolves in 1–2 weeks, no scarring. Lesions unnoticed in 15%. May be multiple chancres, penile edema, phimosis, erosive balanitis, lymphangitis or thrombophlebitis of dorsal vein. Extragenital chancres (especially lips, anoperineal) may occur. Nontender, rubbery regional lymphadenopathy (buboes) in 70% to 80%.

Secondary syphilis (SS): Eruption 3–12 weeks after appearance of chancre; later or before chancre disappears, in up to 15%. Usually recedes in 4–12 weeks. In latent syphilis (LS), 60% do not recall secondary lesions; 25% of these deny appearance of chancre. Skin eruptions in 80% to 95%. Over 95% of eruptions macular, maculopapular, or papular. Nodular and pustular eruptions rare. Malignant syphilis: widespread papulopustules, become necrotic, break down into ulcers covered by layers of thick, dirty-looking crust, associated with toxicity, fever, arthralgias, occasionally hepatitis. Noduloulcerative syphilis more common in HIV-infected persons. Vesicles, bullae only in prenatal syphilis; lesions may be pruritic, especially in blacks, immunocompromised. Condylomata lata and mucous patches commonly accompany eruptions; extremely infectious. Alopecia: patchy or generalized. Other signs: malaise, appetite loss, fever, headache, stiff neck, lacrimation, myalgias, arthralgias, pharyngitis (25%), nasal discharge, lymphadenopathy (50% to 80%).

LS: No lesions; identify by positive results on serologic tests.

Relapsing syphilis (RS): Manifestations as in SS.

Tertiary syphilis (TS): Infiltrates papules and nodules, noduloulcerative lesions, gummas.

Investigations

• Darkfield examination, direct fluorescent antibody tests of lesion exudate or tissue definitive for early syphilis.

• Nontreponemal test (NT): Generally, diagnosis presumptive, by reactive NT (sensitive, inexpensive, good screen, but false-positive in 1% to 2%; must confirm with treponemal tests). NT useful for determining disease relapse, therapeutic response. At least fourfold change in titer, equivalent to a change of two dilutions demonstrates clinically significant difference. After treatment, titers should decline fourfold within 6 months in PS or SS or within 24 months in LS. NTs nonreactive: 60% of PS cases by 4 months; SS in 12–24 months after treatment; in all cases, by 12 months. If therapy administered in early latent stage, low titers may remain up to 5 years. Reactive tests at low titers after 35 years: "serofast reaction."

• Treponemal tests are usually reactive permanently.

Neurosyphilis: Diagnose by combinations of reactive serologic test results, abnormalities of cerebrospinal fluid (CSF) leukocyte count or protein, or reactive VDRL-CSF test.

Skin biopsies: Silver stains help diagnosis if skin lesions present.

Complications

• Any organ. Without treatment, cardiovascular disease in 9.6%; neurosyphilis in 6.5%. Oslo study: death in 11%. Also preterm delivery, stillbirth, prenatal infection, neonatal death.

Differential diagnosis

PS: Chancroid, traumatic ulcers, herpes genitalis, granuloma inguinale, lymphogranuloma venereum, pyoderma, squamous cell carcinoma, basal-cell carcinoma, Behçet's disease, lymphoma, aphthous ulcers, fixed drug eruption, balanitis or vulvitis.

SS: Pityriasis rosea, parapsoriasis, cutaneous T-cell lymphoma, eczema, psoriasis; any cutaneous inflammatory disease.

Etiology

Caused by *Treponema pallidum*. Treponemal strains common in oral, anal cavities; syphilis cannot be diagnosed by dark-field microscopy, but can by specific immunoperoxidase stains.

Epidemiology

In 1998, nearly 38,000 cases reported, mainly ages 20–39; slight male predeliction. Infection after contact with early-S lesion in about one third; chancre develops at site of treponemal penetration; incubation of 10–90 days (average, 21).

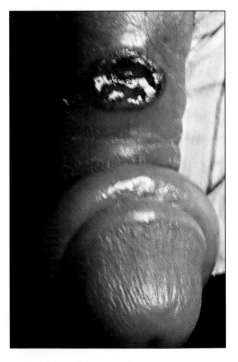

Penile edema and a well-demarcated primary syphilic chancre with raised, rubbery borders and moist, clean base.

Miguel Sanchez and Jacob Lau

Treatment

Pharmacological treatment

PS and SS
•One dose benzathine penicillin G, 2.4 million U, i.m.

Penicillin allergy (PA): If uncomplicated, 2-week course of doxycycline, 100 mg, p.o., b.i.d., or tetracycline, 500 mg, p.o q.i.d., or erythromycin, 500 mg, p.o., q.i.d. Alternative: ceftriaxone, 250 mg/d or 1 g every other day, i.v., 10 days. **Pregnancy**: Desensitize, treat with penicillin. **HIV infection**: Three doses of weekly injections of benzathine penicillin G preferred by some experts. **CSF examination (CSFEx)**: If signs, symptoms of central nervous system (CNS), eye, or hearing involvement; slit-lamp examination if ophthalmologic disease. **Treatment failure**: Re-treat if fourfold or greater increase in rapid plasma reagin (RPR) titer within 6 months. Repeat HIV serology. Unless reinfection definite, CNS examination indicated. If CSF abnormalities indicate neurosyphilis, treat with i.v. penicillin. If neurosyphilis excluded, treat with benzathine penicillin G, 2.4 million U i.m., three doses, 1 week apart. Management unclear if serofast, with RPR titers that do not decline by fourfold factor in 6 months. At least, clinical evaluation, and HIV testing If HIV-seropositive, spinal tap. If HIV-seronegative but adherence to treatment not assured, re-treatment recommended.

Early LS
•One dose of benzathine penicillin G, 2.4 million U i.m.

PA: If neither pregnancy nor HIV-infection, doxycycline, 100 mg, p.o., b.i.d., 4 weeks.
Pregnancy: Desensitize, use penicillin.

" Indeterminate" or late LS
•Benzathine penicillin G, 2.4 million U, i.m., three doses, 1 week apart.

PA : Doxycycline, 100 mg, p.o., b.i.d., 4 weeks. **Pregnancy**, **HIV infection**: Desensitize, use penicillin. **CSFEx** In asymptomatic patients, yield of positive lumbar-puncture findings low, but CSFEx indicated if cardiovascular, neurologic, eye, or auditory symptoms; late benign syphilis; HIV infection; RPR titer of 1:32 or more; treatment failure; nonpenicillin treatment. If CSFEx findings abnormal, unexplainable, treat for neurosyphilis.

TS (cardiovascular, late benign syphilis)
•Benzathine penicillin G, 2.4 million U, three doses, 1 week apart.

PA : If no HIV-infection and negative CSF, treat with doxycycline, 100 mg, p.o., b.i.d., 2 weeks. **CSFEx**: Spinal tap all. If abnormalities, treat for neurosyphilis.

Neurosyphilis
•Aqueous crystalline penicillin G, 18-24 million U; 3.5-4 million U, i.v., q. 4h, 10-14 days. Alternatives (if adherence to regimen assured): procaine penicillin, G, 2.4 million U, i.m., q.d.; probenecid, 500 mg, p.o., q. 6h, 10-14 days.

PA: Desensitize, use penicillin. **Neurosyphilis relapse**: Additional i.v. penicillin, equal or higher doses, usually works.

Treatment of sex partners
•Treat if exposed within 90 days preceding diagnosis of PS, SS, or early LS in a sex partner; infection possible, even if seronegative. Examination and serologic evaluation if exposed after 90 days of partner's diagnosis. Time periods to identify at risk sex partners: 3 months plus duration of symptoms (PS), 6 months plus duration of symptoms (SS), 1 year (early LS).

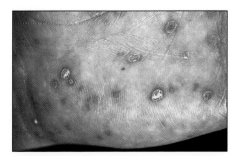

Dusky pink macules and thin papules on a palm, characterisitic of secondary syphilis. Some lesions exhibit hyperkeratotic scaling while others have peripheral collarettes of scales.

Miguel Sanchez and Jacob Lau

Treatment aims
To eradicate infection and prevent complications and prenatal syphilis.

Prognosis
TS: Gummas heal slowly over several months, may require surgical excision after penicillin treatment. Symptomatic cardiovascular syphilis has a poor prognosis; some treat with high-dose i.v. penicillin.
Neurosyphilis: Penicillin cure/improvement rate high.

Follow-up and management
PS, SS: Clinically and serologically reexamine at 6 and 12 months; if HIV-seropositive, reexamine at 3, 6, 9, 12, 24 months.
Early and late LS: Quantitative nontreponemal serologic tests at 6, 12, 24 months; if HIV infected, 6, 12, 18, 24 months. After treatment, reevaluate for neurosyphilis and re-treat accordingly if titers increase fourfold, an initially high titer ($\geq$ 32) fails to decrease fourfold within 12–24 months, or signs, symptoms of TS develop.
Neurosyphilis: Reexamine CSF every 6 months until normal. Cell counts should decrease by 6 months; CSF VDRL and protein levels by 2 years. If not, re-treat with i.v. penicillin. If symptoms worsen during treatment, dose may need to be increased. Blindness due to optic atrophy not reversible with penicillin. Eighth-nerve deafness benefits from combination of long-term penicillin and prednisone.

Special therapeutic considerations
Within 12 hours of treatment with penicillin, Jarisch-Herxheimer reaction (fever, headache, flared skin lesions, etc.) possible; manage with aspirin or nonsteroidal anti-inflammatory drugs. Hoigne syndrome (Pseudo-anaphlyactic reaction) associated with procaine penicillin treatment.

General references
Sanchez MR: Infectious syphilis. *Semin Dermatol* 1994, **31**:134.

Sanchez MR, Luger A: Syphilis. In *Dermatology in General Medicine*, edn 5. Edited by Fitzpatrick TB *et al*. New York, McGraw-Hill; 1999:2551–2580.

The 1998 guidelines for treatment of sexually transmitted diseases. National Center for HIV, STD and TB Prevention, Division of Sexually Transmitted Diseases. Centers for Disease Control and Prevention. *MMWR Morb Mortal Wkly Rep* 1998, **47**:28.

Diagnosis

Signs

• Telangiectasias are dilated capillaries, venules, or arterioles on the skin and mucous membranes. They appear as red, linear, stellate, or punctate macules or patches. Lesions are usually (but not always) blanchable by diascopy. Most telangiectasias are hereditary or secondary to rosacea, photodamage, pregnancy, liver disease, or another condition.

Clinical variants

• Spider angioma (nevus araneus) are characterized by a central, occasionally elevated, sometimes pulsatile (on diascopy) arteriolar punctum, from which vessels radiate symmetrically. They usually appear on the upper half of the body, sun-exposed areas, and occasionally on mucous membranes.

• Matted telangiectasias are red to violaceous macules and are often seen in CREST (calcinosis cutis, Raynaud phenomenon, esophageal motility disorder, sclerodactyly, and telangietasia), and scleroderma.

• Cherry angiomas are bright red to purple, dome-shaped papules up to 8 mm in diameter, that usually begin during middle age and become more numerous with advancing age; they develop on the trunk and extremities.

• Angioma serpiginosum appears as grouped, copper-colored to red or purple puncta, less than 1 mm in diameter, on a background of erythema measuring a few centimeters; develops in girls.

• Generalized essential telangiectasia is a benign condition characterized by sheets of telangiectasias that initially develop on the lower extremities and then spread superiorly to involve the thighs and sometimes the upper extremities and face. It is more common in women, generally begins in late childhood, and may cause bleeding of skin and mucous membranes.

Syndromes associated with telangiectasias

• Hereditary benign telangiectasia: probably autosomal dominant disorder with extensive telangiectasias, usually in light-exposed areas of the skin, beginning in childhood.

• Unilateral nevoid telangiectasia syndrome: present only on one side of the body.

• Hereditary hemorrhagic telangiectasia (Osler-Weber-Rendu disease): multiple macular and papular telangiectasias of mucosa (oral, nasal, conjunctiva, labial), skin (trunk, upper extremities, palms and soles), gastrointestinal tract, and other organs. Epistaxis in childhood is the usual presentation. Complications include pulmonary or gastrointestinal bleeding due to arteriovenous fistulae.

Ataxia-telangiectasia (Louis-Bar syndrome): progressive cerebellar ataxia, recurrent sinopulmonary infections, and telangiectasias.

Symptoms

• Skin telangiectasias are asymptomatic, but they may be considered unattractive and may bleed.

Investigations

• A standard complete medical history and physical examination are performed to determine the cause (primary *vs.* secondary) or to identify as a clinical variant. Systemic evaluation with blood tests may be necessary.

Complications

• Isolated cases are usually benign. Lesions associated with syndromes or other systemic illnesses have complications related to those particular entities.

Differential diagnosis

Angiokeratoma, angioma, vasculitis, venous lake, varicose veins.

Etiology

Secondary telangiectasia can be due to rosacea, actinic damage (often with poikiloderma), hepatic disease, pregnancy, collagen-vascular diseases (scleroderma, CREST, dermatomyositis, systemic lupus erythematosus, mixed connective tissue disease, rheumatoid arthritis, Raynaud phenomenon), Cushing syndrome, diabetes mellitus, genodermatoses (diffuse neonatal hemangiomatosis, Bloom syndrome, Cockayne syndrome, dyskeratosis congenita, Rothmund-Thomson syndrome, pseudoxanthoma elasticum, xeroderma pigmentosum), neoplasms (basal-cell carcinoma, mastocytoma, metastases, carcinoid syndrome, cutaneous T-cell lymphoma), estrogens, topical steroids, radiation therapy, postsurgical trauma, Degos' disease, and HIV infection.

Epidemiology

Spider angiomas are present in about 15% of the population, and occur more frequently in children, pregnant women (nearly two-thirds), and patients with hepatocellular disease.

Angioma serpiginosum occurs predominantly in women (90%) and usually is sporadic.

Hereditary hemorrhagic telangiectasia (autosomal dominant) occurs in about 1–2 persons per 100,000 and affects both sexes equally.

Ataxia-telangiectasia (autosomal recessive) occurs in about one in 40,000 births.

Generalized essential telangiectasia has a female predominance of 2:1.

Brian Jiang and Arielle Kauvar

Treatment

Diet and lifestyle

• Avoid predisposing factors, including excessive sunlight, radiation, trauma, topical corticosteroids, and alcohol.

Surgery

• Pulsed dye laser, frequency doubled neodymium:yttrium-argon-garnet laser therapy, and intense pulsed light sources are the treatments of choice for telangiectasias. These methods are highly effective and well tolerated, with minimal complications. Other options include electrodesiccation, galvanic electrocautery, and sclerotherapy, but these methods are associated with higher risk for adverse effects.

• Electrocautery (voltage should be kept very low, 0.4–0.6 W, to prevent scarring).

• Galvanizing current unit: less effective than laser therapy.

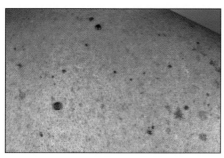

Well demarcated, small, red, acquired superficial hemangioma commonly referred to as "cherry angioma," on the back.

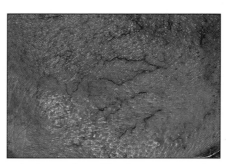

Red, wiry prominent dilated cutaneous vessels (linear telangiectasis) on the face.

Treatment aims

To eliminate vessels with minimal risk for scarring or pigmentary alteration.

Prognosis

Treatment cannot prevent appearance of telengiectasias in untreated sites. Recurrences are fairly common.

Follow-up and management

After cosmetic therapy for telangiectasias, the patient should return in 4–6 weeks for evaluation and possibly re-treatment. In secondary telangiectasias, management of the underlying cause is the primary concern.

General references

Dowd PM, Champion RH: Disorders of blood vessels. In *Textbook of Dermatology*, edn 6, vol 3. Edited by Champion RH, Wilkinson DS, Ebling FJG. Oxford: Blackwell Science; 1998:2091–2097.

Hurwitz S: Vascular disorders of infancy and childhood. In *Clinical Pediatric Dermatology: A Textbook of Skin Disorders of Childhood and Adolescence*, edn 2. Edited by Hurwitz S. Philadelphia: W.B. Saunders; 1993:265–268.

Ross BS, Levine VJ, Ashinoff R: Laser treatment of acquired vascular lesions. *Dermatol Clin* 1997, **15**:385–396.

Diagnosis

Signs

• Papules or papulovesicles 1–3 mm in diameter (may be up to 1 cm), mid-domed to acuminate in shape. Color varies from skin-colored or tan to red or reddish-brown. Lesions may be skin-textured or keratotic, and are frequently excoriated.

• Lesions are usually located on the chest, upper abdomen, and thoracic and lumbar back, with occasional involvement of proximal extremities and neck.

Symptoms

• Itching, often out of proportion to clinical findings.

Investigations

• Skin biopsy shows focal acantholysis and may have features of pemphigus vulgaris, Hailey and Hailey disease, Darier's disease, or spongiosis with acantholysis.

Complications

• Excoriation may be complicated by impetiginization

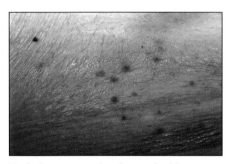

The lesions are excoriated, smooth, shiny, brown-pink papules.

Differential diagnosis

Prurigo papularis (red itchy bump disease), prurigo simplex, papular eczema, irritant dermatitis/asteatotic eczema, excoriated senile pruritus, scabies, *Cheyletiella* dermatitis, miliaria rubra, Darier's disease.

Etiology

Evidence suggests a dissolution of the desmosomal attachment plaque. Similar changes are found in the genodermatoses Darier's disease and Hailey and Hailey disease. Perhaps desmosomal adhesion molecules function ordinarily but are unusually susceptible to injury from ultraviolet light or proteolytic enzymes in sweat. Injury may be fostered by epidermal barrier impairment, thus explaining the prevalence in older patients and the association with asteatotic dermatitis and atopic dermatitis.

Epidemiology

Patients are usually white men.

Age at onset is almost always over 40.

Onset is frequently associated with heat, sweating, or exposure to sunlight. Grover's disease has been associated with asteatotic eczema, atopic dermatitis, and allergic contact dermatitis. It has also been associated with malignancy, but the relevance of this association is unclear. Several cases have been reported in association with use of interleukin-4.

Treatment

Diet and lifestyle

• Avoidance of hot, humid environment; wearing of nonocclusive clothing; protection from ultraviolet radiation are prudent. Soothing baths may relieve symptoms but should be immediately followed by emollients to foster repair of the epidermal barrier and prevent xerosis.

Pharmacological treatment

Topical

• Class I or II topical corticosteroids are often used initially.

• Antipruritic lotions containing menthol or pramoxine may relieve symptoms.

• Tretinoin and calcipotriene have anecdotally been reported to be effective.

Systemic

• Isotretinoin in doses of 0.5 mg/kg, tapering to 10 mg/d for maintenance over several months.

• Systemic corticosteroids in moderate doses, with tapering to low doses upon improvement, can be used for severe or refractory cases.

Nonpharmacological treatment

• Psoralen and ultraviolet A (PUVA) has been reported to be effective, but may initially exacerbate the condition.

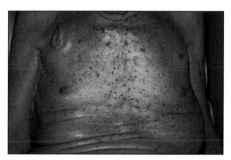

Grover's disease on the chest and upper abdomen of a man.

Treatment aims

Treatment reports are anecdotal or describe uncontrolled studies. Efficacy is particularly difficult to assess because the disease is usually self-limited. However, reported effective treatments include those listed in the following section.

Prognosis

Lesions usually resolve within several months but may persist for years (sometimes they are called persistent acantholytic dyskeratosis). Extent and severity of disease may fluctuate spontaneously.

Follow-up and management

To control symptoms, as required.

General references

Parsons JM: Transient acantholytic dermatosis (Grover's disease): a global perspective. *J Am Acad Dermatol* 1996, **35**:653–666.

Chalet M, Grover R, Ackerman AB: Transient acantholytic dermatosis: a reevaluation. *Arch Dermatol* 1977, **113**:431–435.

Hashimoto K, Fujiwara K, Harada M, *et al.*: Desmosomal dissolution in Grover's disease. *J Cutan Pathol* 1996, **22**:488–501.

Peter Reisfeld

Diagnosis

Signs

Urticaria (U): Erythematous, well-circumscribed, raised, edematous lesions, millimeters to centimeters; usually round or oval; may become confluent plaques; may have halo of pallor, erythema; individual lesions usually last < 24–48 hours; acute (< 6–8 weeks) or chronic. Foci of purpura in wheals of 3–5 days duration suggest urticarial vasculitis. Lesions may be generalized or, especially if due to physical stimuli localized/regional. **Angioedema (A)**: Larger, deeper edema of subcutaneous and submucosal tissues, usually lasting days; usually on eyelids, lips, tongue, extremities, genitalia; less commonly, larynx, gastrointestinal tract. May be acute or chronic. May be accompanied by urticaria.

Symptoms

•Pruritus, burning, occasional tenderness of lesions. Systemic symptoms may include headache, dizziness, "lump in throat," hoarseness, wheezing, dyspnea, nausea, vomiting, abdominal discomfort, diarrhea, arthralgias.

Investigations

History and physical examination: May reveal cause. Special emphasis: food, drugs. **Provocative tests** for physical U: Exercise for cholinergic urticaria; ice-cube test for cold urticaria; brisk mechanical stimulation for dermatographism. **Screening laboratory tests, skin-prick testing**: Generally not helpful or cost-effective, unless indicated by history or physical examination; antinuclear antibodies, erythrocyte and plasma protoporphyrins; phototests (solar U); cryoproteins (cold U); C1-inhibitor (C1INH) and C4 levels (C1INH deficiencies). **Biopsy**: Generally not indicated unless urticarial vasculitis is suspected.

Complications

Both: Systemic manifestations of gastrointestinal, respiratory, cardiovascular systems.

Physical urticaria precipitation by physical events

Dermographism: Arises rapidly after acute mechanical stimuli; usually resolves within 30 minutes. **Pressure U**: Often tender, deep swelling; occurs 2–6 hours after sustained mechanical stimuli; lasts 36 hours; may be accompanied by fever, chills, headache, malaise. **Cold U**: Acquired, idiopathic form, most common; lesions usually appear within minutes of exposure, typically as skin begins to warm; sometimes associated with headache, dyspnea, hypotension, syncope (especially severe cases). **Cholinergic U**: Triggered by rise in body temperature; small (1–2 mm), erythematous lesions with large flare; may be accompanied by bronchoconstriction, syncope, gastrointestinal symptoms. **Adrenergic U**: Tiny wheals with halo, occurring after stress. **Heat U**: Wheals occur within minutes after local heat is applied. **Solar urticaria**: Pruritic, erythematous wheals, occasional angioedema, occur within minutes after exposure to sun or artificial light sources. **Aquagenic U**: Pruritic, small wheals within minutes; pruritus without wheals is more common; may occur in elderly persons with dry skin and in patients with hematologic disorders.

Differential diagnosis

U: Erythema multiforme, bullous pemphigoid, urticaria pigmentosa, erythema annulare centrifugum, erythema chronicum migrans, systemic lupus erythematosus, serum sickness, urticarial vasculitis. **A**: Cellulitis, congestive heart failure, renal insufficiency, panniculitis, lymphangitis, thrombophlebitis, myxedema, superior vena cava syndrome.

Etiology

Urticaria and angioedema mediators
IgE, IgE-receptors: Atopy; specific antigens (eg, food, drugs, aeroallergens); physical U or A; contact U (eg, latex proteins); autoimmune U. **Complement and other plasma effector systems**: Hereditary angioedema—autosomal dominant deficiency of C1INH, activation of complement system with production of anaphylatoxins (C3a, C4a, C5a) spontaneously or after trauma; angioedema with acquired C1INH deficiency—one form associated with malignancy, eg, B-cell lymphoma; another form associated with autoantibody-necrotizing venulitis, angiotensin-converting enzyme inhibitors, infections (eg, hepatitis B); blood product transfusions; serum sickness. **Direct mast-cell degranulation**: Opiates, radiocontrast media, polymyxin B, curare, D-tubocurarine. **Abnormal arachidonic acid metabolism**: Aspirin, nonsteroidal anti-inflammatory drugs, azo dyes (especially tartrazine), benzoates (eg, preservatives), salicylates. **Idiopathic**: At least 70% of chronic cases; approximately one third of these may have circulating IgG autoantibodies against high-affinity IgE-receptor.

Epidemiology

Urticaria affects 20% of population, at some point. More common in women; any age, but mostly after adolescence; highest incidence in young adults. In children, more frequently associated with infection.

Treatment

Diet and lifestyle

•Identification and avoidance of known triggering agents, including physical precipitants in physical U, is most effective treatment. Sunblock, protective clothing for solar U.

Pharmacological

Topical

•Topical antipruritic agents may provide temporary relief.

Systemic

Antihistamines: Treatment of choice. Begin with second-generation H_1-antihistamines (*eg*, cetirizine, loratadine, fexofenadine) May also try first-generation H_1-antihistamines (*eg*, hydroxyzine, cyproheptadine). Start at low dose, increase as tolerated; use regular dosing, not as-needed. If agent from one therapeutic group ineffective, try agent from another therapeutic group; agents from different groups may be combined. **Standard dosage**: Hydroxyzine HCl, 25 mg, orally, every 4–6 hours; cyproheptadine, 4 mg, orally, every 4–6 hours; cetirizine, 10 mg, orally, once daily; loratadine, 10 mg, orally, once daily; fexofenadine, 120 mg, orally, once daily. **Contraindications**: Monoamine oxidase inhibitors (prolong, augment anticholinergic effects); pregnancy (limited guidelines; mostly category B and C); prostatic hypertrophy. **Combination**: In some cases of chronic idiopathic U, a combination of H_1- and H_2-antihistamines may be helpful. **Main drug interactions**: Advise patients to use caution with central nervous system (CNS) depressants (*eg*, alcohol, benzodiazepines); cimetidine: many drug interactions, especially warfarin, quinidine, nifedipine, theophylline, phenytoin. **Main side effects**: CNS (*eg*, drowsiness) and anticholinergic (*eg*, dry mouth), gastrointestinal (*eg*, nausea).

•:Other pharmacologic agents are available. **Systemic glucocorticoid therapy**: Rare use in refractory U; use alternate-day regimen. **Epinephrine**, 0.01 mL/kg, up to 0.3 mL; reserve for laryngeal edema and cardiovascular collapse. **Stanozolol**, 0.5–2 mg/d, and **danazol**, 50–400 mg/d are widely used to prevent attacks of hereditary and acquired C1INH deficiencies; may double or triple dose for 5 days before anticipated trauma (*eg*, dental procedures); may result in irregular menstruation in nonpregnant women. **Anecdotal, novel treatments**: Cyclosporine, sulfasalazine, nifedipine, i.v. immune globulin, colchicine, plasmapheresis, thyroxine, nalmefene, aminophylline, terbutaline, propanolol, phototherapy.

Treatment aims

To relieve itching; reduce swelling, systemic features; prevent recurrence.

Prognosis

Of patients with U alone, 50% free of lesions after 1 year; 20% of all patients affected for > 20 years. Only 25% of patients with chronic U and A or A alone free of lesions after 1 year; 20% of all patients affected for > 20 years.

General references

Greaves MW, Sabroe RA: ABC of allergies. Allergy and the skin. I—Urticaria. *BMJ* 1998, **316**:1147–1150.

Kozel MM, Mekkes JR, Bossuyt PM, *et al.*: The effectiveness of a history-based diagnostic approach in chronic urticaria and angioedema. *Arch Dermatol* 1998, **134**:1575–1580.

Poon E, Seed PT, Greaves MW, *et al.*: The extent and nature of disability in different urticarial conditions. *Br J Dermatol* 1999, **140**:667–671.

Sabroe RA, Greaves MW: The pathogenesis of chronic idiopathic urticaria. *Arch Dermatol* 1997, **133**:1003–1008.

Sabroe RA, Seed PT, Francis DM, *et al.*: Chronic idiopathic urticaria: comparison of the clinical features of patients with and without antiFc*epsilon*RI or anti-IgE autoantibodies. *J Am Acad Dermatol* 1999, **40**:443–450.

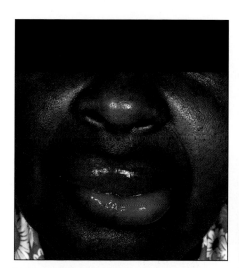

Acute swelling of the lips in a patient with hereditary angioedema.

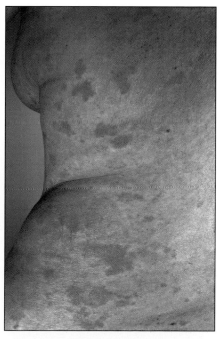

Discrete pink edematous papules and plaques (wheals) in a woman with urticaria.

Edwin Joe and Nicholas Soter

Diagnosis

Signs

Arterial ulcers: Sharp, punched out ulcerations, often with deep edges. Usually over site of pressure, trauma. Common on distal points (*ie*, toes, bony prominences); may develop above ankle or on feet. Arterial ischemic findings possible. Hyperpigmentation unusual. Pain with leg elevation.

Venous insufficiency ulcers: Irregularly shaped ulcerations, usually with shallow pink edges. Size, depth vary from small erosions with weeping, crusting to ulcerated skin across entire width of leg, down to subcutaneous tissue. Induration, edema, lipodermatosclerosis (sclerosing panniculitis) commonly associated. May be scattered islands of healthy epidermis. Ulcers typical on medial malleolus, lower aspect of calf; rarely, feet. Pain in dependent position.

Venous stasis dermatitis: Hyperpigmented, scaly, erythematous patches on lower legs, ankles; associated with venous insufficiency. Occasionally pruritic.

Investigations

•Diminished pulses indicate arterial ischemia. Simultaneous presence of varicose veins or history of venous thrombosis with typical ulcer usually diagnostic of venous ulceration.

Doppler ultrasonography to assess blood flow. Ankle brachial indices (normal > 0.9) by Doppler, blood pressure cuff to evaluate arterial ischemia.

Arteriography if diminished blood flow in vascular surgery candidate.

Cultures can exclude infection with bacteria or fungus.

Radiographic examinations, magnetic resonance imaging indicated if osteomyelitis suspected.

Biopsy indicated if malignancy suspected or cause unknown.

Complications

Infection: Most common pathogenic bacteria are *Staphyloccocus, Pseudomonas, Streptococcus* species; *Escherichia coli, Proteus* species. In hospitalized patients, penicillin-resistant staphylococci, *Pseudomonas* species very common. Consider anaerobes *ie, Bacteroides* species.

Lymphedema: Superficial lymphatics often absent around ulcers. Hyperkeratosis, dermal fibrosis, fibroplasia of muscular fascia may occur. Chronic lymphedema may lead to significant epidermal hyperplasia, known as elephantiasis nostras verrucosa. Malignant change rare; poor prognosis.

Bone: Periostitis common beneath ulcer. Osteoporosis can occur later.

•Cellulitis may accompany stasis dermatitis. Contact dermatitis frequent in venous stasis dermatitis, skin around vascular ulcers. Most common allergens: neomycin, parabens, colophony, balsam of Peru.

Differential diagnosis

Vascular ulcers: Pyoderma gangrenosum, deep fungal infection, neoplasia (basal-cell carcinoma, squamous-cell carcinoma, leukemia, lymphoma), trauma, necrobiosis lipoidica diabeticorum, sickle cell anemia or thalassemia ulcerations, rheumatic disease, vasculitis, cryoglobulinemia.

Stasis dermatitis: Allergic contact dermatitis, asteatotic eczema, irritant dermatitis, nummular eczema, psoriasis.

Etiology

Arterial ulcers: Poor tissue perfusion from decreased arterial flow leads to tissue ischemia, breakdown.

Venous ulcers: Increased venous pressure from incompetent superficial, communicating veins or venous thrombosis; causes leakage of fluid, electrolytes. Fibrinolytic abnormality or trapping of macromolecules (cytokines) may be contributory.

Epidemiology

Arterial-related ulcers associated with atherosclerosis, high cholesterol levels, hypertension, diabetes, obesity, cigarette smoking, family history of ischemic heart disease; sedentary lifestyle contributes. Venous ulcers in 1% of world population; 2.5 million, US. Incidence increases with age; higher in women than men. Of vascular leg ulcers, 75% venous, 10% arterial, 15% mixed arterial-venous.

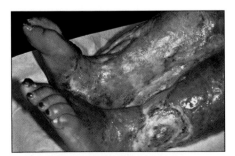

Bilateral, large, chronic ulcers with exuberant granulation tissue in a patient with venous insufficiency and lymphedema.

Treatment

Diet and lifestyle

Arterial ulcers: Cessation of smoking, control of other risk factors (hypertension, diabetes, hyperlipidemia), exercise extremely important.

Venous ulcers: Low plasma zinc levels reported in patients with venous ulcer; accelerated healing with oral zinc sulphate controversial. Vitamins A and C, protein, iron, calcium may promote wound healing. Exercise increases venous drainage; weight loss relieves pressure on legs. Leg elevation at rest. Important to avoid trauma.

Pharmacological treatment

Antibiotics for infection; analgesics for pain.

Nonpharmacological treatment

Venous ulcers

Compression: Determine adequacy of arterial flow. Unna boots excellent; can be used with bandage wraps, support dressings. In venous stasis without arterial insufficiency, use graduated elastic compression stockings that deliver pressure of 30 mm Hg or more, to prevent dermatitis, ulcer formation.

Occlusion: Promote formation of granulation tissue, enhance debridement; nonadherent, adherent cotton, impregnated dressings. Hydrocolloids (impermeable to water and vapor) absorb moisture, improve wound healing by at least 40%; especially advantageous in ulcers covered with dried fibrinous exudate. Dressing should cover at least 3 cm of intact skin around ulcer. Polyurethane films: adhesive, oxygen-permeable but impermeable to bacteria and water; transparency allows wound visualization; increase healing more than 20%. Dressings should be changed every 3–7 days, should not exert tension, because increased shearing forces may increase skin breakdown. Hydrogels keep moisture in; excellent for dried out ulcers. Alginates, foams especially beneficial if copious exudate. Ulcers can be packed under dressings with foam, hydrophilic, or alginate granules.

Debridement is imperative; enhances epithelialization. Mechanical: scalpel, scissors, curettage. Chemical: zinc chloride, collagenase, fibrinolysin, trypsin, streptokinase; follow manufacturer's directions carefully to avoid inactivation by other agents commonly used in ulcer wound care. Hydrocolloid dressings enhance autolytic debridement. Maggot debridement, although not standard therapy, is very effective.

Surgery

•In either venous or arterial disease, surgery, pinch graft, full-thickness graft, bovine graft, Apligraft (Organogenesis, Canton, MA; bioengineered graft; may be tried if ulcer resistant to standard therapy) may be indicated if necrotic tissue is extensive.

Arterial ulcers: Blood flow to affected area must be increased; bypass surgery, endarterectomy; surgical debridement of larger areas of necrosis.

Venous ulcers: Split-thickness grafting, pinch grafts may aid in closure; especially helpful in burn ulcers.

Special therapeutic considerations

•Measure ulcer and update drawing of outline or photograph at each visit.

General references

Falanga V: Apligraf treatment of venous ulcers and other chronic wounds. *J Dermatol* 1998, **25**:812–817.

Choucair M: Compression therapy. *Dermatol Surg* 1998, **24**:141–148.

Alguire PC: Chronic venous insufficiency and venous ulceration. *J Intern Med* 1997, **12**:374–383.

Phillips T: Leg ulcers. *J Am Acad Dermatol* 1991, **25**:965–983.

Diagnosis

Classification

Cutaneous necrotizing venulitis (CNV): Autoimmune disorder–associated: Systemic lupus erythematosus, rheumatoid arthritis, Sjögren's syndrome, antiphospholipid syndromes. Paraneoplastic: Lymphoma, leukemia, myelofibrosis, multiple myeloma, solid tumors. Cryoglobulinemia-associated: Hepatitis, cystic fibrosis, inflammatory bowel disease, Behçet's disease. Complement deficiency–associated: C2, C4, C4b. Drug-induced: Penicillin, sulfonamides, thiazides, allopurinol, phenytoin, nonsteroidal anti-inflammatory drugs. Infection-triggered: Group A *Streptococcus; Staphylococcus aureus; Mycobacterium leprae;* hepatitis A, B, and C; meningococcus, Rocky Mountain spotted fever. Idiopathic: Henoch-Schönlein purpura (HSP), **acute hemorrhagic edema of childhood (AHEC), urticarial vasculitis (UV), erythema elevatum diutinum (EED), necrotizing vasculitis (NV), livedoid vasculitis (LV). Systemic necrotizing arteritis (SNA): Polyarteritis nodosa (PAN),** classic and microscopic; **allergic angiitis and granulomatosis of Churg-Strauss (CS); polyangiitis overlap syndrome; Wegener's granulomatosis (WG); giant-cell (temporal) arteritis; Takayasu's arteritis; Kawasaki's disease; thromboangiitis obliterans (Buerger's disease); Behçet's disease.**

Signs

CNV: Palpable purpuravesicles/bullae/pustules, ulcers/necrosis. **UV:** Persistent wheals, with or without foci of purpura. **PAN:** Livedo reticularis, erythematous nodules. **AHEC:** Edematous petechiae and ecchymoses. **EED:** Erythematous plaques. **LV:** Livedo reticularis, ulcerations, atrophie blanche.

Distribution

CNV: Lower extremities, dependent areas. **Systemic vasculitis:** Extremities. **EED:** Overlying joints of extensor extremities, gluteal area. **Nodular vasculitis:** Posterior lower legs. **AHEC:** Head, distal extremities. **LV:** Lower extremities. **TA:** Temporal, scalp regions.

Symptoms/complications

Skin Mild pruritus, burning or pain (all). **Constitutional:** Fever, malaise, arthralgias, or myalgias (all); weight loss, nausea, vomiting, abdominal pain, peripheral and central neurologic symptoms (systemic vasculitis); jaw claudication (temporal arteritis; TA). **Upper respiratory tract:** Sinus pain, rhinorrhea, cough, hemoptysis, otitis media, saddle nose deformity (WG), laryngeal edema (UV). **Lower respiratory tract:** Wheezing, dyspnea (CS); hemoptysis, pleuritic chest pain, pulmonary nodules (WG, lymphomatoid granulomatosis); diffuse pneumonitis, hemorrhage (microscopic PAN). **Ocular:** Retinal vasculitis (PAN); episcleritis, scleritis, scleromalacia perforans, or proptosis (WG); hemianopsia, visual disturbance (TA). **Cardiovascular:** Hypertension, heart failure, myocardial infarction, or pericarditis (CS > PAN > WG); jaw claudication (TA). **Neurologic:** Mental status change, seizures, hemiparesis (PAN, WG, CS; Sneddon's syndrome); pseudotumor cerebri (UV); headache, scalp tenderness (TA), peripheral neuropathy (PAN). **Renal:** Hematuria, proteinuria (PAN > WG > CS > UV); focal necrotizing glomerulonephritis (microscopic PAN). **Gastrointestinal:** Cholecystitis, bleeding, perforation, or infarction. **Musculoskeletal:** Arthritis, myositis, polymyalgia rheumatica (TA).

Investigations

Blood tests: Complete blood count with differential, erythrocyte sedimentation rate, hepatitis serologic testing (all); complement levels, antinuclear antibody, rheumatoid factor, cryoglobulins, immune complexes, HIV serologic testing, rapid plasma reagin test, coagulation profile, antineutrophil cytoplasmic antibody (ANCA) levels, serum protein electrophoresis. **Biopsy:** Punch biopsy of skin (CNV), deep excisional skin biopsy (SNA), temporal artery biopsy (TA). **Angiography:** Indicated for brain, intestinal, or large-vessel involvement. **Other:** Chest radiography (select cases), urinalysis and culture (all).

Differential diagnosis

Nonpalpable purpura: Thrombocytopenia, trauma, hypercorticism, pigmented purpuric dermatoses. **Palpable purpura:** Kaposi's sarcoma, scurvy, infections (purpura fulminans/disseminated intravascular coagulation/septic emboli, Rocky Mountain spotted fever, viral infections), cholesterol emboli. **Purpuric nodules:** Erythema nodosum, panniculitis, thrombophlebitis.

Etiology

CNV: Immune complex deposition in postcapillary venules, complement activation, inflammatory cell infiltration, neutrophil leukocytoclasis, and fibrinoid necrosis of venules. Triggers of immune complex formation include autoimmune disorders, paraneoplastic disease, cryoglobulinemia, infections, and drugs.
SNA: Immune complex formation, complement fixation, tissue deposition and inflammation involving multiple organ systems; small to large arteries (**PAN**); venules, arterioles, small and medium-sized arteries (microscopic PAN); small and medium-sized arteries, veins, and venules, most prominently in pulmonary vasculature (**CS**); upper and lower respiratory tracts, glomerulae, and disseminated small vessels (**WG**); or large and medium-sized arteries, branches of carotid artery (**TA**). The latter three involve intra- and peri-vascular granulomatous inflammation. ANCAs have been associated with **WG** (cytoplasmic ANCA), **PAN**, and **CS** (p-ANCA), and, to a lesser degree, **CNV**. Antiendothelial cell antibodies have been associated in various vasculitic syndromes.

Macrene Alexiades-Armenakas and Andrew Franks, Jr.

Treatment

Pharmacological treatment

Topical

Class I corticosteroids for mild cutaneous cases of CNV.

Systemic

CNV: First-line (usually used in combination): H_1 antihistamines, NSAIDs, colchicine, hydroxychloroquine sulfate, dapsone; second-line: prednisone, azathioprine, cyclophosphamide, intravenous γ-globulin, cyclosporine, plasmapheresis.

LV: Aspirin, dipyridamole, colchicine, low-dose heparin, prednisone, nicotinic acid, low-molecular-weight dextran, pentoxifylline. **PANL**: Prednisone, 1 mg/kg/d, and cyclophosphamide, 2 mg/kg/d; vidarabine, plasmapheresis, with or without glucocorticoids, interferon-α, plasmapheresis for hepatitis B–associated PAN.**CS**: Systemic corticosteroids, cyclophosphamide and alternate-day prednisone (for glucocorticoid failure or fulminant disease). **WG**: First-line: Cyclophosphamide, 2 mg/kg/d (maintain leukocyte count at 3000 cells/μL; monitor for cystitis, bladder cancer; continue therapy 1 year after complete remission with subsequent gradual taper; pulse therapy less effective than daily dosing and should not be used as first-line); prednisone, 1 mg/kg/d during first month of induction phase, then alternate-day dosing within 3 months, followed by taper after 6 months, discontinuation within 6–12 months. Second-line: Prednisone (as above) and methotrexate, 0.3 mg/kg per week initially, with 15 mg per week maximum, for 1–2 weeks; then increase by increments of 2.5 mg per week to 20–25 mg per week (maintenance dosage). As maintenance therapy after cyclophosphamide induction, prednisone (as above) and azathioprine, 1–2 mg/kg/d (in patients with cyclophosphamide toxicity—neutropenia, cystitis, or bladder cancer). **TA**: Prednisone, 40–60 mg/d for 1 month, followed by taper to maintenance dose of 7.5–10 mg/d for 1–2 years. Monitor erythrocyte sedimentation rate for disease activity and during taper. **Takayasu's arteritis**: Prednisone, 40–60 mg/d, combined with surgical therapy, with or without angioplastic therapy. **HSP**: Prednisone, 1 mg/kg/d, followed by taper. Immunosuppressants and plasmapheresis for rapidly progressive glomerulonephritis. Treatment helpful for marked edema, arthralgias, abdominal pain; not for skin or renal disease or shortening duration or preventing recurrence. **Lymphomatoid granulomatosus (LG)**: Cyclophosphamide and prednisone (if no systemic symptoms), multi-agent chemotherapy (if systemic symptoms).

Surgery

Vascular surgery, angioplasty in select cases, particularly in Takayasu's arteritis.

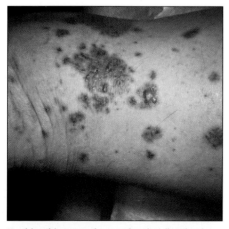

Nonblanching, purple macules that develop into papules (palpable purpura) and blisters due to cutaneous necrotizing venulitis.

Treatment aims

To prevent complications.

Prognosis

SNA: Five-year survival: 80% (PAN, WG). Highest mortality: pulmonary hemorrhage, renal failure. Disease-free remission in small percentage; 50% relapse within 5 years. **CS**: Poor prognostic indicators: 5-factor score: proteinuria > 1 g/d, creatinine level > 1.58 mg/dL, cardiomyopathy, gastrointestinal and central nervous system involvement; 5-year mortality rates: 12% (score = 0), 26% (score = 1), 46% (score ≥ 2). **Takayasu's arteritis**: Five-year survival: 83%; 10-year, 58%; cause of death usually myocardial infarction, congestive heart failure, or cerebrovascular accident. **LG**: Up to 90% mortality; most patients die within 2 years. **CNV**: Most patients have single episode that resolves spontaneously within weeks to months; 10% recurrences at intervals of months to years.

Follow-up and management

Frequent relapses require long-term follow-up. Hemorrhagic cystitis (50%) and bladder cancer (8%) occur in patients treated with daily cyclophosphamide.

General references

Jeanette JC, Falk RJ: Medical progress: small-vessel vasculitis. *N Engl J Med* 1997, **337**:15121523.

Jayne DRW, Rasmussen N: Treatment of antineutrophil cytoplasm autoantibody-associated systemic vasculitis: initiatives of the European community systemic vasculitis clinical trials study group. *Mayo Clin Proc* 1997, **72:737–747**.

Diagnosis

Signs

• Well-demarcated, depigmented macules; chalky white or off-white. Off-white macules are transitional to complete depigmentation. Macules may coalesce to form patches. Depigmented skin forms convex border; vitiliginous skin appears to extend into normal skin. Hair in macules may depigment with time. Border may rarely be erythematous with thin zone of partial depigmentation. **Trichrome vitiligo**: Lesion borders may be hypopigmented, center depigmented, resulting in three color appearance.

Symptoms

• Lesions are asymptomatic; inflammatory lesions may be pruritic.

Distribution, depigmentation patterns

Focal: One to a few isolated macules. **Segmental**: Unilateral macules or patches, distribution often dermatomal; early onset; stable, nonfamilial, not associated with autoimmune diseases. **Generalized**: Most common; bilateral distribution often symmetrical; frequently involves face, axillae, groin, areolas, genitalia. Perioral, periorbital areas frequently involved. Dorsal hands, elbows also common.

Investigations

Wood's-light examination in darkened room improves contrast between normal and depigmented skin. **Laboratory**: If history suggests endocrine abnormalities, laboratory tests appropriate. Potassium hydroxide preparation helps differentiate vitiligo from tinea versicolor. **Biopsy**: May be needed to rule out other conditions. Long-standing lesions: complete loss of melanocytes; evolving lesions: partial loss.

Complications

Sunburn of depigmented skin is easy. **Disfigurement**: Serious psychosocial implications possible; in some cultures, associated social stigma because of previous confusion with leprosy. **Association** with alopecia areata, halo nevi, thyroid, diabetes mellitus, Addison's disease, pernicious anemia, myasthenia gravis.

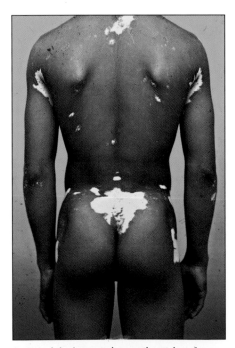

Scattered depigmented, smooth patches characteristic of vitiligo.

Differential diagnosis

Postinflammatory hypopigmentation: Asymptomatic, poorly demarcated macules, tan or off-white, at sites of a previous dermatosis, eg, psoriasis, atopic dermatitis, lichen planus.

Idiopathic guttate hypomelanosis: Asymptomatic, well-demarcated hypopigmented macules; round or angular; typically 2 to 10 mm; usually on sun-exposed areas, especially forearms, dorsal hands, anterior legs; spares face.

Pityriasis alba: Common on faces of darkly pigmented children; multiple, poorly demarcated hypopigmented macules; fine scale. Lesions may be mildly pruritic, respond to topical corticosteroids.

Other leukodermic conditions: Chemical depigmentation (occupational), lichen sclerosus et atrophicus, tinea versicolor, nevus anemicus, nevus depigmentosus, Futcher's lines, mycosis fungoides, piebaldism, leprosy, tuberous sclerosis.

Etiology

Unknown, but three hypotheses.

Autoimmune: Autoantibodies cause melanocyte destruction.

Self-destruction: Substance produced in synthesis of melanin results in cell death.

Neurogenic: Nerve endings release substance, such as acetylcholine, that destroys melanocytes; this theory helps explain segmental vitiligo.

Epidemiology

Affects all skin types. Approximately 1% of the population is affected; 50% of cases begin before age 20. There is a genetic predisposition with 30% of patients having a family history.

Samuel Beck and Thomas Meola

Treatment

Pharmacological treatment

Topical

Sunblocks, sunscreens: To preventing burning of involved skin and koebnerization (tanning) of uninvolved skin, resulting in increased contrast between tanned normal skin and depigmented skin.

Cosmetics (DyoDerm, Vitadyne stain, Dermablend, Covermark): Acceptable to many patients. Self-tanning products with dihydroxyacetone especially useful; they do not rub off and may not contain sunscreen.

Topical glucocorticoids: May be useful in treating small areas; must be used several months before significant repigmentation. Only 30% to 50% of patients respond. Monitor for development of atrophy, telangiectasias, acne, striae essential.

Systemic

•Skin bleaching with 20% monobenzyl ether of hydroquinone; option for patients with extensive depigmentation and only residual pigment. Must be applied twice daily for 9 to 12 months. Over 90% achieve complete depigmentation within 1 year. Depigmentation permanent. Patients must use appropriate sun protection to avoid repigmentation, sunburn. Beta-carotene 30–60 mg may be useful, to give the skin color.

Nonpharmacological treatment

Surgery

•Surgical minigrafts: some success, but risk of koebnerization. Best used in segmental or stable vitiligo.

Physical modalities

Phototherapy: Narrow-band ultraviolet B (UVB) used with some success. UVA (without psoralens); in combination with topical corticosteroids, is more effective than either modality alone.

Topical photochemotherapy (PUVA): Useful for limited involvement; 8-methoxypsoralen 0.1% applied 1 hour before UVA treatment. May need 100 or more treatments for complete repigmentation. Frequently, repigmented areas are darker than surrounding skin; usually blends in, with time.

Systemic photochemotherapy: For more extensive involvement and areas difficult to treat with topical psoralen.

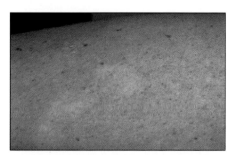

Round and oval hypopigmented patches, with very fine scaling, on the forearm of a patient with pityriasis alba. The subtle pink hue has almost entirely faded.

Treatment aims

Treatment is difficult and requires a motivated patient. The face is most responsive to therapy, whereas acral areas are least responsive.

Prognosis

Chronic, progressive, recurrent, unpredictable condition. Complete spontaneous repigmentation rare; significant spontaneous repigmentation unusual. After successful treatment, may recur, even in areas of previous involvement. Life stressors may exacerbate condition.

Segmental vitiligo: Stable; rarely progresses beyond area involved.

Follow-up and management

Encourage sun protection

Support organizations

National Vitiligo Foundation, 611 South Fleishel Ave. Tyler, TX 75701; Phone: (903) 531-0074; fax: (903) 525-1234; email: vitiligo@trimofran.org.

Diagnosis

Signs

Lichen sclerosus et atrophicus (LSA): Atrophic pink or hypopigmented to depigmented patches; telangiectasia, purpura, erosions, fissures, scarring; on vulva, perianal skin (often figure-of-eight pattern).

Lichen planus (LP): Violaceous, flat-topped papules with white surface scale or bright red erosions with occasional white reticulate pattern.

Vulvodynia (V): Occasionally vulvar erythema.

Symptoms

LSA: Can be asymptomatic but often pruritic, with pain, burning.

LP: Pruritus, discomfort, pain.

V: Itching, discomfort, pain, dyspareunia, apareunia, inability to have intercourse. Three types: vulvar vestibulitis (VV), pain to pressure in vestibule; dysesthetic vulvodynia (DV), diffuse pain; cyclic vulvitis (CV), symptoms worsen around menses.

Investigations

• Skin biopsy.

LSA: Epidermal atrophy, dermal sclerosis, telangiectasia.

LP: Band-like, lichenoid, lymphohistiocytic infiltrate at dermo-epidermal junction; jagged saw-toothed epidermal hyperplasia with wedge-shaped hypergranulosis, parakeratosis.

Complications

LSA: Apareunia, dyspareunia, superinfection with bacteria and yeast, secondary squamous-cell carcinoma.

LP: Squamous-cell carcinoma, dyspareunia, apareunia.

V: Dyspareunia, apareunia.

Differential diagnosis:

LSA: Lichen simplex chronicus, vitiligo, bullous diseases, lichen planus.

LP: Lichen sclerosis, plasma cell vulvitis, cicatricial pemphigoid, pemphigus vulgaris, erythema multiforme, lupus erythematosus.

V: Lichen sclerosis; lichen planus; lichen simplex chronicus; yeast, bacterial, viral infection; irritant or allergic contact dermatitis.

Etiology

LSA: Unknown. Few cases with familial clustering. May be associated with other autoimmune diseases.

LP: Unknown. Some cases may be associated with positivity for hepatitis C virus antibody or drug reaction (antimalarial agents, gold, penicillamine most likely; also quinine, β-blockers, hydroxyurea, captopril).

V: Unknown. May be type of neuropathy. Can occur after trauma. Previously thought to be associated with candidiasis and human papillomavirus (HPV) infection, but symptoms persist despite anticandidal therapy, negative cultures, and same incidence of infection with HPV as asymptomatic population.

Epidemiology

LSA: Unknown incidence. Typically affects postmenopausal women, prepubescent girls.

LP: Increased human leukocyte antigen (HLA)-DR1 and HLA-B7. Peak incidence: 30 to 60 years.

VV: Usually premenopausal, sexually active women; 75% nulliparous; white predeliction.

DV: Usually past third decade, but at any age.

CV: Usually premenopausal.

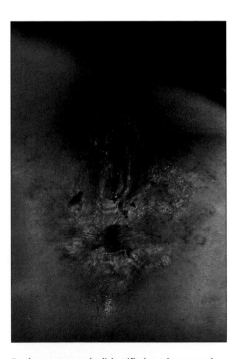

Well demarcated, atrophic, depigmented patches, pink hue; due to lichen sclerosus (kraurosis vulvae) covering anogenital areas and causing scarring of vulva, anus of a young girl. Petechiae present within; milia visible around lesions.

Erythematous, scaly, lichenified patches, excoriations involving anogenital area in extramammary Paget's disease. Untreated lesions become atrophic, possibly ulcerated. Resembles perianovulvar psoriasis, lichenified eczema.

Rebecca Baxt and Miriam Pomeranz

Treatment

Diet and lifestyle

• In vulvodynia, discontinue all currently used topical products, soaps, creams, douches; they may contribute to irritation or be causing allergic reaction.

Pharmacological treatment

Topical

LSA: 3–5 months of class-1 (high-potency) steroids, twice daily; maintenance: three-times-weekly application. For children, class-3 agent may work, in 2-month to 3-month course. Second line: estrogen, progesterone; 2% testosterone in petrolatum results disappointing. Tretinoin may be helpful.

LP: Class-1 steroids, twice daily for 1 month, then taper dose; long-term use may be necessary. May be improvement with metronidazole or clindamycin alone, or intravaginal corticosteroids, such as hydrocortisone acetate suppository.

V: White petrolatum or zinc oxide paste, lidocaine cream.

Systemic

LSA: Nighttime antihistamines or tricyclic antidepressants against pruritus; oral antibiotic if superinfected; consider fluconazole, 150 mg per week, to prevent candidal infection.

LP: For severe disease, prednisone, 40–60 mg/d for 2 weeks or until control of symptoms, then taper. Oral antibiotics (*eg*, clindamycin, cephalexin, dicloxacillin, doxycycline, minocycline), in standard doses may help. Also minocycline, 100 mg/d, plus nicotinamide, up to 2 g/d; dapsone, griseofulvin, cyclosporine, etretinate.

DV: Tricyclic antidepressants, *eg*, amitriptyline, 10 mg/d, increased to 100 mg or until resolution (several weeks) or serotonin reuptake inhibitors. Psychological evaluation may help.

VV: Local injections of interferon-α, 1 million U, three times per week, for 12 injections.

CV: Fluconazole, various regimens (*eg*, 150 mg twice weekly for 6 months, then taper), or topical antifungal creams. Itraconazole, 100 mg/d, during premenstrual week.

Surgery

VV: Vestibulectomy, vestibuloplasty, local excision, if condition unresponsive to pharmacological treatment.

Special therapeutic considerations

• Fluconazole, 150 mg/week, can be administered to prevent yeast infection in patients given systemic corticosteroid or antibiotic treatment.

V: Supportive methods include psychological counseling, pelvic-floor physical therapy, biofeedback.

Treatment aims

To relieve symptoms and reverse skin changes.

Prognosis

LSA: Chronic, but can be controlled with topical steroids; recurs if therapy is stopped. Clears in two-thirds of prepubescent girls at puberty.

LP: Usually resolves within 2 years; can be chronic in erosive disease.

V: Chronic. Symptoms can be relieved with supportive medical care and appropriate treatment.

Follow-up and management

LSA: Follow closely; squamous-cell carcinoma occurs in up to 5%; consider complete blood count, thyroid screening, diabetes screening.

LP: Monitor; squamous-cell carcinoma occurs in 5% with chronic erosive lichen planus.

V: Follow closely to monitor progress, offer support, rule out irritant dermatitis, allergic contact dermatitis, bacterial infections, yeast infections.

General references:

Ball SB, Wojnarowska F: Vulvar dermatoses: lichen sclerosus, lichen planus, and vulvar dermatitis/lichen simplex chronicus. *Semin Cut Med Surg* 1998, **17**:182–188.

Bohl TG: Vulvodynia and its differential diagnoses. *Semin Cut Med Surg* 1998, **17**:189–195.

Davis GD, Hutchinson CV: Clinical management of vulvodynia. *Clin Obstet Gynecol* 1999, **42**:221–233.

Rebecca Baxt and Miriam Pomeranz

Diagnosis

Signs

Xanthoma striatum: Yellow, pinkish, orange-brown macules that arise in skin folds and especially along the creases of the palms.

Xanthoma eruptivum: Small soft yellow papules that usually erupt on the buttocks, posterior aspects of thighs, or axillae.

Xanthoma tuberosum: Large nodules and plaques present on the elbows, knees, buttocks, and fingers.

Xanthoma tendineum: Yellow-orange plaques most commonly located along the Achilles tendons and the extensor tendons of the fingers

Xanthelasma palpebrarum: Soft, yellow or yellow-orange polygonal, planar papules that surround surrounding eyelids.

Xanthoma planum: Diffuse orange-yellow pigmentary areas with recognizable borders, in patients with normal lipid values. These lesions may be idiopathic or associated with leukemia or multiple myeloma.

Symptoms

• Lesions are asymptomatic.

• Chest pain and shortness of breath, when associated with atherosclerotic disease or abdominal pain associated with pancreatitis.

Investigations

• Fasting serum lipid profile, glucose.

• Skin biopsy: Dermal collections of foamy macrophages filled with lipid droplets (xanthoma cells). In tuberous xanthomas, many fibroblasts and some Touton giant cells are also present.

• If diffuse planar: Serum protein electrophoresis (SPEP) and urine protein electrophoresis.

Complications

• Atherosclerotic cardiovascular disease, pancreatitis.

Differential diagnosis

Xanthoma: Nevus sebaceum, Fox-Fordyce disease, adnexal tumors,

Xanthelasma: Milia, syringomata, conglomerates of comedones

Etiology

Xanthelasma palpebrarum: Normolipemic (90%). Usually develops in persons over 50 years of age. Those associated with familial hypercholesterolemia or familial dysproteinemia tend to develop in children or young adults.

Xanthoma tendineum: Familial hypercholesterolemia type 2: increased low density lipoproteins (LDL); very low density lipoproteins (VLDL) is normal)

Xanthoma tuberosum: Familial dyslipoproteinemia, familial hypetriglyceridemia,

Hypercholesterolemia: Type 3 presence of beta-VLDL, increased cholesterol, increased triglycerides; type 4, increased VLDL; type 2a, increased LDL, VLDL.

Xanthoma papuloeruptivum: Familial dyslipoproteinemia, familial hypertriglyceridemia, familial lipoprotein lipase deficiency. Type 2, increased LDL; type 4, increased VLDL; type 5, chylomicrons present; type 6, Massive chylomicronemia, VLDL, normal, LDL, HDL normal or decreased.

Xanthochromia and **xanthoma striatum palmare**: Familial dyslipoproteinemia: Type 3, presence of beta-VLDL; Tangier disease, decreased HDL levels.

Dina Began

Treatment

Diet and lifestyle
• Exercise and low-fat diet for hyperlipidemia.

Pharmacological treatment

Topical
• **Xanthelasma**: Trichloroacetic acid, 50%–100%
• **Xanthelasma**: Bichloracetic acid, 100%.

Systemic
• For elevated LDL-cholesterol: Bile acid sequestrant resins, nicotinic acid, the 3-hydroxy-3-methylglutaryl (HMG) coenzyme A reductase inhibitors (or statins), and estrogen (in postmenopausal women). For elevated triglyceride levels: Nicotinic acid, gemfibrozil, and the statins. Atorvastatin and simvastatin are particularly effective.

• For dysbetalipoproteinemia: Nicotinic acid, gemfibrozil, and clofibrate, in addition to modifications in diet and additional exercise.

• For elevated HDL levels: Nicotinic acid and estrogen (in postmenopausal women).

Surgery
• Excision for individual xanthomas and xanthelasmas.

• **Xanthclasma**: Pulsed CO_2, erbium, or pulsed dye laser; electrocautery.

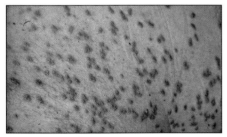

Small, reddish orange papules (eruptive xanthomas) on the buttock of a woman with diabetes mellitus and hypertriglyceridemia.

Treatment aims
To lower levels of cholesterol and triglycerides and to prevent atherosclerotic heart disease and pancreatitis.

Prognosis
Good with proper lifestyle, diet, exercise, and pharmacologic interventions.

Follow-up and management
Internal medicine and cardiology consultation recommended.

General references

Raulin C, Schoenermark MP, Werner S, *et al.*: Xanthelasma palpebrarum: treatment with the ultrapulsed CO2 laser. *Lasers Surg Med* 1999, 24:122–127.

Haygood LJ. Bennett JD. Brodell RT: Treatment of xanthelasma palpebrarum with bichloracetic acid. *Dermatol Surg* 1998, 24:1027–1031.

Bickley L: Yellow papules on a middle-aged woman. Eruptive xanthomatosis (EX). *Arch Dermatol* 1989, 125:288–289.

Yamamoto A, Hara H, Takaichi S, *et al.*: Wakasugi J, Tomikawa M: Effect of probucol on macrophages, leading to regression of xanthomas and atheromatous vascular lesions. *Am J Cardiol* 1988, 62:31B–36B.

Introduction

Alternative therapies include potentially effective medical treatments that are not widely taught to medical students or physicians, usually prescribed or recommended in traditional medicine, or generally available in US hospitals.

"Alternative and complementary medicine" (ACM) is a loose term that includes numerous treatments, ranging from apitherapy (treatment using bee venom) to yoga. The popularity of ACM is enormous. In 1990, about 60 million Americans spent an estimated $13.7 billion on ACM therapies, and Americans made more visits to ACM providers (425 million) than to primary care physicians (388 million).

However, perhaps as many as 70% of the persons receiving ACM therapies do not disclose this to their physicians. Increasingly, patients are asking their physicians' advice about ACM treatments, but are often disappointed when their requests are dismissed without consideration. Although serious complications from most treatments are remarkably uncommon, deaths have been attributed to the consumption of herbs, such as Herba ephedra (ma huang) and pennyroyal, and cases of kidney failure and urinary tract cancer have been blamed on dietary supplements containing herbs. Over time, more is being learned about the safety, efficacy, mechanism of action, and cost-effectiveness of individual alternative treatments.

Certainly, dermatology has a tradition of using many treatments that are "natural" and currently would be classified as "alternative" or "complementary." These include acetic acid compresses for *Pseudomonas* infection, leeches for wound debridement, capsaicin for neuralgia and psoriasis, sulfur for acne and rosacea, oatmeal (*Avena sativa*) and menthol for itching, and honey for wound healing. Studies of Manuka honey found enhanced wound healing of ulcers and burns, decreased pain, reduced infection and diminished malodor.

ACM methods

Acupuncture has been disappointing in improving skin disease, but it may be beneficial against pruritus and neuralgia.

Curcumin, the yellow pigment of turmeric (*Curcuma longa*), is a potent anti-inflammatory agent that has been shown to inhibit leukotriene formation and platelet aggregation, and to stabilize neutrophilic lysosomal membranes. At higher doses, it stimulates cortisone secretion by the adrenal glands. The usual dose is 250–400 mg, three times daily.

Glycorrhetic acid, a metabolite of licorice root (*Glycyrrhiza glabra*), inhibits the activity of leukotrienes, prostaglandins E-2, and phospholipase A-2. This agent has anti-inflammatory effects, with clinical efficacy comparable to that of topical corticosteroids, against contact dermatitis, seborrheic dermatitis, and psoriasis. Additionally, it enhances the effect of topical corticosteroids. Topical preparations are not currently available, but compresses can be made by adding 3 gm (1 teaspoon) of the extract to 150 mL of water. The oral dose is 1 gm of the powder, 1 teaspoon of the fluid extract, or one half teaspoon of the solid extract, three to four times daily, before meals. It is recommended for eczema, lichen simplex chronicus, and seborrheic dermatitis.

Salicin, a product in the bark of the willow tree (*Silix alba*), relieves pruritus and pain, and is available in topical preparations. A tea can be made by brewing 1–2 teaspoons of powdered bark in 1 cup of boiling water for 10 minutes; as much as five cups per day can be consumed. Tincture is also used, commonly in the amount of 1–2 mL, three times per day. The daily intake of salicin is typically 60–120 mg per day. Like salicylates, possible complications include Reye's syndrome in children and gastrointestinal ulcers.

Chamomile (*Matricaria* or *Chamaemelum*) contains terpenoids, with anti-inflammatory and soothing effects against a number of inflammatory dermatosis, when used in creams or compresses. A tea can be made with 3 gm of whole flower head, and can be taken 3 to 4 times daily, between meals. It is especially beneficial for dry, eczematous lesions.

Aloe vera has been found to enhance wound healing and to improve psoriasis. It can be applied directly from the cut leaves or from topical preparations.

Bromelain, a mixture of proteolytic enzymes derived from the pineapple plant, has anti-inflammatory activity related to inhibited production of pro-inflammatory prostaglandins and induced production of anti-inflammatory (Series I) prostaglandins. It also reduces capillary permeability. This agent appears to reduce pain and swelling following skin surgery, and to speed healing. The dose is 80–320 mg, two to three times daily, for 8 to 10 days.

Calendula (*Calendula officinalis*) is derived from the marigold plant, and has soothing and anti-inflammatory effects due to flavonoids and saponins. As a tincture or ointment, it is used topically, three times a day. It may also be applied for 3 days before elective skin surgery, because it is an antiseptic and enhances wound healing.

Witch hazel (*Hamamelis virginiana*) reduces inflammation. When topically applied, twice daily, in a cream, ointment or compress, it has soothing antipruritic and astringent effects, which are particularly beneficial in acute eczema.

Yarrow (*Achillea millefollum*) contains anti-inflammatory ingredients, such as chamazulene, and has anti-pruritic and astringent effects when used externally in compresses or baths. It is especially beneficial for chronic eczema. A tea can be prepared by steeping 1–2 teaspoons (5–10 grams) of yarrow in 250 mL (1 cup) of boiling water for 10–15 minutes. Three cups a day can be consumed, or the tea can be applied topically. Also, 3–4 mL of tincture can be ingested three times daily.

Oak bark (*Quercus alba*) contains tannins, such as proanthocyanidins and ellagitannins, which give it astringent, vasoconstrictive, and cooling properties. In compresses (20 gm of cut herb per liter of water, boiled for 15 minutes and allowed to cool), it provides symptomatic relief of inflamed, oozing skin lesions, such as those of acute contact dermatitis.

Quercetin and **hesperidin** are bioflavinoids, which inhibit histamine release from mast cells and basophils, as well as phospholipase A-2 and lipoxygenase. They are beneficial against eczema and possibly urticaria. The dose of quercetin is 400 mg, two or three times daily, with vitamin C.

Other anti-inflammatory herbs include **walnut leaf** (*Juglans regia*), containing ellagitannins, which have soothing and astringent effects when applied to weeping lesions in compresses; **chickweed** (*Stellaria media*), which is antipruritic when used in baths, lotions or creams; **plantain** (*Plantago species*) **juice**, which can be topically applied against pruritus; **St. John's Wort** (*Hypericum perforatum*); and **Coleus forskolii**, which is a potent herb with anti-histaminic activity.

Comfrey (*Symphytum officinale*) contains the cell-proliferating agent allantoin, which debrides fibrinous exudate and promotes granulation tissue of skin ulcers. It can be used as a gel, plaster or solution.

Gingko biloba, two capsules, three times daily, enhances circulation and may be helpful in healing of chronic vascular ulcers.

Gotu kola or Indian pennywort *Centella asiatica* improves collagen synthesis, enhance connective tissue repair, and improves healing of skin wounds and ulcers.

Emollients include **comfrey** (*Symphytum officinalis*), **marshmallow** (*Althaea officinalis*), **mallow** (*Malva sylvestris*) and **slippery elm** (*Ulmus fulva*).

Antimicrobial agents: Most notable of the essential oils, which are all antimicrobial, are **thyme** (*Thymus vulgaris*), **eucalyptus** (*Eucalyptus globus*); **tea tree** (*Melalucca* species); **myrrh** (*Commiphora mol-mol*) and **goldenseal** (*Hydrastis canadensis*).

Essential fatty acids: Eicosapentanoic acid (EPA), gamma-linoleic acid (GLA; present in primrose oil), and docosahexanoic acid (DHA; present in fish oils) are the most effective essential fatty acids because they bypass the desaturation enzyme steps. Of these, flaxseed, borage, black currant, and evening primrose oils are usually recommended in dermatology. These oils increase levels of anti-inflammatory prostaglandins; supplementation for several months may improve atopic dermatitis and psoriasis. Anecdotal reports indicate that evening primrose oil (linoleic acid) improves chapped, irritated skin. For psoriasis, an alternative medicine practitioner may recommend flaxseed oil, 1 tablespoon, three times daily, in addition to glucosamine sulfate, 500 mg, two to three times, daily, and fumaric acid, 100–200 mg, three times daily, and topical salicylic acid and glucosamine sulfate.

Immunoenhancers: **Astragalus** enhances the immune response by promoting the activity of T lymphocytes and interferon. **Garlic** may stimulate the activity of natural killer cells. **Goldeneal** stimulates white blood cells and has antimicrobial effects.

L-lysine, at a dose of 1000 mg, three times daily, between meals, is often (despite the lack of scientific support) recommended for herpes simplex, in addition to topical application of either lemon balm (*Melissa officianalis*), licorice balm, or red Alaskan dulse, three times daily. Vitamin C, 1000 mg, two to three times a day, and tinctures of echinacea, Siberian ginseng, stinging nettles (*Urtica dioica*)and goldenseal, orally, may also be added to the regimen.

Vitamins and minerals: **Vitamin A** is beneficial against acne, psoriasis, pityriasis rubra pilaris, ichthyosis, and other disorders of keratinization, but prolonged use of doses greater than 50,000 IU causes multiple complications. **Beta carotene** may be less toxic. **Vitamin C** is an anti-oxidant that decreases histamine levels and may retard aging. **Vitamin E** is an antioxidant that may retard aging and also inhibits the arachidonic acid pathway and decreases pro-inflammatory prostaglandins. **Zinc picolinate**, at a daily dosage of 150 mg,

has been used to enhance wound healing, but lower amounts (30–60 mg) may be equally effective. Zinc may also possibly be beneficial as a supplement in the treatment of acne, dermatitis and psoriasis. When recommending high amounts of zinc, copper, 2–3 mg daily, and selenium, 200, μg, should be supplemented. **Vitamins** are often recommended by alternative medicines practitioners for eczema (Vitamin A, 50,000 IU/day; vitamin E, 400 IU/day; zinc picolinate, 50 mg/day, decreased as conditions clears; quercetin, one eighth to one quarter teaspoon, 3 times a day; and evening Primrose oil; two to four capsules, 3 times a day) and for acne (vitamin A, 100,000 IU/day for 3 months; vitamin, E 400 IU/day; vitamin, C 1000 mg/day; zinc picolinate, 50 mg/day; selenium, 200 μg/day; and Brewer's yeast, 1 tablespoon, twice a day)

Dietary changes, despite the lack of scientific substantiation, are often recommended by practitioners of alternative medicine for eczema (elimination of cows' milk, eggs, cheese, fish, sugar, food additives), acne (elimination of margarine, shortening, milk products, saturated fats in red meats, refined sugars; institution of high-fiber diet), herpes simplex (elimination of nuts, chocolates), psoriasis (avoidance of alcohol, wheat, nuts, citrus foods, spicy foods together; institution of high-fiber diet).

Other regimens: In addition to anti-inflammatory, astringents, antimicrobial and antipruritic substances, practitioners of alternative medicine may prescribe regimens that include agents considered to be **lymphatic tonics** (*Galium aparine, Urtica dioica*; alternatives: *Arctium lappa, Galium aparine, Rumex crispus, Urtica dioica*); **nerve relaxants** (*Valeriana officinalis, Verbena officinalis*); **diuretics** (*Arctium lappa, Galium aparine, Urtica dioica*); **bepatics** (*Arctium lappa, Galium aparine, Rumex crispus, Verbena officinalis*), or **vulneraries** (topical herbs that enhance wound healing). For example, a regimen for **eczema** may include *Fumaria officinalis, Galium aparine, Scrophularia nodosa, Trifolium pratense, Viola tricolor, Urtica dioica, Arctium lappa, Berberis aquifolium, and Hydrastis canadensis*), while a regimen for acne may include *Iris versicolor, Arctium lappa, Echinacea species, Galium aparine* (equal parts to 5 mL of tincture, three times a day), Urtica dioica (an infusion drunk 2 or 3 times a day), *Calendula officinalis* (applied topically as a wash or an infusion mixed with distilled Witch Hazel, and green clay or betonite clay masks).

General references

Evans FQ: The rational use of glycyrrhetinic acid in dermtology. *Br J Clin Pract* 1958, **12**:269–274.

Seamon KB, Padgett W, Daly JW: Forskolin: unique diterpine activator of adenylate cyclase in membranes and intact cells. Proc Natl Acad Sci 1981, **78**:3363–3367.

Berth-Jones J, Thompson J, Graham-Brown RA: Evening primrose oil and atopic eczema. Lancet 1995, **342**:520.

Teelucksingh S, Mackie AD, Burt D, *et al*,: Potentiation of hydrocortisone activity in skin by glycyrrhetinic acid. Lancet 1990, **335**:1060–1063.

Graf J. Herbal anti-inflammatory agents for skin disease. Skin Therapy Lett 1999 **3**:1–4.

Jeannette Graf and Miguel Sanchez

Appendix B: Compounding

Introduction

The scientific art of prescribing a compound is now almost exclusively practiced by dermatologists. Compounding permits the formulation of tailor-made products for a skin condition that is difficult to treat or has been recalcitrant to commercially available topical medications. Although insurance does not often reimburse for compounded products, patients may be willing to purchase a product formulated especially for them. Many pharmacists are willing to prepare prescribed compounds, also known as extemporaneous prescriptions, but it is important to find a pharmacist with experience in compounding.

A compounded medication contains two to three parts:

Basis: Principal drug that gives the prescription its chief activity.

Adjuvant: Drug that aids or increases the action of the principal ingredient.

Vehicle: Ingredient used as a solvent, to increase the bulk, or to dilute the mixture.

When abbreviated Latin terms are used in the body (inscription) of the prescription, they are directions for the pharmacist; when used in the label (signature), they are directions for the patient. See Table 1.

Commonly used ingredients in compounds include ethyl and isopropyl alcohol (antiseptic and usually used as a vehicle for tinctures), benzoic acid (keratolytic, preservative, antiseborrheic, antiseptic, antifungal agent), camphor (antipruritic and anti-inflammatory), corticosteroids (antipruritic and anti-inflammatory), menthol (antipruritic and anti-inflammatory), phenol (bactericidal and antipruritic), resorcinol (antipruritic, keratolytic, bactericidal, and fungicidal), salicylic acid (keratolytic), sulfur (keratolytic, antifungal, antiscabetic), tars (keratoplastic and antipruritic, faintly antiseptic and antiparasitic), urea (proteolytic and keratolytic).

Medications are incorporated into bases, which are important because they affect the penetration of the active ingredients as well as the ease with which they are applied.

Bases

Oleaginous vehicle (petrolatum, mineral oil).

Absorptive (water absorbable) vehicle (Aquaphor ointment, Anhydrous lanolin ointment, Polysorb Hydrate cream).

Oil-in-water emulsion (Acid Mantle cream, Dermabase cream, hydrophilic ointment, Lubriderm lotion, Nutraderm cream and lotion, Vanicream): produces a cooling sensation; generally marketed as lotions.

Water-in-oil emulsion (Eucerin cream): allows some heat retention; generally marketed as creams.

Shake lotions (*eg*, calamine lotion): suspensions of relatively inert powders in water.

Water-soluble vehicle (PEG ointment, Polybase).

Liquid vehicle (Cetaphil lotion, C-Solve, Vehicle/N Mild, isopropyl alcohol, ethyl alcohol).

The following compounds have been used to treat the diseases listed:

Scalp acne

Salicylic acid 1% to 5%.

    Resorcinol 3% to 6%.

    Isopropyl alcohol.

    Water a.a. q.s.a.d. 8 ounces.

• Percentages of active ingredients may be varied; water may be omitted. Other ingredients, such as menthol, can be added depending on the area to be treated. Resorcinol can stain blond hair and may be omitted in scalp preparations.

Acne

Salicylic acid 1% to 5%, with isopropyl alcohol (70%) q.s.a.d. 240 mL

Clindamycin phosphate, 150 mg: dissolve contents of 4 capsules in isopropyl alcohol (70%) q.s.a.d. 240 mL

Pruritic dermatitis

Triamcinalone cream 0.5% (or fluocinonide cream 0.05%) 15.0 g.

    Menthol 0.5%.

    Phenol 0.5%.

    Cetaphil moisturizing cream q.s.a.d. 120 g.

(0.5% camphor or 2% to 5% liquor; carbonis detergens may be added).

Recalcitrant hand eczema

Crude coal tar or liquid carbonis detergens 5.0%.

Triamcinolone acetonide cream 0.5%, 15.0 g.

Cold cream q.s.a.d., 120 g.

Psoriasis

Lidex cream 0.05% 30.0 g.

    Lubriderm lotion q.s.a.d., 120.0 g

Coal tar solution 5%, with Lubriderm lotion, q.s.a.d. 120.0 g.

Scalp psoriasis

Salicylic acid 5%, with olive oil q.s.a.d., 120 mL.

Drying lotions

Sulfur precipitate 5%.

    Resorcinol 6%.

    Calamine lotion q.s.a.d., 120 mL.

Warts

Salicylic acid 15%

Lactic acid 15%

Flexible collodion q.s.a.d., 60 mL.

Hyperkeratotic tinea pedis

Salicylic acid 5%–10%.

Benzoic acid 5%–10%.

Petrolatum q.s.a.d., 120 g.

Palmoplantar keratosis

Urea 20%.

Salicylic acid 5%.

Petrolatum q.s.a.d., 120 g.

Paronychia

Thymol 3.0 %.

70% alcohol q.s.a.d., 60 mL.

Table 1. Abbreviated Latin terms

Abbreviation	Latin	English
ana	ana	equal part of each
a	ante	before
a.c.	ante cibum	before meals
gtt	gutta, guttae	drop, drops
p.c.	post cibum	after meals
q.s.a.d.	quantum sufficiat	sufficient amount to make

General references

Practical Pediatric Dermatology Edited by Leider M. St. Louis: C.V. Mosby; 1956,

The Pharmacologic Bases of Therapeutics, edn 4. Edited by Goodman L, Gilman A. New York: Macmillan; 1970.

Textbook of Dermatology. Edited by Rook A, Wilkinson DS. London: Blackwell Scientific Publications; 1968.

Introduction

Cryosurgery uses cryogenic agents to treat benign, premalignant, and malignant cutaneous lesions by causing local destruction of tissue through rapid freezing and slow thawing (minimum tissue temperatures, –25 °C to –60 °C). Malignant lesions require repeated freeze-thaw cycles.

It is particularly useful for patients who are receiving anticoagulants, are allergic to local anesthetics, or have a pacemaker. Liquid nitrogen (the most commonly used cryogen) is applied using an open spray (OS), cotton-tipped dipstick applicator (D), or cryoprobe (P).

Treatment methods

Open spray method: By use of a spray gun, liquid nitrogen is sprayed with the nozzle held 1 cm from skin surface on the center of lesion until ice ball that encompasses lesion and margin forms. If more than one freeze-thaw cycle (FTC) needed, complete thawing should occur before next cycle. Feathering (F) is a technique used for lesions in which the freeze required for cure may induce permanent hypopigmentation. Border is sprayed until beginning of ice formation to produce mild hypopigmentation, thereby diminishing contrast between treated and untreated areas.

Cotton-tipped dipstick applicator: Used to treat superficial, benign, or flat lesions. Dip cotton wool bud into cup containing liquid nitrogen and firmly apply bud to lesion until narrow halo of ice forms around bud. Reapplication may be necessary.

Cryoprobe: Probe is attached to liquid nitrogen spray gun and applied directly to the lesion. Once the ice forms, the probe and lesion are gently retracted to prevent further injury.

Relative contraindications

Blood dyscrasias of unknown origin, cold intolerance, Raynaud's phenomenon, cold urticaria, cryoglobulinemia, cryofibrinogenemia, pyoderma gangrenosum, collagen and autoimmune disease. Hypopigmentation is common in dark-skinned patients. Inner canthus of eye, nasolabial and retroauricular folds, hair-bearing areas, skin with superficial nerves, and pretibial area are less favored treatment sites.

Complications

Pain, erythema, edema, blisters, weeping, eschar formation, infection, scarring, hypopigmentation, alteration of sensation, alopecia.

Postoperative care

Wash lesion with soap and water once to twice daily. Leave treated area open to the air until blister ruptures. If inflamed, may use antibiotic ointment. Drain vesicles with sterile needle if vesicles are bothersome.

Table 1. Indications and suggested freeze times

Condition	Technique	Freeze time (seconds)	FTC	Session/intervals	Margin response
Benign lesions					
Acne scarring					
Face	OS	5	1	1–3/4–8 wks	1 mm; good/excellent
Back	OS	5–15	1	1–3/4–8 wks	1 mm; good/excellent
Cherry angioma	P	10	1	1	1 mm; good
Chondrodermatitis nodularis helices	OS or P	15	1	2–3/4–8 wks	2 mm; 20% improved
Dermatofibroma	OS or P	30	1	1–3/4–8 wks	2 mm; 90% improved
Keloid	OS or P	15–30	1	5–10/4–8 wks	1 mm; variable
Lentigo simplex	OS or P	Light	1	1	Feathering; good
Sebaceous hyperplasia	OS or P	5–15	1	1	1 mm; good
Seborrheic keratosis	OS, D, or P	Flat, 8–15; thick, 15–30	1	1	1 mm; excellent
Solar lentigo	OS or P	5–10	1	1	Feathering; good
Skin tag	OS	5–10	1	1	1 mm; excellent
Tattoo	OS	30	2	variable/4–6 wks	1 mm; 54% improved
Verruca vulgaris	OS or D	10–60 (per thickness)	1	1	1–2 mm; excellent
Premalignant lesions					
Actinic keratosis	OS or D	5–10	1	1	2 mm; 98.8% improved
Hypertrophic actinic keratosis	OS or D	20	1	1	2 mm; excellent
Skin cancer					
Kaposi's sarcoma	OS	10–30	2	3/3wks	3 mm; 80% improved
Keratoacanthoma	OS	30	2	1	5 mm; variable
Nodular, superficial basal cell carcinoma	OS or P	30–60	2	1	3–4 mm; 96% improved
Squamous cell carcinoma (depth less than 3 mm)	OS or P	30–60	2	1	5 mm; 94% improved

General references

Drake LA, Ceilley RI, Cornelison RL, et al.: Guidelines of care for cryosurgery. *J Am Acad Dermatol* 1994, **31**:648–653.

Thai KE, Sinclair RD: Cryosurgery of benign skin lesions. *Australas J Dermatol* 1999, **40**:175–184.

Sinclair RD, Tzermias C, Dawber RPR: Cosmetic cryosurgery. In *Textbook of Cosmetic Dermatology*. Edited by Baran R, Maibach HI. London: Martin Dunitz; 1998:691–700.

Sinclair RD, Dawber RPR: Cryosurgery of malignant and pre-malignant diseases of the skin: a simple approach. *Australas J Dermatol* 1995, **36**:133–142.

Kuflik EG: Cryosurgery updated. *J Am Acad Dermatol* 1994, **31**:925–944.

Immunofluorescence

Test conducted on blood and/or tissue specimens to determine if, present in the blood or fixed in skin, there are autoantibodies that react against skin antigens. These tests are useful to confirm diagnoses and help in the management of autoimmune blistering diseases, including pemphigus, bullous pemphigoid, herpes gestationis, cicatricial pemphigoid, linear IgA bullous dermatosis, epidermolysis bullosa, and paraneoplastic pemphigus. They are also very useful in the evaluation and management of patients with lupus erythematosus, immune complex disease and porphyria.

Indirect immunofluorescence

This test is used to detect circulating anti-skin antibodies and is performed on serum. The serum is incubated with sections of fresh tissue containing stratified squamous epithelium (monkey or guinea pig esophagus). Antibodies in the serum that react to antigens in the skin are visualized with flourescein-labeled anti-human IgG and/or IgM or IgA. The test is positive for circulating antibodies to intercellular (IC) antigens in approximately 70% to 80% of patients with active pemphigus. There is a relation between the level of antibody and the activity of the disease. Approximately 5% of normal individuals will have low levels of antibodies to ABO blood group antigens, which give a staining pattern indistinguishable from that seen in pemphigus. Low levels of intercellular antibodies can also be seen in patents with drug reactions or fungal infections.

Circulating antibodies to basement membrane zone (BMZ) are present in approximately 70% of patients with active bullous pemphigoid, in approximately 1/3 of those with cicatricial pemphigoid, and in approximately 50% of patients with acquired epidermolysis. Patients with herpes gestationis have complement-fixing BMZ antibodies, which may be visualized in a modification of complement-fixing indirect immunofluorescence.

Combinations of both intercellular and BMZ antibodies can be seen in mixed bullous disease and paraneoplastic pemphigus. The specific antigens to which these antibodies are directed can be determined by immunoblotting techniques, but these procedures are still experimental.

Direct immunofluorescence

This test is conducted to detect abnormal deposits of antibodies or other proteins in the skin. The best site to conduct this test is at the edge of blisters or in the center of urticarial lesions. When biopsing normal skin to evaluate systemic lupus, the best location is sun-exposed extensive surface of the forearm or the deltoid area.

The biopsy specimen must by immediately frozen in liquid nitrogen or placed in a special transport medium. The specimen cannot be preserved in the standard formaldehyde solution used to preserve specimens for histology.

In the laboratory, the specimen is cut on a cryostat, and incubated with fluorescein-labeled antibodies to human IgG, IgM, IgA, complement and/or fibrin.

Abnormal intercellular deposits of any Ig and/or complement will be present in approximately 90% of lesions of pemphigus. This test is more sensitive than indirect immunofluorescence.

Abnormal deposits of any Ig and/or complement will be present in approximately 90% of lesions of pemphigus. This test is more sensitive than indirect immunofluorescence.

Abnormal deposits of any Ig and/or complement can be found at the BMZ in 80-90% of patients with bullous pemphigoid, cicatricial pemphigoid or herpes gestationis. Linear deposits at the BMZ consisting only of IgA are diagnostic of linear IgA bullous dermatosis. Granular or broad homogenous deposits of any immunoglobulin and/or complement at the BMZ are present in 80% to 90% of lesions of discoid or systemic lupus, and in 50% of normal skin of patients with SLE, but not DLE. These deposits can be present in sun-damaged facial skin of otherwise normal patients, or in the facial skin of patients with rosacea. Combinations of deposits at the BMZ and around blood vessels can be seen in porphyria and in vasculitis. In porphyria, these deposits are very broad and homogenous. In vasculitis they are sparser, thinner and granular.

Microscopic examination for fungi

The direct examination of cutaneous material is the most important laboratory procedure available to determine if a skin lesion is caused by a fungus. Correct selection of the specimen is important. If possible, the active borders of a skin lesion should be scraped, nail material abutting normal-appearing nail obtained, or obviously damaged hair plucked. The specimen should be placed on a slide, a drop or two of 10% KOH (or NaOH) added, and the specimen covered with a cover slip. The purpose of the KOH is to soften the keratin and to dissolve the intracellular cement, changing the mass of horny cells into a more-or-less unicellular preparation, making visible any fungi present. This process of "clearing" can be hastened by gentle warming of the KOH preparation and by applying pressure onto the coverslip, flattening the specimen. It is not possible to give the length of time that it takes before a KOH prep is ready to be read, but this combination of chemical, thermal and physical manipulation clears almost all preparations rapidly.

Once a scraping has been cleared, it is ready for microscopic examination. Making sure that the microscopic light is low and diffuse (too much light is detrimental) and that you are focused on the specimen between the slide and coverslip, the search for fungi can begin. Scan the entire area under the coverslip for suspicious fields using the low-power (10X) lens. Confirm any suspicious fields by examination under high-dry (40X) lens.

Ringworm fungi in skin and nails can be recognized by the fact that they form only filaments and arthroconidia in vivo. The filaments grow by elongation, with the subsequent formation of septa (cross-walls). The filaments are of various lengths and my branch. Eventually the filaments disarticulate at the septa forming arthroconidia. At first the arthroconidia retain the linear arrangement of the filaments from which they were derived, but later may become scattered in a haphazard manner. Under suitable conditions, the arthroconidia may germinate to form new filaments, completing the life cycle of ringworm fungi in skin and nails.

Candida species (especially *C. albicans*) can be differentiated from ringworm fungi in KOH preparations by the fact that they do not form filaments and arthroconidia, but rather grow in the form pseudofilaments (false filaments), which bear blastoconidia (buds) as well as free, budding yeast cells in varying numbers. Another fungal disease that lends itself to rapid diagnosis by the KOH examination is tinea versicolor, caused by *Malassezzia furfur*.

Culturing of clinical material complements the KOH test in the mycological examination of skin, hair and nails.

Four simple steps must be employed to maximize the yield of cultures:

Use of a standard medium: Since the gross morphology of fungi growing on a culture medium may be dramatically influenced by the composition of the medium, it is important that a medium of standard composition be employed in different laboratories so that the description of fungal morphology given in one laboratory can be recognized in another. The medium developed by Dr. Raimond Sabouraud in Paris at the beginning of the 20th century has generally been accepted as the standard by mycologists throughout the world. It is a simple medium, consisting of peptone (1%), dextrose (2% to 4%) and agar (1.5% to 2.0%) called Sabouraud Dextrose Agar (SDA). Although most pathogenic fungi grow well on this medium, it is also supports the growth of fast-growing bacteria and saprophytic fungi, which may inhibit the growth of the pathogens which are of interest to clinicians. In order to make SDA more selective, antibiotics, such as chloramphenicol (to inhibit bacteria) and cycloheximide (to inhibit saprophytic fungi) are added to SDA. This medium is available commercially under a number of trade names. These selective media are strongly recommended for office use. Although no dermatophyte is inhibited by these media, certain other pathogenic fungi, such as *Cryptococcus neoformans*, are markedly inhibited so it cannot be used indiscriminately. Another medium in wide use for the isolation of dermatophytes is Dermatophyte Test Medium (DTM). DTM is also a selective medium (containing antibacterials and cycloheximide) but, in addition, also contains the pH indicator, phenol red. The phenol red turns red when the medium becomes alkaline, as when dermatophytes grow on it, but remains yellow (usually) when saprophytic fungi grow on it. Thus the change of DTM from yellow (uninoculated) to red usually heralds the growth of a dermatophyte.

Access to oxygen: Fungi are aerobic organisms and growth may be inhibited if there is not free access to air. Once culture media are inoculated, any caps on the containers must remain loosened to allow for the diffusion of air into the culture bottle and the diffusion of metabolic gasses out.

Temperature: Fungi grow best at temperatures in the range of 25–30°C (room temperature). Most dermatophytes are inhibited at body temperature. Incubation of culture media on a shelf (protected from light) or in a drawer is satisfactory.

Time of incubation: Experience has shown that two weeks of incubation is usually sufficient to allow characteristic growth of dermatophytes to develop, although some laboratories prefer longer periods.

The cultures that develop on the culture medium can often be identified by gross examination of the colonies which form (texture, color of the surface and undersurface, formation of convolutions, rate of growth) as well as by microscopic examination of the colonies (culture mount). At times, ancillary tests, such as nutritional studies or hair perforation tests, must be performed for definitive identification.

Broad-band ultraviolet B (UVB) light

1. Determine the skin phototype (SPT).
2. Determine the minimal erythema dose (MED).
3. For SPT I or II, start at 50% of the MED and increase the exposure by 50%, 40%, 30%, 20%, and 10 % of previous dose, on each successive treatment.
4. For SPT III to VI, start at 60% of the MED and increase the exposure by 50%, 40%, 30%, 20%, and 10 % of previous dose, on each successive treatment.
5. After the fifth treatment, increase the doses by 5% to 15%, as tolerated by the patient.
6. Begin facial exposure at 20 mJ/cm^2 and increased by 2.5mJ/cm^2. Do not exceed two MEDs.
7. Extra exposure can be given to the upper and lower extremities, if necessary.
8. Adjust treatment if the patient develops erythema or tenderness.
9. Participant should wear ultraviolet protective goggles during therapy.
10. Shield the male genitalia, when possible.
11. The ideal treatment frequency is three times per week.
12. Applying mineral oil to the skin helps with light absorption.
13. A significant beneficial response should be seen by 25 treatments.
14. After an adequate response has been achieved, the treatment frequency can be decreased to twice a week and then to once a week.

Narrow-band ultraviolet B light

This treatment modality uses a narrow portion of the spectrum of the UVB spectrum, located around 311 nm. It has been found to be more efficacious in the treatment of psoriasis than broad band UVB. The protocol for narrow band differs from broad band in the increments by which the light is increased after the first treatment.

1. Obtain the narrow-band MED.
2. For SPT I or II, start at 50% of the MED, and increase the exposure by 20% of previous dose, on each of the next four successive treatments.
3. For SPT III to VI, start at 60% of the MED, and increase the exposure by 20% of previous dose, on each of the next four successive treatments.
4. After the fifth treatment increase the doses by 5%–15% as tolerated by the patient.

Psoralen with ultraviolet light A (UVA) photochemotherapy (PUVA)

1. Prior to initiation of therapy, the patient's eyes must be examined.
2. The dose of 8-methoxypsoralen is 0.4mg/kg, to be administered 1 hour prior to phototherapy.
3. Determine skin type by history.
4. The initial dose of UVA is one half of the SPT in J/cm^2, for example, if the patient's skin is type III, start at 1.5 J/cm^2.
5. Erythrodermic and vitiliginous skin is considered to be SPT I.
6. Increase the dose by 0.25–0.5 J/cm^2.
7. Extra exposure can be provided to the upper and lower extremities.
8. Initially, patients should be treated at a maximum of three times per week and at a minimum of two times per week, but not on successive days.
9. Participants should wear UV goggles during the treatment.
10. The male genitalia should be shielded during procedure.
11. Patients should have a significant response by 20 treatments.
12. UV protective eyewear should be worn for 24 hours following the ingestion of 8-methoxypsoralen.
13. If the patient develops erythema, blisters, or tenderness she or he should be evaluated by a physician prior to any further treatment.
14. The maximum dose depends on the SPT; however, these doses my be exceeded when necessary.
15. After an adequate response has been achieved. the treatment frequency can be decreased to twice a week, once a week, and then discontinued.

For skin phototypes I and II, the maximum recommended dosage is 8 J/cm^2; for types III and IV, 12 J/cm^2; for types V and VI, 20 J/cm^2.

Topical hand/foot PUVA therapy

1. The initial dose is 0.25 J/cm ^{2}; it should be increased by 0.25 J/cm^2.
2. The maximum exposure should not exceed 20 J/cm^2.
3. If the patient develops erythema, blisters, or tenderness, he or she should be evaluated by a physician.

Changes in dose if treatments are missed (for all UV therapy modalities)

One or two treatments: maintain previous dose.

One or two weeks: decrease by 33%

Two to four weeks: decrease by 66%

More than one month: start over at initial dose

- If a patient is placed on an oral retinoid, the dosage should be reduced by 25%.

* Adapted from the *Ronald O. Perelman Department of Dermatology Resident Handbook*. New York: New York University School of Medicine; 2000.

Disease	Infectious agent	First choice(s) for therapy	Alternative choice(s) for therapy	Comments
Bacterial Infections				
Actinomycosis	*Actinomyces israelii*	Ampicillin, 50 mg/kg/d, i.v., 4–6 weeks, followed by amoxicillin, 500 mg, p.o., t.i.d., 6–12 months. Penicillin G, 10–20 million units/d, i.v., 4–6 weeks, followed by penicillin V, 2–4 g/d, p.o., 6–12 months.	Doxycycline, 100 mg, p.o. or i.v., b.i.d. Ceftriaxone, 2.0 g, i.v., q. 12h. Clindamycin, 900 mg, i.v., q. 8h. Chloramphenicol, 50–60 mg/kg/d, p.o. or i.v., divided, q. 6h.	Duration: 4–6 weeks, i.v., then 6–12 months, p.o. May need surgical drainage and excision of sinus tracts, necrotic or fibrotic tissues.
Wound infection, contaminated in fresh water	*Aeromonas hydrophila*	Ciprofloxacin, 500–750 mg, p.o., b.i.d.	Trimethoprim/sulfamethoxazole, double-strength tablet, p.o., b.i.d.	Duration: 7–10 days.
Anthrax	*Bacillus anthracis*	Penicillin G, 20 million units/d, divided q. 6h.	Ciprofloxacin, 750 mg p.o., b.i.d., or 400 mg, i.v., b.i.d. Doxycycline, 100 mg, p.o. or i. v., b.i.d.	Duration: up to 6 weeks. Occupational risk: immunize.
Oroya fever, Verruga peruana	*Bartonella bacilliformis* (frequent *Salmonella* super-infection)	Chloramphenicol, 500 mg, p.o. or i.v., q.i.d.	Tetracycline, 500 mg, p.o. or i.v., q.i.d.	
Bacillary angiomatosis	*Bartonella henselae*, *Bartonella quintana*	Clarithromycin, 500 mg, p.o., b.i.d. Azithromycin, 250 mg, p.o., qd. Ciprofloxacin, 500–750 mg, p.o., b.i.d.	Erythromycin, 500 mg, p.o., q.i.d. Doxycycline, 100 mg, p.o. or i.v., b.i.d.	Duration: up to 8 weeks; longer in HIV patients.
Trench fever Cat scratch disease	*Bartonella quintana* *Bartonella henselae*	Doxycycline, 100 mg p.o., b.i.d. No treatment: generally self-resolving.	Azithromycin, 500 mg, p.o., single dose, then 250 mg, p.o., qd, x4d. **Children:** 10 mg/kg, single dose, then 5 mg/kg/d, 5d.	Duration: 5 days.
Lyme borreliosis, cutaneous	*Borrelia burgdorferi*	Doxycycline, 100 mg, p.o. or i.v., b.i.d. Amoxicillin, 500 mg, p.o., t.i.d. Cefuroxime axetil, 500 mg, p.o., b.i.d. Clarithromycin, 500 mg, p.o., b.i.d.		Duration: 14–21 days.
Brucellosis	*Brucella* species	Doxycycline, 100 mg, p.o. or i.v., b.i.d., plus gentamicin, 2.0 mg/kg, i.v., then 1.7 mg/kg, i.v., q. 8h. Streptomycin, 1.0 g, i.m., qd.	Doxycycline, 100 mg, p.o. or i.v., b.i.d., plus rifampin, 600–900 mg, p.o. qd. Trimethoprim/sulfamethoxazole, double-strength tablet, p.o., b.i.d., plus gentamicin, 2.0 mg/kg, i.v., then 1.7 mg/kg, i.v., q. 8h.	Duration: up to 6 weeks.
Meliodosis	*Burkholderia pseudomallei*	Ceftazidime, 2.0 g, i.v., q. 8h.		
Granuloma inguinale	*Calymmatobacterium granulomatis*	Doxycycline, 100 mg, p.o. or i.v., b.i.d. Trimethoprim-sulfamethoxazole, double-strength tablet, p.o., b.i.d.	Erythromycin, 500 mg, p.o., q.i.d. Ciprofloxacin, 750 mg, p.o., b.i.d.	Duration: 6–20 weeks. Duration: 3–4 weeks.
Lymphogranuloma venereum	*Chlamydia trachomatis* types L1, L2, L3	Doxycycline, 100 mg, p.o., b.i.d.	Erythromycin, 500 mg, p.o., q.i.d.	Duration: 3 weeks.

Continued on next page

Continued from previous page

Disease	Infectious agent	First choice(s) for therapy	Alternative choice(s) for therapy	Comments
Gas gangrene	*Clostridium perfringens*	Clindamycin, 900 mg, i.v., q. 8h, plus penicillin G 24 million units/d, i.v., divided, q. 4–6h.	Ceftriaxone, 2.0 g, i.v., q. 12h. Erythromycin, 1.0 g, i.v., q. 6h.	Surgical debridement is primary.
Diphtheria, cutaneous	*Corynebacterium diphtheriae*	Antitoxin plus erythromycin, 20–25 mg/kg, i.v., q. 12h.		Duration: 7–14 days.
Erythrasma	*Corynebacterium minutissinum*	Erythromycin, 250 mg, p.o., q.i.d.	Erythromycin solution, b.i.d. Benzoyl peroxide, 2.5% gel, b.i.d.	Duration: 14 days, p.o. Duration: 7 days, topical. Shave hair.
Trichomycosis axillaris	*Corynebacterium* species	Benzoyl peroxide gel, topically.		
Ehrlichiosis	*Ehrlichia* species	Doxycycline, 100 mg, p.o. or i.v., b.i.d.	Tetracycline, 500 mg, p.o., q.i.d.	Duration: 7–14 days.
Erysipeloid	*Erysipelothrix rhusiopathiae*	Benzathine penicillin G, 1.2 million units, i.m., single dose.	Erythromycin, 250–500 mg, p.o., q.i.d.	Duration: 7 days, p.o.
Tularemia	*Francisella tularensis*	Streptomycin, 7.5–10 mg/kg, i.v. or i.m., q. 12h.	Gentamicin, 3–5 mg/kg/d, i.v., divided q. 8h. **If meningitis,** add chloramphenicol, 500 mg, p.o. or i.v., q.i.d.	Duration: 7–14 days.
Chancroid	*Haemophilus ducreyi*	Ceftriaxone, 250 mg, i.m., single dose. Azithromycin, 1.0 g, p.o., single dose.	Ciprofloxacin, 500 mg, p.o., b.i.d., x3d. Erythromycin, 500 mg, p.o., q.i.d., 7d.	
Rhinoscleroma	*Klebsiella pneumoniae* sp. *rhinoscleromatis*	Fluoroquinolone.	Trimethoprim/sulfamethoxazole plus rifampin.	
Leptospirosis	*Leptospira* species	Surgical debridement. Penicillin G, 20–24 million units, i.v., qd, divided, q. 4–6h.	Doxycycline, 100 mg, p.o. or i.v., b.i.d.	Duration: Until lesions heal.
Listeriosis	*Listeria monocytogenes*	Ampicillin, 2.0 g, i.v., q. 4h.	Ampicillin, 0.5–1.0 g, i.v., q. 6h.	
Pitted keratolysis	*Micrococcus sedentarius*	Topical benzoyl peroxide or erythromycin, qd.		Reduce sweating with aluminum chloride, talcum powder
Gonococcemia	*Neisseria gonorrhea*	Ceftriaxone, 1.0 g, i.v., qd. Cefotaxime, 1.0 g, i.v., q. 8h. Ceftizoxime, 1.0 g, i.v., q. 8h.	Spectinomycin, 2.0 g, i.m., q. 12h. Ciprofloxacin, 500 mg, i.v., q 12h.	
Meningococcemia	*Neisseria meningitidis*	Penicillin G 24 million units, i.v., divided, q. 4h.	Ceftriaxone, 2.0 g, i.v., q. 12h. Cefotaxime, 2.0 g, i.v., q. 8h.	Duration: 2 days.
Meningococcemia (contact prophylaxis)	*Neisseria meningitidis*	Rifampin, 600 mg, p.o., b.i.d., x4d.	Ciprofloxacin, 500 mg, p.o., single dose.	
Nocardiosis	*Nocardia asteroides* *Nocardia brasiliensis*	Sulfisoxazole, 2 g, p.o., q. 6h. Trimethoprim-sulfamethoxazole, double-strength tablet, p.o., b.i.d.	Minocycline, 200 mg, p.o., b.i.d. **Serious infection**: Cefotaxime, 1 g, i.v., q. 8h, plus imipenem, 500 mg, i.v., q. 6h.	Duration: 6 months.
Cat bite	*Pasteurella multocida,* *Staphylococcus aureus*	Amoxicillin, 875 mg, plus clavulanate, 125 mg, p.o., b.i.d., or Amoxicillin, 500 mg, plus clavulanate, 125 mg, p.o., t.i.d.	Cefuroxime axetil, 0.5 g, p.o., q. 12h. Doxycycline, 100 mg, p.o., b.i.d.	

Narayan S. Naik and Miguel Sanchez

Appendix F: Treatment of cutaneous infections

Disease	Infectious agent	First choice(s) for therapy	Alternative choice(s) for therapy	Comments
Dog bite	Streptococcus viridans, Pasteurella multocida, Staphylococcus aureus, Eikenella corrodens, Fusobacterium species, Bacteriodes species, Capnocytophaga species	Amoxicillin, 875 mg, plus clavulanate, 125 mg, p.o., b.i.d., or Amoxicillin, 500 mg, plus clavulanate, 125 mg, p.o., t.i.d.	Clindamycin, 300 mg, p.o., q.i.d.	
Rat bite	Streptobacillus moniliformis	Amoxicillin, 875 mg, plus clavulanate, 125 mg, p.o., b.i.d.	Doxycycline, 100 mg, p.o., b.i.d.	Duration: 10 days.
Seal bite	Mycoplasma phocidae	Tetracycline, 500 mg, p.o., q.i.d.		Duration: 10 days.
Human bite	Streptococcus viridans, Bacteriodes, Staphylococcus aureus, Corynebacterium species, Eikenella species, Staphylococcus epidermidis	**Early, uninfected:** Amoxicillin, 875 mg, plus clavulanate, 125 mg, p.o., b.i.d. **Late, infected:** Ampicillin/sulbactam, 1.5 g, i.v., q. 6h. Cefoxitin, 2.0 g, i.v., q. 8h.	**Late infection, penicillin-allergy:** Clindamycin, 900 mg, i.v., q. 8h, plus Ciprofloxacin, 400 mg, i.v., b.i.d.	
Whirlpool (hot tub) folliculitis	Pseudomonas aeruginosa	**No treatment needed; generally self limited.**		Chlorinate water.
Ecthyma gangrenosum	Pseudomonas aeruginosa	Ceftazidime, 2.0 g, i.v., q. 8h. Imipenem, 0.5 g, i.v., q. 6h. Cefipime, 2.0 g, i.v., q. 8h.	Antipseudomonal penicillin plus antipseudomonal aminoglycoside.	
Rocky Mountain spotted fever	Rickettsia rickettsii	Doxycycline, 100 mg, p.o. or i.v., b.i.d.	Chloramphenicol, 500 mg, p.c. or i.v., q.i.d.	Duration: 7 days.
Typhus, epidemic	Rickettsia prowazekii	Doxycycline, 100 mg, p.o. or i.v., b.i.d.	Chloramphenicol, 500 mg, p.c. or i.v., q.i.d.	Duration: 7 days.
Typhus, endemic	Rickettsia typhi	Doxycycline, 100 mg, p.o. or i.v., b.i.d.	Chloramphenicol, 500 mg, p.c. or i.v., q.i.d.	Duration: 7 days.
Typhus, scrub	Orientia tsutsugamushi	Doxycycline, 100 mg, p.o. or i.v., b.i.d.	Chloramphenicol, 500 mg, p.c. or i.v., q.i.d.	Duration: 7 days.
Rickettsialpox	Rickettsia akari	**Self limited,** but doxycycline or chloramphenicol shortens course.		
Typhoid fever	Salmonella typhi, Salmonella paratyphi	Ciprofloxacin, 500 mg, p.o., b.i.d., x10d Ceftriaxone, 2.0 g, i.v., qd, x5d	Chloramphenicol, 500 mg, p.o. cr i.v., q.i.d., x14d. Cefixime, 10–15 mg/kg, p.o., q. 12h, x8d. Azithromycin, p.o. Clarithromycin, p.o.	Duration: 5–14 days.
Scarlet fever	Streptococcus pyogenes	Benzathine penicillin G, 1.2 million units, i.m., single dose. Penicillin V, 250 mg, p.o., q.i.d., 10d.	Erythromycin estolate, 20–40 mg/kg/d, p.o. Erythromycin ethylsuccinate, 40 mg/kg/d, p.o.	
Staphylococcal scalded skin syndrome	Staphylococcus aureus (exfoliative toxin)	Nafcillin, 2.0 g, i.v., q. 4h. **Children:** 150 mg/kg/d, divided, q.i.d.		Duration: 5–7 days. Supportive skin care and hydration measures.
Toxic shock syndrome (Staphylococcal)	Staphylococcus aureus (TSST toxin)	Nafcillin, 2.0 g, i.v., q. 4h	Cefazolin, 1–2 g, i.v., q. 8h	

Continued on next page

Appendix F: Treatment of cutaneous infections

Disease	Infectious agent	First choice(s) for therapy	Alternative choice(s) for therapy	Comments
Toxic shock syndrome (streptococcal)	*Streptococcus pyogenes*, *Streptococcus* groups B, C, G	Penicillin G, 24 million units/d, i.v., divided, q. 4–6h, plus clindamycin, 900 mg, i.v., q. 8h.	Erythromycin, 1.0 g, i.v., q. 6h, Ceftriaxone, 2.0 g, i.v., q. 24h, plus clindamycin, 900 mg, i.v., q. 8h.	
Furunculosis (prevention of recurrence)	*Staphylococcus aureus*	Mupirocin (topical) 2%, intranasally, b.i.d.	Rifampin, 600 mg, p.o., qd, plus dicloxacillin, 500 mg, p.o., q.i.d.	Duration: 10 days.
Cellulitis, lower extremity	*Streptococcus pyogenes*, *Streptococcus* groups B, C, G	Nafcillin, 2.0 g, i.v., q. 4h. Cefazolin, 1.0 g, i.v., q. 8h. **Less severe infections:** Dicloxacillin, 500 mg, p.o., q.i.d.	Erythromycin, 500 mg, p.o., q.i.d. First-generation cephalosporin. Clarithromycin, 500 mg, p.o., b.i.d. Azithromycin, 500mg, p.o., single dose, then 250 mg, p.o., qd.	
Cellulitis, facial and erysipelas	*Streptococcus pyogenes*, *Staphylococcus aureus*	Nafcillin, 2.0 g, i.v., q 4h.	First-generation cephalosporin. Vancomycin, 1.0 g, i.v., q. 12h. **If not severe:**Amoxicillin, 875 mg, plus clavulanate, 125 mg, p.o., b.i.d., or amoxicillin, 500 mg, plus clavulanate, 125 mg, p.o., t.i.d.	
Wound infection, postoperative	*Staphylococcus aureus*, *Streptococcus pyogenes*	Amoxicillin, 875 mg, plus clavulanate, 125 mg, p.o., b.i.d., or Amoxicillin, 500 mg, plus clavulanate, 125 mg, p.o., t.i.d. First-generation cephalosporin, p.o.	Dicloxacillin, 500 mg, p.o., q.i.d.	
Wound infection, extremity (post-injury)	*Staphylococcus aureus*, *Streptococcus pyogenes*, anaerobic streptococci	Amoxicillin, 875 mg, plus clavulanate, 125 mg, p.o., b.i.d., or Amoxicillin, 500 mg, plus clavulanate, 125 mg, p.o., t.i.d. First-generation cephalosporin, p.o.	Azithromycin, 500 mg, p.o., single dose x1 then 250 mg, p.o., qd. Clarithromycin, 500 mg, p.o., b.i.d. Erythromycin, 500 mg, p.o., q.i.d.	
Nonbullous impetigo, ecthyma	*Streptococcus pyogenes*	Penicillin V K. 250 mg, p.o., q.i.d. First-generation cephalosporin, p.o.	Mupirocin (topical), t.i.d. Azithromycin, 500 mg, p.o., single dose, then 250 mg, p.o., qd. Clarithromycin, 500 mg, p.o., b.i.d. Erythromycin, 500 mg, p.o., q.i.d. Second-generation cephalosporin.	Duration: 10 days.
Bullous impetigo	*Staphylococcus aureus*	Dicloxacillin, 500 mg, p.o., q.i.d.	Mupirocin (topical) Amoxicillin, 875 mg, plus clavulanate, 125 mg, p.o., b.i.d., or Amoxicillin, 500 mg, plus clavulanate, 125 mg, p.o., t.i.d. Azithromycin, 500 mg, p.o., single dose, then 250 mg, p.o., qd Clarithromycin, 500 mg, p.o., b.i.d.	
Paronychia, bacterial (manicuring, nail-biting)	*Staphylococcus aureus*	Clindamycin, 300 mg, p.o., q.i.d.	Erythromycin, 500 mg, p.o., q.i.d.	Duration: 2–5 days.
Fish-farm cellulitis	*Streptococcus iniae*	Penicillin, cefazolin, ceftriaxone,	Erythromycin, clindamycin.	Duration: 10 days.

Narayan S. Naik and Miguel Sanchez

Disease	Infectious agent	First choice(s) for therapy	Alternative choice(s) for therapy	Comments
Syphilis, primary or secondary	*Treponema pallidum*	Benzathine penicillin, G 2.4 million units, i.m., single dose.	Doxycycline, 100 mg, p.o., b.i.d., 14d. Tetracycline, 500 mg, p.o., q.i.d., 14d. Ceftriaxone, 125 mg, i.m., qd, 10d, or 250 mg, i.m., q.o.d, 5 doses, or 1000 mg, i.m., q.o.d, 4 doses.	Consider penicillin desensitization of pregnant women, HIV-positive patients.
Pinta	*Treponema carateum*	Benzathine penicillin G, 1.2 million units, i.m., single dose.	Same as syphilis	
Yaws	*Treponema pallidum pertenue*	Benzathine penicillin G, 1.2 million units, i.m., single dose.	Same as syphilis	
Endemic syphilis	*Treponema pallidum endemicum*	Benzathine penicillin G, 1.2 million units, i.m., single dose.	Same as syphilis	
Wound infection, contaminated by sea water	*Vibrio vulnificus*	Ceftazidime, 2.0 g, i.v., q. 8h., plus doxycycline, 100 mg, i.v. or p.o., b.i.d.	Cefotaxime, 2.0 g, i.v., q. 8h. Ciprofloxacin, 750 mg, p.o., b.i.d., or 400 mg, i.v., b.i.d.	
Plague	*Yersinia pestis*	Streptomycin, 1.0 g, i.v. or i.m., q. 12h. Gentamicin, 2.0 mg/kg, i.v., then 1.7 mg/kg, i.v., q. 8h.	Doxycycline, 100 mg, p.o. or i.v., b.i.d. Chloramphenicol, 500 mg, p.o. or i.v., q.i.d.	
Tuberculosis, cutaneous	*Mycobacterium tuberculosis*, *Mycobacterium bovis*	**Low resistance** (< 4% strains): isoniazid, 5mg/kg/d, plus rifampin, 10 mg/kg/d, plus pyrazinamide, 25 mg/kg/d; p.o., qd, 2 months; followed by isoniazid and rifampin, 4 months. **High resistance** (> 4% strains): as above, but add streptomycin, 1.5 mg/kg, i.m., and ethambutol, 25 mg/kg/d, 2 months, then 15 mg/kg/d, p.o., qd, to above drugs, until susceptibilities available.	**Multi-drug resistant strains:** Isoniazid, plus rifampin, plus pyrazinamide, plus ethambutol, plus streptomycin, plus amikacin (7.5–10 mg/kg /d), plus quinolone (ciprofloxacin, levofloxacin, sparfloxacin) *Mycobacterium bovis:* Isoniazid, plus rifampin, plus ethambutol (resistant to pyrazinamide).	Duration: 6 months, up to 18 months if resistant to isoniazid or rifampin. Duration for multi-drug strains not known. Pyridoxine, 25–50 mg, p.o., qd, while on isoniazid. May consider directly observed therapy in patients who are unreliable, non-compliant, or who have resistant strains.
Leprosy, paucibacillary	*Mycobacterium leprae*	Dapsone, 100 mg, p.o., qd, unsupervised, plus rifampin, 600 mg, p.o., 1 month, supervised		

Continued on next page

Continued from previous page

Disease	Infectious agent	First choice(s) for therapy	Alternative choice(s) for therapy	Comments
Leprosy, multibacillary	*Mycobacterium leprae*	Dapsone, 100 mg, p.o., qd, plus clofazimine, 50 mg, p.o., qd, unsupervised, plus rifampin, 600 mg, p.o., 1 month, and clofazimine, 300 mg, p.o., 1 month, supervised.		Prednisone or thalidomide for erythema nodosum leprosum.
	Mycobacterium chelonei	Surgical excision.	Clarithromycin, 500 mg. p.o., b.i.d.	Duration: 6 months.
	Mycobacterium fortuitum	Surgical excision.		Duration: 6–12 months.
	Mycobacterium kansasii	Amikacin plus cefoxitin plus probenecid, 6 weeks, then trimethoprim/sulfamethoxazole or doxycycline, p.o.		Duration: 12–18 months.
"Fish-tank" granuloma	*Mycobacterium marinum*	Isoniazid, 300 mg, p.o., qd, plus rifampin, 600 mg, p.o., qd, plus ethambutol, 25 mg/kg/d, p.o., qd. Clarithromycin, 500 mg, p.o., b.i.d. Minocycline, 100 mg, p.o., qd Doxycycline, 100 mg, p.o., qd.	Trimethoprim, 160 mg; sulfamethoxazole, 800 mg; p.o., t.i.d. Rifampin plus ethambutol.	Duration: 3 months.
Scrofuloderma	*Mycobacterium scrofulaceum*	Surgical excision.		
Buruli ulcer	*Mycobacterium ulcerans*	Rifampin plus amikacin; 7.5 mg/kg, i.m., q. 12h, b.i.d. Ethambutol plus trimethoprim/sulfamethoxazole, 160 –800 mg, p.o., t.i.d. Surgical excision.		Duration: 4–6 weeks.
Varicella (chicken pox), immunocompetent host	Varicella zoster virus	**Not routinely treated.** **If increased risk of severe disease: Children:** Acyclovir, 20 mg/kg/d; **Adults:** Acyclovir, 800 mg, p.o., q.i.d.; started within 24h of rash onset.		Duration: 5 days (if treated).
Varicella (chicken pox), immunosuppressed host	Varicella zoster virus	Acyclovir, 10–12 mg/kg, i.v., q. 8h.		Duration: 7 days.
Herpes Zoster; immunocompetent host	Varicella zoster virus	Acyclovir, 800 mg, p.o., five times daily. Famciclovir, 500 mg, p.o., t.i.d. Valacyclovir, 1000 mg, p.o., t.i.d.		Duration: 7–10 days.
Herpes Zoster; immunosuppressed host	Varicella zoster virus	Acyclovir, 800 mg, p.o., five times daily. **Severe infection:** Acyclovir, 10–12 mg/kg, i.v. q 8h.		Duration: 7–14 days.
Herpes Primary Gingivostomatitis	Herpes simplex virus 1,2	**Children:** Acyclovir, 15 mg/kg, p.o., five times daily.		Duration: 7 days.
Herpes, genital; first episode	Herpes simplex virus 1,2	Acyclovir, 400 mg, p.o., t.i.d. Famciclovir, 250 mg, p.o., t.i.d. Valacyclovir, 1000 mg, p.o., b.i.d.		Duration: 10 days.

Disease	Infectious agent	First choice(s) for therapy	Alternative choice(s) for therapy	Comments
Herpes, genital; recurrence	Herpes simplex virus 1,2	Acyclovir, 400 mg, p.o., b.i.d. Famciclovir, 125 mg, p.o., b.i.d. Valacyclovir, 250 mg, p.o., b.i.d. or 500 mg, p.o., qd or 1 g, p.o., qd.		Duration: 5 days
Herpes, genital; chronic suppression (> 10 recurrences per year)	Herpes simplex virus 1,2	Acyclovir, 400 mg, p.o., b.i.d. Famciclovir, 250 mg, p.o., b.i.d. Valacyclovir, 250 mg, p.o., b.i.d. or 500 mg, p.o., qd or 1 g, p.o., qd.		Chronic.
Herpes, orolabial; immunocompetent host	Herpes simplex virus 1,2	Usually not treated. Penciclovir, 1% cream, q. 2h. Acyclovir (topical), q. 2h.		Duration: 4 days.
Herpes, orolabial; immunosuppressed host	Herpes simplex virus 1,2	Acyclovir, 5.0 mg/kg, i.v., q. 8h. Famciclovir, 500 mg, p.o., b.i.d.		Duration: 7 days.
Aspergillosis, invasive	Aspergillus species	Amphotericin B, 1.0 mg/kg/d, i.v. Itraconazole, 200 mg, i.v., t.i.d., 4d, followed by 200 mg, p.o., b.i.d.	Amphotericin B: Liposomal, lipid complex or cholesteryl complex	
Blastomycosis	Blastomyces dermatitidis	Itraconazole, 200–400 mg, p.o., qd. Serious infections: Amphotericin B, 0.5–1.0 mg/kg/d, i.v.	Fluconazole, 400–800 mg, p.o., qd.	Duration: 6 months.
Balanitis or vaginitis	Candida species	Fluconazole, 150 mg, p.o., single dose. Itraconazole, 200 mg, p.o., b.i.d., single dose. Topical miconazole, clotrimazole, butoconazole, tioconazole. Terconazole, t.i.d.-q.i.d.	Nystatin (topical).	Keep area dry.
Paronychia, fungal (prolonged water contact)	Candida species	Topical clotrimazole, t.i.d.-q.i.d.		Keep area dry.
Candidiasis, cutaneous	Candida species	Topical miconazole, clotrimazole, econazole, nystatin, t.i.d.-q.i.d. Topical ciclopirox olamine, b.i.d. Ketoconazole, 400 mg, p.o., qd.		Duration: 2 weeks. Keep area dry.
Candidiasis, disseminated	Candida species	Amphotericin B, 0.5–1.0 mg/kg/d, i.v. Fluconazole, 400 mg, i.v, qd, 7d, then 400 mg, p.o., qd, 14d after eradication of candidemia.		
Candidiasis, chronic mucocutaneous	Candida species	Ketoconazole, 400 mg, p.o. qd.		
Thrush	Candida species	Fluconazole, 200 mg, p.o., single dose. Itraconazole solution, 200 mg (20cc), qd, 7d.	Nystatin lozenges or swish and swallow, q.i.d. Nystatin, 2 tablets, t.i.d., 14d. Clotrimazole troches, five times daily, 14d.	Duration: 3–9 months.

Continued on next page

Narayan S. Naik and Miguel Sanchez

Continued from previous page

Disease	Infectious agent	First choice(s) for therapy	Alternative choice(s) for therapy	Comments
Phaeohyphomycosis	*Exophiala jeanselmei; Wangiella dermatitidis*	Surgery plus itraconazole, 400 mg, p.o. qd.		Duration: 6 months.
Chromoblastomycosis	*Fonsecaea* species, *Cladosporium* species, *Phialophora* species, *Wangiella dermatitidis*	Few lesions: Surgical excision, cryotherapy. Many lesions: Itraconazole, 100 mg, p.o., qd.		Duration: 18 months, p.o.
Coccidioidomycosis	*Coccidioides immitis*	Fluconazole, 400–800 mg, p.o., qd. Serious infections: Amphotericin B, 1 mg/kg/d, i.v.	Itraconazole, 200 mg, p.o., b.i.d.	Duration questionable: 12–18 months, p.o.
Cryptococcosis	*Cryptococcus neoformans*	Amphotericin B, 0.5–0.8 mg/kg/d,i.v. Fluconazole, 400 mg/d, i.v. or p.o.	Amphotericin B, 0.3 mg/kg/d, i.v., plus flucytosine, 37.5 mg/kg, p.o., q.i.d., 6 weeks.	Duration: 8–10 weeks, p.o.
Histoplasmosis	*Histoplasma capsulatum*	Itraconazole, 400 mg, p.o., b.i.d. Serious infections: Amphotericin B, 0.5–1.0 mg/kg/d, i.v.		Duration: 12 weeks.
Tinea versicolor	*Malassezia furfur Pityrosporum orbiculare*	Ketoconazole 2% cream, qd, 2 weeks. Ketoconazole, 400 mg, p.o., single dose.	Fluconazole, 400 mg, p.o., single dose. Itraconazole, 400 mg, p.o., qd, 3–7d. Selenium sulfide, 2.5% lotion, qd, 7d.	
Paracoccidioidomycosis	*Paracoccidiodes brasiliensis*	Itraconazole, 200 mg, p.o., qd. Ketoconazole, 400 mg, p.o., qd.	Amphotericin B, 0.5mg/kg/d, i.v.	Duration: 6–18 months.
Lobomycosis	*Paracoccidiodes loboi*	Surgical excision, clofazimine. Amphotericin B.		
Penicilliosis	*Penicillium marneffei*	Amphotericin B, 0.5–1.0 mg/kg/d, i.v., 2 weeks, then itraconazole, 400 mg, p.o., qd, 10 weeks, then 200 mg, p.o., qd.	Itraconazole, 200 mg, p.o., t.i.d., 3d, then 200 mg, p.o., b.i.d., 12 weeks, then 200 mg, p.o., qd.	Duration indefinite for HIV patients.
Mycetoma/Madura foot	*Pseudoallescheria boydii*	Surgery plus itraconazole, 200 mg, p.o., b.i.d.	Miconazole, 600 mg, i.v. q. 8h.	Duration: until healthy.
Mucormycosis/zygomycosis	*Rhizopus* species	Amphotericin B, 0.8–1.0 mg/kg/d, i.v., plus surgical debridement.		Treat underlying conditions: Diabetic ketoacidosis.
Sporotrichosis	*Sporothrix schenckii*	Itraconazole, 100–300 mg, p.o., qd, 6 months, then 200 mg, p.o., b.i.d., long term.	Saturated solution potassium iodide (1 g/cc) Slowly increase to 50 drops, t.i.d., 6–12 weeks.	
Onychomycosis, toenails	*Trichophyton* species, *Microsporum* species, *Epidermophyton* species	Terbinafine, 250 mg, p.o., qd, 12 weeks. Itraconazole, 200 mg, p.o., qd, 3 months. Itraconazole (pulse), 200 mg, p.o., b.i.d., 1week/month, 2 months Fluconazole, 150–300 mg, p.o., weekly, 3–6 months.		

Narayan S. Naik and Miguel Sanchez

Disease	Infectious agent	First choice(s) for therapy	Alternative choice(s) for therapy	Comments
Onychomycosis, fingernails	Trichophyton species, Microsporum species, Epidermophyton species	Terbinafine, 250 mg, p.o., qd, 6 weeks. Itraconazole, 200 mg, p.o., qd, 3 months. Itraconazole (pulse), 200 mg, p.o., b.i.d., 1 week/month, 3–4 months. Fluconazole, 150–300 mg, p.o., weekly, 6–12 months.	Ketoconazole, 200 mg, p.o., qd.	
Tinea capitis	Trichophyton tonsurans, Microsporum canis, other species	Terbinafine, 250 mg, p.o., qd, 2–8 weeks.	**Children:** Ketoconazole, 3.3–6.6 mg/kg, p.o., qd, 4 weeks. Itraconazole, 3–5 mg/kg/d, 30d. Terbinafine, 250 mg, p.o., qd Ketoconazole, 200 mg, p.o., qd. Fluconazole, 150 mg, p.o., every week.	Duration: 2–4 weeks.
Tinea corporis, cruris, or pedis	Trichophyton rubrum, Trichophyton mentagrophytes, Epidermophyton floccosum	Topical miconazole, ketoconazole, butenafine, ciclopirox, clotrimazole, econazole, naftifine, oxiconazole, fluconazole, terconazole, b.i.d.		
Acanthamebiasis, cutaneous	Acanthamoeba species	**No proven therapy.**		
Cutaneous larval migrans (creeping eruption)	Ancyclostoma braziliense	Ivermectin, 150 µg/kg, p.o., single dose.	Albendazole, 200 mg, p.o., b.i.d., 3d. Topical thiabendazole.	
Hookworm disease	Ancyclostoma duodenale Necator americanus	Albendazole, 400 mg, p.o., single dose. Mebendazole 100 mg p.o. b.i.d. x 3 d	Pyrantel pamoate, 1 mg/kg, p.o., qd, 3d.	
Ascariasis	Ascaris lumbricoides	Albendazole, 400 mg, p.o., single dose. Mebendazole, 100 mg, p.o., b.i.d., 3d.	Pyrantel pamoate, 1 mg/kg, p.o., single dose.	
Dirofilariasis	Dirofilaria species	Surgical extraction.		
Guinea worm	Dracunculus medinensis	Surgical extraction.	Metronidazole, 250 mg, p.o., t.i.d., 10d (to decrease inflammation and facilitate removal).	
Hydatid cyst disease	Echinococcus granulosus	Percutaneous drainage, surgical resection, plus albendazole, p.o., 3 cycles (each cycle is 28d, with 14 d between cycles).		Hypertonic saline or ethanol at time of excision.
Amebiasis, cutaneous	Entamoeba histolytica	Metronidazole, 750 mg, p.o., t.i.d., 10d, followed by iodoquinol, 650 mg, p.o., t.i.d., 20d.	Tinidazole, 600 mg, p.o., b.i.d. or 800 mg, p.o., t.i.d; 5d.	
Enterobiasis (perianal pruritus)	Enterobius vermicularis (pinworm)	Albendazole, 400 mg, p.o., single dose; repeat in 2 weeks. Mebendazole, 100 mg, p.o., single dose; repeat in 2 weeks.	Pyrantel pamoate, 11 mg/kg, p.o., single dose, repeat in 2 weeks; repeat again in 2 weeks.	
Gnathostomiasis	Gnathostoma species	Surgical removal, plus albendazole, 400 mg, p.o., qd or b.i.d.		Duration: 21 days.
Leishmaniasis, cutaneous	Leishmania species	Antimony (stibogluconate), 20 mg/kg/d, i.v., divided, b.i.d. Pentamidine, 2mg/kg, i.v., qod, 7 doses.	Topical 15% paromomycin, plus 15% methylbenzethonium chloride in paraffin, b.i.d., 10d.	Duration: 28 days.

Continued on next page

Continued from previous page

Disease	Infectious agent	First choice(s) for therapy	Alternative choice(s) for therapy	Comments
Loiasis	*Loa Loa*	Diethylcarbamazine, over 21d: 50 mg, p.o., t.i.d. (days 1 and 2); 100 mg, p.o., t.i.d. (day 3); 2 mg/kg/d, p.o., t.i.d., (days 4–21).		Surgical removal, if possible
Filariasis, cutaneous	*Mansonella streptocerca*	Ivermectin, 150 µg/kg, p.o., single dose. Diethylcarbamazine, over 21 d: 50 mg, p.o., t.i.d. (days 1 and 2); 100 mg, p.o., t.i.d. (day 3); 2 mg/kg/d, p.o., t.i.d., (days 4–21).		
Onchocerciasis (river blindness)	*Onchocerca volvulus*	Ivermectin, 150 µg/kg, p.o., single dose; repeat every 6 months		Prednisone, p.o., several days before Ivermectin, if eye involvement.
Paragonimiasis	*Paragonimus westermani*	Praziquantel, 25 mg/kg, p.o., t.i.d.		Duration: 2 days.
Lice (body)	*Pediculus humanus, var. corporis*	Discard or treat clothing with malathion powder or 10% DDT.		
Lice (head, pubic)	*Pediculus humanus, var. capitis, Phthirus pubis*	Permethrin 5% or 1% lotion: Wash hair, apply for 10 minutes, rinse; apply second treatment 7–10d later.	Ivermectin, 200 µg/kg, p.o., single dose. Pyrethrin (over-the-counter). Lindane 1%.	Treat sexual partners. Discard or wash clothing.
Scabies	*Sarcoptes scabiei*	Permethrin 5% cream: Apply to entire skin; leave on 8–10h; repeat in 1 week. **Norwegian scabies:** Permethrin 5% on day 1, then 6% sulfur in petrolatum, qd, days 2–7; repeat every several weeks.	Lindane 1% lotion. **Children** (< 2 months) and **pregnant:** Precipitated sulfur, 6% to 10%, in petrolatum, qd, 3d. **Norwegian scabies:** Ivermectin, 200 µg/kg, p.o., single dose.	Wash all clothes and linens. Treat close contacts; isolate if necessary.
Schistosomiasis	*Schistosoma species*	Praziquantel, 20–25 mg/kg, p.o., b.i.d.–t.i.d.		
Cercarial dermatitis (swimmer's itch)	*Schistosoma species, Trichobilharzia species, other fluke species*	**No specific treatment; self-resolving.**		
Sparganosis	*Spirometra species*	Surgical resection		
Strongyloidiasis	*Strongyloides stercoralis*	Ivermectin, 200 µg/kg/d, p.o., 2 d. Albendazole, 400 mg, p.o., qd, 3 d	Thiabendazole, 25 mg/kg, p.o., b.i.d, 2d.	Duration: 1–2 days.
Cysticercosis	*Taenia solium*	Praziquantel, 10 mg/kg, p.o., single dose.	Albendazole, (dosing by weight), p.o., b.i.d.	

Narayan S. Naik and Miguel Sanchez

Continued from previous page

Disease	Infectious agent	First choice(s) for therapy	Alternative choice(s) for therapy	Comments
Visceral larval migrans	*Toxocara canis*	Diethylcarbamazine, 2 mg/kg, p.o., t.i.d., 10d.	Albendazole, 400 mg, p.o., b.i.d. Mebendazole, 100–200 mg, p.o., b.i.d., 5d	Duration: 10–14 days. Give with prednisone, 40–60 mg/kg, p.o., qd
Trichinosis	*Trichinella spiralis*	Albendazole, 400 mg, p.o., b.i.d.	Mebendazole, 5 mg/kg, p.o., b.i.d.	Prednisone, p.o., may decrease post-treatment encephalopathy (occurs in 10% of cases).
African trypanosomiasis (sleeping sickness)	*Trypanosoma brucei*, subtypes *gambiense* and *rhodesiense*	**Early infection:** Suramin (after test dose of 0.2 g, i.v.) 20 mg/kg, i.v., on days 1, 3, 7, 14, 21 (max dose 1.0g). **Late infection:** Melarsoprol, 2–3.6 mg/kg, i.v., 3 doses; repeat after 1 week, and then after 10–21d. **Prophylaxis (gambiense only):** Pentamidine isethionate, 3mg/kg, i.m., every 6 months.	**Early infection:** Pentamidine isethionate, 4mg/kg, i.m., qod, 10 doses. **Gambiense only:** Eflornithine, 100 mg/kg, i.v., q. 6h, 14d. then 75 mg/kg, i.v., 21–30d. **Late infection:** Suramin, 0.2 g/d, i.v., 2 d, then start Melarsoprol.	
American trypanosomiasis (Chagas' disease)	*Trypanosoma cruzi*	Nifurtimox, 8–20 mg/kg/d, (depending on age), divided, q.i.d., after meals.	Benznidazole, 7.5 mg/kg/d, p.o., divided, b.i.d., 60d.	Duration: 90–120 days.
Elephantiasis (lymphatic filariasis)	*Wuchereria bancrofti* *Brugia* species	Ivermectin, 100–440 µg/kg, single dose.	Diethylcarbamazine, over 21d: 50 mg, p.o., t.i.d., (days 1,2); 100 mg, p.o., t.i.d. (day 3); 2 mg/kg/d, p.o., t.i.d., (days 4–21).	

General references

The Sanford Guide to Antimicrobial Therapy edn 25. Edited by Gilbert DN, Moellering RC, Sande MA. Hyde Park, VT: Antimicrobial Therapy, Inc.; 1999

Pocket Guide to Medications Used in Dermatology edn 6. Edited by Scheman AJ, Severson DL. Philadelphia: Lippincott, Williams and Wilkins; 1999

Dermatology in General Medicine edn 5. Edited by Freedberg IM. New York: McGraw-Hill; 1999

Color Atlas and Synopsis of Clinical Dermatology edn 3. Edited by Fitzpatrick TB. New York: McGraw-Hill; 1997

Narayan S. Naik and Miguel Sanchez

Dapsone

Class: Potent antioxidant, neutrophil response inhibitor and antibacterial sulfone, with antimetabolite effect against para-aminobenzoic acid in folate synthesis.

Dose: 50 mg, once daily, initially (available in 25- and 50-mg tablets), increased by 50 mg every 1 to 2 weeks, up to 300 mg daily.

Adverse effects: Nausea, vomiting, dose related dyspnea, hemolysis (may drop 25% in 3–4 weeks, even if G-6-PD positive with dose of 300 mg); hemolysis with acute tubular necrosis (most common in blacks); dose-related methemoglobinemia; distal motor neuropathy (usually hands); acute psychosis, potentially fatal mononucleosis-like hypersensitivity syndrome, hypoalbuminemia; leukopenia; agranulocytosis (0.01 to 0.1% of cases, almost always during first 3 months of therapy); toxic epidermal necrolysis.

Monitoring: CBC with differential and glucose-6–phosphate dehydrogenase levels (which must be present in order to decrease the risk of severe hemolysis) before initiation of therapy; then CBC with differential every week for the first month and then twice a month during the next 2 months. Thereafter, CBCs should be ordered every 3 to 6 months. Liver and renal function should be tested initially, every month for 3 months and then every 3 to 6 months. Urinalysis at the start of treatment, monthly for 3 months and then every 3 to 6 months. Reticulocyte counts are ordered as indicated.

Sulfapyridine

Class: Sulfone

Dose: 1 to 1.5 mg, four times daily, with lots of water.

Adverse effects: Similar to dapsone, but less risk of hemolysis and hepatotoxicity and greater risk of leukopenia (5%), photosensitivity (10%) and nephrotoxicity due to renal precipitation.

Mycophenolate mofetil

Class: Immunomodulator that inhibits lymphocyte proliferation and antibody production by inhibiting type II inosine monophosphate dehydrogenase in lymphocytes, thus inhibiting purine synthesis.

Dose: 1g every 12 hours (available in 250-mg capsules and 500-mg tablets).

Adverse effects: Nausea, abdominal pain, vomiting, diarrhea, infection (including sepsis), increased incidence of lymphoproliferative diseases and lymphoma, severe leukopenia (< 3%). May be prescribed with cyclosporine or glucocorticosteroids, since there is no increase in nephrotoxicity, hepatotoxicity, hypertension, or neurotoxicity.

Monitoring: CBC initially, every 2 weeks for 2 months, then every month.

Herpes antivirals

Class: Viral thymidine reductase inhibitors.

Dose: *See* Herpes simplex chapter.

Size: Acyclovir: 200-mg caspsule, 400-mg and 800-mg tablets, 200-mg/5cc suspension; Valacyclovir: 500-mg, 1000-mg tablets; Famcyclovir: 125-mg, 250-mg, 500-mg tablets. Pencyclovir: 1% cream applied q. 2 h for four days; reduces time to clearance by an average of 10%.

Adverse effects: Well tolerated. Nausea/vomiting (8%), diarrhea (9%), headaches and rarely, rashes, vertigo, dizziness, fatigue, anorexia. Obstructive nephropathy (with intravenous doses) that can be decreased by hydration.

H₁ antihistamines

Classes: Ethylenediamines (pyrilamine antazoline, mepyramine, tripelennamine), ethanolamines (diphenhydramine [25–50 mg, q. 4–6h], bromodiphenhydramine, carbinoxamine, clemastine [1.34-2.68 mg, q. 8–12h], diphenhydramine, doxylamine, phenyltoloxamine), alkylamines (brompheniramine [4 mg, q. 4–6h, dexbrompheniramine, tripolidine [2.5 mg, q. 4–6h], dexchlorpheniramine, chlorpheniramine [4 mg, q. 4–6h], dimethindene, pheniramine), phenothiazines (promethazine [25 mg, h.s.], methdilazine, trimeprazine), piperazines (chlorcyclizine, hydroxyzine [10–25 mg, q. 4–6h], meclizine, thiethylperazine), piperidines (cyproheptadine [4 mg, q. 4–6h],azatadine [1-2 mg, q. 12h]), nonsedating (astemizole, 10 mg, q.d.; loratadine,10 mg, q,d,; cetirizine, 10 mg, q.d.; fexofenadine, 60 mg, b.i.d.).

Adverse effects: Sedation, gastrointestinal symptoms; cholinergic effects (may worsen prostatic obstruction and glaucoma); central nervous system symptoms.

Methotrexate

Class: Immunosuppressant.

Dose: An oral test dose of 2.5 to 5 mg (available in 2.5-mg tablets) may be given initially to evaluate bone marrow suppression. Usual doses for psoriasis are 7.5 to 15 mg per week, preferably without food, either in a single dose or 3 equally divided doses 12 hours apart. If necessary, increased by weekly increments of 2.5 mg; if tolerated, up to 30 mg. Higher doses occasionally needed. Intramuscular methotrexate may be given if poor absorption is suspected or to decrease gi intolerance. Folic acid, 5mg daily, or folinic acid, 2.5-5.0 mg daily, or 3 days after methotrexate dose, may reduce adverse reactions.

Contraindications: Pregnancy (drug should be discontinued 90 days before), lactation, renal, pulmonary, hepatic disease, high alcohol intake, blood dyscrasias.

Adverse effects: Nausea or vomiting (10% to 30%), which may be reduced with food, antacids (may reduce absorption), H2-blockers; diarrhea, fever; gastric ulceration, reduced male fertility, oral and skin ulcers (may herald bone marrow toxicity), elevated transaminases (8% to 67% of cases, but not indicative of progress to cirrhosis), cirrhosis (rare with total cumulative doses less than 1.5 g); leukopenia; anemia; thrombocytopenia; pruritus; reversible hair loss; lymphoma; rare anaphylaxis.

Drug interactions: NSAIDs and salicylates increase toxicity. Ethanol, sulfonamides, azathioprine , trimethoprim, co-trimoxazole, phenytoin, probenecid, diuretics, colchicine, retinoids, barbiturates may also increase adverse effects.

Monitoring: Baseline CBC with differential, urinalysis, biochemical profile with hepatic enzymes, BUN and creatinine; creatinine clearance; hepatitis B and C markers (optional). Repeat CBC weekly for one month and 7 days after dose escalations; then every month thereafter; biochemistry profile every 1 to 2 months; and urinalysis every 3 to 4 months; chest radiograph yearly, creatinine clearance annually. Liver biopsy should be considered at baseline and after every 1.5 g of drug (or 1 g if risk factors for liver disease or persistently elevated transaminases).

Overdose: Folinic acid, 10 mg/m³ (usually 15–20 mg), i.v., then 20 mg, p.o., q. 6 h, 36–48 h, until blood level of methotrexate decreases.

Etanercept

Description: A dimeric fusion protein that binds specifically to tumor necrosis factor (TNF), and blocks its interaction with cell surface TNF receptors. Approved for rheumatoid arthritis.

Dose: 25 mg, twice weekly, s.c., 72–96 h apart. Methotrexate, glucocorticoids, salicylates, nonsteroidal anti-inflammatory drugs, or analgesics may be continued during treatment.

Adverse effects: Injection site reactions, infections including sepsis, headaches.

Cyclosporine

Description: Immunosuppressant that inhibits helper T-cells without significant bone marrow suppression.

Dose: Begin with 1.25 mg/kg, p.o., b.i.d., four weeks, with food but not grapefruit juice. If improvement is not sufficient, increase dose, at 2-week intervals, by 0.5 mg/kg daily, to a maximum of 4.0 mg/kg/d. Discontinue treatment if improvement is not achieved after 6 weeks at 4 mg/kg/d. Once benefit is observed, decrease dose by 25% every 2 to 4 weeks (doses less than 2.5 mg/kg/d may be effective).

Size: Capsules: 25-mg, 100-mg, 250-mg; Injection: 50 mg/mL; Solution: 100 mg/mL.

Adverse effects: Hypertension that precedes nephrotoxicity, edema, headaches, nausea, diarrhea, gum hyperplasia, anorexia, gastritis, hiccoughs, peptic ulcer, pancreatitis, constipation, oral sores, difficulty in swallowing, leukopenia, thrombocytopenia, anemia, microangiopathic hemolytic anemia syndrome, rarely anaphylaxis chest pain, cramps, mild tremors, fever, rarely seizures, lethargy, acne, hirsutism, brittle finger nails, hair breaking, pruritus, rare hepatotoxicity, flushing, paresthesia, sinusitis, gynecomastia, conjunctivitis, hearing loss, tinnitus, muscle pain, infections, immunosuppression, hematuria, blurred vision, weight loss, joint pain, night sweats, tingling, hypomagnesemia with seizures, increased risk of malignancy.

Monitoring: Blood pressure and serum creatinine, BUN, liver function tests, serum potassium, uric acid, magnesium, CBC, cholesterol every 2 weeks for 3 months and then monthly. Reduce dose by 25% to 50% if abnormalities occur.

Drug interactions: Levels are decreased by anticonvulsants (phenytoin, barbiturates, carbamazepine, valproate); antibiotics (isoniazid, rifampin Bactrim). Levels are increased by antibiotics (macrolides, imipenem-cilastin, ketoconazole, fluconazole, itraconazole, terbenafine, amphotericin B, cephalosporins, doxycycline, acyclovir and other thymidine kinase inhibitors, HIV-protease inhibitors); diuretics (thiazides, furosemide); others (amiodarone, bromocriptine, warfarin, calcium channel blockers, H_2 antihistamines). Nephrotoxicity is increased by antibiotics (aminoglycosides, Bactrim, amphotericin, vancomycin); ranitidine; nonsteroidal antiinflammatory drugs; melphalan; tacrolimus. Other increased toxicity: Imuran, high dose corticosteroids, colchicine, verapamil.

Azothioprine

Description: Purine analog that inhibits DNA metabolism predominantly in the S phase.

Dose: Usual initial dose is 1 mg/kg/d, 25-mg tablets; can be increased by 0.5 mg/kg/d, every 6 to 8 weeks, then every 4 weeks, as long as it is well tolerated, to a maximum dose of 2.0 mg/kg/d.

Adverse effects: Dose related leukopenia, thrombocytopenia, macrocytic anemia, nausea and vomiting (10%), oral ulcers, pancreatitis, hepatotoxicity (< 1%), opportunistic infections, alopecia, morbilliform eruption, reduced fertility.

Drug interactions: Allopurinol (increases effect), succinylcholine.

Monitoring: Baseline CBC with differential and platelets, serum chemistry panel, urinalysis, tuberculin test, and routine screening for malignancy (Stool for heme, breast exam, Pap smear, physical examination, prostatic antigen, yearly colonoscopy); then complete CBC weekly for 1 month, biweekly for 2 months and then every 1 to 2 months; Chemistry profile in one and two months and then every 2 months; examination for malignancy every six months.

Cyclophosphamide

Description: Alkylating agent with preferential B-cell over T-cell (mainly suppressor) depression and inhibition of nuclear DNA replication.

Dose: 1–2 mg/kg/d, 25- or 50-mg tablets, in one morning dose or 2–3 doses during daytime. Effect may not be evident for 6 weeks.

Adverse effects: Hemorrhagic cystitis (5 to 40%); leukopenia; anemia; thrombocytopenia; increased risk of lymphoma, leukemia, bladder carcinoma and skin squamous cell carcinomas; anorexia (up to 70%); nausea, vomiting, stomatitis, hemorrhagic colitis, azospermia, amenorrhea, rare cardiomyopathy, pneumonitis and pulmonary fibrosis (with doses higher than recommended above); reversible anagen effluvium (5% to 30%); rarely urticaria; hyperpigmentaion of skin and nails.

Drug interactions: Allopurinol (increases toxicity), chloramphenicol, doxorubicin, other immunosuppressive agents (increase risk for malignancy and opportunistic infections).

Monitoring: Baseline CBC with differential and platelets, serum chemistry profile, urinalysis, tuberculin test and evaluation for malignancy; then complete CBC, urinalysis weekly for 1 month, biweekly for 3 months and, then monthly. Serum chemistry profile monthly. Malignancy evaluation every 6 months.

Isotretinoin and acitretin

Class: Synthetic retinoids.

Dose: Isotretinoin: usually 1 mg/kg, daily for 20 weeks, or 120–150 mg/kg per treatment course, regardless of daily dose (available in 10-, 20-, and 40-mg tablets) for acne; Acitretin: 25 to 50 mg, q.d. (available in 10- and 25-mg tablets).

Adverse effects: Teratogenicity (CNS, craniofacial, cardiac and thymus abnormalities in half of first-trimester isotretinoin exposures), cheilitis, skin eruption, telogen effluvium, hypertriglyceridemia, hypercholesterolemia, increased transaminases, hepatitis, musculoskeletal pains, phototoxicity, paronychia, hyperostosis, osteoporosis, premature epiphyseal closure, xeropthalmia, depression, decreased night vision, corneal opacities, gastrointestinal distress, inflammatory bowel disease, and a rare acute retinoid syndrome (fever, respiratory distress, weight gain, lower extremity edema, pleural or pericardial effusions, hypotension), which is treated with systemic corticosteroids. Use cautiously in sexually active women of child-bearing age, even on oral contraceptives and in patients at risk for coronary artery disease or severe liver disease.

Monitoring: Baseline complete blood count, chemistry profile with hepatic transaminases, lipid profile, and creatinine, pregnancy test; then liver function studies and trigyceride levels in 2 weeks, chemistry profile including lipids and hepatic enzymes and pregnancy test monthly thereafter. CBC in one month.

Appendix G: Selected dermatologic formulary

Thalidomide

Class: Antiinflammatory and immunomodulator. Suppressor of tumor necrosis factor-α.

Dose: Usually 50 to 200 mg daily, taken at night (available in 50-mg tablets).

Adverse effects: Potent teratogen (fetal phocomelia), somnolence (37%), dizziness, leukopenia, peripheral edema, neuropathy, paresthesias, peripheral sensory neuropathy, rashes (including erythroderma and toxic pustuloderma), fever.

Monitoring: Contraception is mandated in all potentially fertile women; pregnancy testing within 24 hours prior to initiating therapy, then weekly for one month, monthly thereafter. Warn patients that several drugs, including griseofulvin, rifampin, phenytoin, carbamazepine, rifabutin, HIV-protease inhibitors, and some antibiotics, may decrease the efficacy of hormonal contraceptives.

Potassium iodide

Class: Anti-inflammatory, immunomodulator and antifungal.

Dose: A supersaturated solution (1 gm/mL of water) of potassium iodide (SSKI), is diluted in water, or preferably juice to disguise the taste, and sipped with a straw to prevent dental discoloration. A starting dose of 0.6 cc (600 mg), p.o., t.i.d., is gradually increased up to 2.4 to 3.0 cc (3 gm) per dose. The dose needed for anti-inflammatory effects is usually smaller (900 mg daily) than for antifungal activity (3 to 12 g daily). Enteric coated tablets (300-mg) cause small-bowel lesions, with potential obstruction and perforation. The tablets should be swallowed whole (not crushed or chewed) with 240 cc of fluid. Improvement may be slow and treatment needs to continue for 4–6 weeks after apparent clinical cure. The starting dose in erythema nodosum is 300 mg, t.i.d.

Adverse effects: Nausea, vomiting, epigastric pain, rash, iodism with prolonged use. If iodism develops, discontinue treatment temporarily and restart at a lower dose after symptoms resolve. Hypothyroidism (may become apparent after discontinuationof drug), thyroid adenoma, goiter, gastrointestinal bleeding and pulmonary edema and hypersensitivity reaction are more serious side effects. Skin eruptions may be maculopapular, urticarial or purpuric. Pustular, cystic and carbuncular acneiform eruptions and vegetating and ulcerative nodules and plaques may require isotretinoin and/or oral corticosteroids.

Contraindication: Hypersensivity to drug, pregnancy (risk of fetal abnormal thyroid and goiter), renal failure and other potential causes of hyperkalemia, cystic fibrosis and thyroid disease.

Colchicine

Class: Antiinflammatory and immunomodulatory.

Dose: Usual dose 0.6 mg two or three times daily. Maximum dose is 1.2 mg three times daily. Available in 0.5-mg and 0.6-mg tablets. Do not take with acid drinks (juices or colas) or alcohol.

Adverse effects: Diarrhea, abdominal pain, nausea, and vomiting are especially common. Less common are skin rash, purpura, alopecia, elevated hepatic enzymes and creatine kinase, dysuria, urinary frequency, reversible azospermia, myopathy and peripheral neuropathy With toxic doses, patients may develop mental confusion, convulsions, coma, vascular collapse and nephrotoxicity. Especially problems are bone marrow depression with aplastic anemia, agranulocytosis and thrombocytopenia, so blood counts should be closely followed during prolonged therapy. Because colchicine arrests cell division at the metaphase stage, spermatogenesis may be depressed. Vitamin B12, which is suppressed, may need to be supplemented.

Drug interactions: Sympathomimetics, CNS suppressants, and sulfapyrazone (may increase the risk of leukemia).

Contraindications: Serious gastrointestinal, renal and cardiac disorders, pregnancy and lactation.

Monitoring: Monthly CBC and chemistry profile monthly for three months then every 3 months

Itraconazole

Class: Triazole antifungal.

Dose: Usually 200 mg daily, with food. Pulse doses of 200 mg, b.i.d., 7 days every month for 3 months (available in 100-mg capsules).

Adverse effects: Nausea, vomiting, diarrhea, rash, edema, fatigue, dizziness, liver function test elevations, fulminant hepatitis, and hypertension.

Drug interactions: Cisapride, astemizole, triazolam, or midazolam.

Lamisil

Class: Synthetic allylamine antifungal.

Dose: One 250-mg capsule daily.

Adverse effects: Gastrointestinal symptoms, liver function test abnormalities, rash, urticaria, pruritus, reversible taste disturbances, malaise, fatigue, lens and retinal changes, vomiting, arthralgia, myalgia, and hair loss, symptomatic idiosyncratic hepatobiliary dysfunction, toxic epidernmal necrolysis, severe neutropenia, thrombocytopenia and anaphylaxis.

Drug interactions: Cyclosporine

Miguel Sanchez

Tetracyclines, doxycycline, and minocycline

Dose: Doxycycline or minocycline: 50 to 100 mg, b.i.d.; tetracycline: 250-500 mg, b.i.d.–q.i.d.

Adverse effects: Photosensitization (predominantly with doxycycline), dizziness and vertigo (predominantly minocycline), gastrointestinal distress (especially tetracycline), esophagitis (never take before lying down), blue pigmentation of lower extremities, and gingiva (minocycline), tooth discoloration (tetracycline, minocycline), headache, rarely hepatitis and pseudotumor cerebri, hyperesensitivity reaction with eosinophilia.

Drug interaction: Accutane (increased risk of pseudotumor cerebri).

Fluconazole

Class: Triazole antifungal.

Dose: 150 to 300 mg, once weekly; at least three months for fingernails, six to 12 months for toenails. For candidal vaginitis, a single 150-mg dose.

Adverse effects and drug interactions: Similar to itraconazole.

Corticosteroids

Class: Antiinflammatories and imunosuppressants.

Dose: Prednisone (24–36 hours) is usually prescribed; less often: methylated methylprednisolone (24–36 hours) and long acting dexamethasone (36–48 hours), which have decreased mineralocorticoid activity.

Adverse effects: Ventricular arrhythmias and death with high doses; fluid retention; immunosuppression; diabetes; venous thrombosis; urolithiasis; cataracts; glaucoma; myopathy; agitation, depression; psychosis; aseptic bone necrosis; osteoporosis; menstrual irregularities, depressed wound healing; iatrogenic Cushing's syndrome; striae; weight gain; hypertension.

Topical corticosteroid classes

Class 1: superpotent

Clobetasol propionate (cream/ointment/gel, 0.05%). Betamethasone dipropionate in augmented base (gel/ointment/cream, 0.05%). Diflorasone diacetate (cream/ointment, 0.05%). Halobetasol propionate (cream/ointment, 0.05%).

Class 2: potent

Amcinonide (ointment, 0.1%). Betamethasone dipropionate (cream/ointment, 0.05%). Desoximetasone (cream/ointment, 0.25%; gel 0.05%). Diflorasone diacetate (cream/ointment, 0.05%). Fluocinonide (cream/ointment, 0.05%). Halcinonide (cream, 0.1%).

Class 3: upper mid-strength

Betamethasone dipropionate (cream/ointment, 0.05%). Betamethasone valerate (ointment, 0.1%). Mometasone furoate (ointment, 0.1%). Triamcinolone acetonide (cream/ointment, 0.5%).

Class 4: mid-strength

Desoximetasone (cream, 0.05%). Fluocinolone acetonide (cream, 0.2%; ointment, 0.025%). Flurandrenolide (ointment, 0.05%). Triamcinolone acetonide (ointment, 0.1%).

Class 5: lower mid-strength

Betamethasone dipropionate (lotion, 0.05%). Betamethasone valerate (cream/lotion, 0.1%). Fluocinolone acetonide (cream, 0.025%). Flurandrenolide (cream, 0.05%).

Class 5: nonfluorinated lower mid-strength

Hydrocortisone butyrate (cream, 0.1%). Hydrocortisone valerate (cream, 0.2%). Prednicarbate (emollient cream, 0.1%).

Class 6: mild

Alclometasone dipropionate (cream/ointment, 0.05%). Triamcinolone acetonide (cream, 0.1%). Desonide (cream, 0.05%). Fluocinolone acetonide (cream/solution, 0.01%). Desonide (cream, 0.05%). Betamethasone valerate (lotion, 0.1%).

Class 7: very mild

Hydrocortisone, 1 % and 2.5%.